Scottish Herbs and Fairy Lore

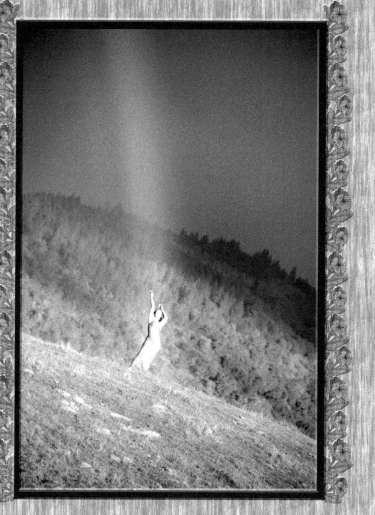

Ellen Evert Hopman

Scottish Herbs and Fairy Lore

Ellen Evert Hopman

PENDRAIG Publishing
Los Angeles, CA 91040

Scottish Herbs and Fairy Lore
Ellen Evert Hopman
First Edition © 2010
by PENDRAIG Publishing
All rights reserved.

Edited by: Tony Mierzwicki

Cover Design & Interior Images
Typeset & Layout   Jo-Ann Byers Mierzwicki

Photographer   Cat Crawford
Model   Lasára Allen

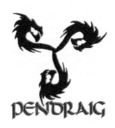

PENDRAIG Publishing
Los Angeles, CA 91040
www.PendraigPublishing.com
Printed in the United States of America

ISBN: 978-1-936922-01-7

Dedication

This book is dedicated to
Alexei Kondratiev
without whose constant advice
I could never have completed the work.
He was my Druid.

Further Acknowledgements and Thanks

To the Evert (Evet/Eviot/Eviotte) clan, Marcia for endless boxes of supplies to tide me over in my writing career, Jackie for funding a recent trip to Scotland, and to David for keeping my computer programs up to snuff. Many thanks to Tom Hutcheson for Scots language help, to Stacey Weinberger for Gaelic tree names, and to Daibhidh MacGilleathain (Dave MacLean), who grew up in the Highlands, for invaluable advice on history and lore. To Iain MacKenzie for enthusiastic support and advice, to Leona Stonebridge Arthen for advice on weaving with nettles, to Michael Dunning for choice historical tidbits, to Joyce Sweeney for her kind assistance, and to Dr. Kenneth Proefrock for herbal suggestions. As always a big thank you is owed to Alexei Kondratiev for help with the Gaelic and other arcane languages and a special thank you to Ellen Waff for her editorial advice. My grateful thanks to Dr. Jane Sibley for comments about Norse language.

Foreword

"Earth, water, fire and air met together in a garden fair" and magic was born! The kind of magic that happens every day, the kind of magic you can carry in your pocket, or see happening all around you if you have eyes to look in the right places: the kind of magic that happens when you're with the right people in the right place at the right time.

Here, all around my home in Scotland, magic can be discovered throughout the year, and in an often skeptical twenty-first century we are amply aided in our search for that greater certainty through Ellen Evert Hopman's remarkable book "Scottish Herbs and Fairy Lore". It shines with a clear and insightful light on Auld Scotia's culture of folk lore, folk magic and folk traditions.

Although for 300 years Scotland has been a part of the United Kingdom of Great Britain and Northern Ireland, she has retained an independence of identity through the great institutions of Law, Education, and Religion. Now, since 1999, the devolved Scottish Parliament has brought with it a renewed spirit of Scottish self confidence, and connectedness with the rest of the world, as a sovereign nation.

What is more, throughout Scotland's great history, up to the vibrant present day, the undercurrent of tradition has pulsated through the nation's heart, ever-changing over time, as all living traditions do, but built on solid foundations as old as the mountains and glens carved by the retreating ice-age 10,000 years ago, when human feet first walked fresh and free on the Caledonian landscape.

Layer upon layer of custom and belief have rooted into the Scottish cultural landscape. From before the time 5,000 years ago when early Orcadians built a temple to the returning midwinter sun, Maes Howe, just as the sapling

Fortingall Yew tree began its new growth on a hillside near Loch Tay, to the present day, when twelve thousand people come to share the spectacular procession of the annual Beltane Fire Festival on Calton Hill in Edinburgh. Just as the same Fortingall Yew tree continues to survive into old age.

The ethnic sources of Scottish lore are many and varied, and, more often than not, interconnected. A profusion of lore and wisdom, tradition and practicality has been left to us by the Crannog and Broch builders, Picts, Romans, Scots, Britons, Vikings, the Irish, and even the English.

And from these ancestral backgrounds the Spey Wives, Druids, Seers, Skalds, Witches, Diviners, Storytellers and all the ordinary folk of Alba have kindly left us the fruits of their knowledge and craft to use, if only we know where to look. It is to these traditions, that Ellen Evert Hopman turns her attentions in this book.

No newcomer to the world of folk wisdom, plant lore, healing and magic, Ellen is a priestess in the modern Druidic Tradition, and her many years of study and practice are reflected in this information packed volume. With great care and attention to detail she has gathered for our benefit a work of great significance in keeping alive the folk culture of Scotland's past.

What we find here includes festivals, rites of passage, recipes, healing, divination and a cornucopia of Caledonian herb and plant know-how, all clearly presented and structured, so that readers can dip in and partake of the wisdom contained here at their own measure.

Ellen Evert Hopman is a Master Herbalist and as such has listed exact dosages, preparation methods, cautions, and so on for the herbs and preparations so that readers can actually use them and work with them safely. Many comparable books fail to contain this kind of professional advice.

Her grasp of fairy and folk magic, earth energies, the ancient revels, the lore of land, sea and sky is impeccable, and the reader will surely return often and eagerly to reference "Scottish Herbs and Fairy Lore".

I for one will not only have this book with me out on the hills and heaths of my homeland, but also by me on my bedside table. It is a source book to experience and enjoy wherever you may be in this magical mystical world!

Iain Mackenzie,
musician and folklorist,
and member of Historic Scotland,
Lanarkshire, Scotland.
February 2010

A Note to My Readers

*T*his book contains folklore, magic, and traditional practices from all areas of Scotland; from the Highlands and Lowlands to the Hebrides, Orkney and Shetland. It is unlikely that any Scottish magical practitioner or herbalist would have practiced all these traditions.

Readers should feel free to pick the customs that speak to them personally, keep them and use them, and pass them along to future generations.

Table of Contents

Introduction – Ancient Roots   13
   Caledonia ~ A Thumbnail Ancient History

The Druids   19

The Old Gods   23

Lore of the Elements   33
   Honoring the Sun and Moon
   Farming by the Moon
   The Winds and Directions (The Airts)
   Water Magic
   Fire Magic
   Earth Magic

Stones, Bones, and Talismans   49
   Minerals, Crystals and Fairy Stones
   Healing Threads and Knots
   Bone Magic
   Stones of Power

Holy Days and Holidays   63
   The Fire Festivals:
   The Year in Scotland

Life Passages   89
   Courtship and Marriage
   Conception and Childbirth
   Death Rites

Divination Practices   107
   Second Sight
   Famous Seers

A Highland Herbal   113
   Medicinal Plants and Trees

Fishing Magic, Boats, and the Lore of the Sea   191
   The Lore of Boats
   Magical Protection of Boats and Ships
   Fishing Magic

Farming, Fertility, and Harvest Customs   195
   The Plow, the Seed and the Grain
   Wheat Weavings and Corn Dollies
   Straw Men and Scare-Crows
   Harvest Home
   Dairy Magic

Domestic Life   201
   Money
   Food and Whisky
   House and Home

Sacred Birds and Animals   205
   Sacred Birds
   Sacred Animals

Magical Practices   219
   Prayers, Rituals, and Incantations
   Quarter Days and Fire Festivals
   Love Spells and Moon Magic
   Magic and Luck
   Protective Magic
   Healing Magic
   Curses

Elves, Spirits, Witches and Monsters   239

The Fairies   247

Conclusion   253

Appendix   255
   Pronounciation Guide

Bibliography   269

Index   273

Introduction
Ancient Roots

Caledonia
A Thumbnail Ancient History

Early Inhabitants

*T*his book explores the herbal wisdom, Fairy lore, and magical lore that have been passed down to us from the peoples who inhabited Caledonia for millennia. The land that we now call Scotland was settled after the last ice age by several major groups: the Picts, Britons, the Celts, Scandinavians, and Angles. These varied cultures are reflected in the Fairy lore and magic of Scotland whose indigenous Spirits and sacred places may have Celtic, English or Norse names.

Orkney and Shetland still have strong Norse and Danish ties while the cultures of more southern areas are primarily Anglo-Saxon or Celtic. Orkney did not become a part of Scotland until 1468 when the impoverished king of Denmark, Norway and Sweden, Christian I, gave Orkney to the Scottish King James III as part of a marriage settlement between Christian's daughter Margaret and the Scottish King. Orkney was held as a pledge redeemable by 50,000 Rhenish Florins, and when Christian failed to live up to his agreements, Orkney, and later Shetland, were annexed by the Scottish crown.

The Picts

Once known as *"Alba"* the name *"Caledonia"* was given to the area by the Romans, named after the *Caledonii*, the largest and strongest Pictish tribe, whose territory stretched from the Valley of the Tay to the Great Glen. Caledonia once encompassed all lands north of the Antonine Wall, built by the Romans to contain Pictish raiders. The entire island was called *Britannia* (Britain) by the Romans. Caledonia was North Britain and the rest (modern England) was South Britain, with the Wall as the separating line.

The mountain called Shiehallion on the moor of Rannoch is known as *"The Fairy Mound of the Caledonians"* (and is the reputed home of the Fairy Queen).

Dunkeld hill is *"The Fort of the Caledonians"*. Tribes allied to the *Caledonii* were the *Taezali* of the North East, the *Lugi* of Sutherland, the *Decantae* of Easter Ross, and the *Smertae* and *Caereni* of Sutherland. These tribes spoke *"British"*, an ancestor language of modern Welsh.[1]

The *Maetae* and *Caledonii* were alliances of Pictish tribes North of Hadrian's Wall that were never fully subdued and were a constant source of irritation to Rome.[2] The *Atecotti* were a fierce tribal alliance based in the Western Isles and North to Caithness (there is some evidence that they were cannibals) who were never fully conquered, either.

The Picts were named *"Picti"* (Painted Ones) by the Romans, probably due to their bodies being painted with woad (Isatis tinctoria) and marked by blue tattoos. They were dominant until about 500 BCE when the Gaels arrived. Politically the Picts were a free people who elected their leaders, even accepting foreigners as kings if they found them worthy. Their territory once stretched from the Forth to the Pentland Firth and they retained their strongholds in Orkney and North East Scotland until the Viking presence gradually took hold. Their language is still unknown.

The Romans never completely dominated Caledonia, largely due to the fierce resistance of her native Pictish tribes.

Arrival of the Celts

The *Hallstatt* Celts (named for a region of Austria where their culture originated) were the earliest Celtic group to reach Caledonia. This first wave of Celts migrated into Britain around 600 BCE, probably from Gaul and Iberia.

A second wave of Celtic settlers arrived in 250 BCE (the late Iron Age, La Téne, Gaulish culture). This second Celtic group brought with it the two wheeled chariot and specially bred ponies, along with their heroic myths and legends, and may have introduced the Druids to Britain. However, it is also possible that the Druids were already there courtesy of the earlier *Hallstatt* Celts, or even as a remnant of earlier Bronze Age religions.

The *Scotti* were Gaelic speaking Celts from Ireland who settled in during the latter stages of Roman occupation.

Many Languages

Before the fourth century CE the main languages spoken in Caledonia were *Pictish, Cumbric,* and *Norse. Gaelic* arrived later with the Irish. The *P-Celtic* language was still spoken in Strathclyde in the eleventh century CE. *P-Celtic* and *Q-Celtic* languages have the same roots but pronunciation differences, for example the *Q-Celtic Irish* "mac" for "son" and "ceann" for "head" become "map" and "pen" in Welsh P-Celtic. Pictish may have been an archaic form of P-Celtic.

It is probable that by the fifth and sixth centuries Gaelic was the dominant language. It is after all only ten miles from Ireland to Scotland near Arran, meaning that travel and commerce made it easy for the language to migrate over through trade and intermarriage.

---

1. Ross, Anne, *Folklore of the Scottish Highlands, P. 21*
2. Ross, Anne, *Pagan Celtic Britain, PP. 14-16*

Hadrian's Wall

The Romans built Hadrian's Wall to hold back the Picts, and to more easily extract tolls from travelers. The forts constructed near the wall provided baths, food, spas, and livery services for toll takers and weary travelers. The majority of the "*Roman*" soldiers serving at the Wall were in fact locals who had joined the legions in hopes that after thirty years of service they might become Roman citizens with all the attendant rights and privileges. After the Romans left Caledonia in the fifth century CE, Britons, who were fast returning to their Pre-Roman Celtic ways, still complained about Pictish raiders. As the wall was intact, the Picts were probably raiding from the coasts in boats and coracles.[3]

Viking Influence

The Norse Vikings were an important group in the settlement of Scotland and their cultural presence is still felt in areas such as Sutherland, Shetland and Orkney. The Norse were certainly trading with the Caledonians from ancient times, but the first Viking "*raid*" on record was the attack on Iona in 795. Within a few years, the Vikings were moving into Orkney and the Outer Hebrides, establishing their "*jarldoms*" (earldoms) and answering to the King of Norway in Bergen.

The Vikings were consummate merchants who sailed from Iceland to Istanbul, and as far West as Newfoundland. Norwegian rule in Scotland ended with the Viking defeat at Largs in 1263 when Scotland was given the Isle of Man, the Shetlands, and the Hebrides.

Caledonian traders navigated the world to exchange goods with Greeks, Phoenicians, and other Mediterranean and North African peoples making Scotland a cosmopolitan place from early times.

Lifestyle of the Indigenous Peoples

The pollen record shows that Willow, Hazel, and Birch were important trees for the earliest inhabitants of Scotland – one reason why they feature strongly in traditional lore. Willow provided medicine and material for thatching, baskets, and harps. Hazel was an important food source, and Birch provided medicine, thatching and wood for household implements.

Barley (the native grain) and Oats (introduced by the Romans) were grown and Red Deer were hunted. There were dogs for guarding and cats, both wild and domestic, whose skins may have been used for clothing. They fashioned plows, querns (stones used for grinding grain), whalebone hoes and mattocks (pick axes for loosening soil), dug peat for fuel and burned the ubiquitous Heather. Seaweeds such as Dulse were a food staple and were also burned, used to compost fields and given to domestic animals as fodder.[4]

Flax was grown for cloth fiber and seed oil. Lesser Celandine (*Chelidonium majus*) made a remedy for piles and a gargle for sore throats, Juniper (*Juniperus communis*) was a digestive aid and antiseptic with diuretic properties, Puffball (*Bovista nigrescens*) was a styptic and a burn remedy.[5]

---

3. Davies, Norman, *The Isles – A History, P.162*
4. Hunter, John, *A Persona for the Northern Picts, P. 19*
5. Hunter, P. 19

Cattle, sheep (the tough wild mountain variety), and pigs were eaten, especially when the numbers of Red Deer fell or when the deer were monopolized by the elites. Gannet, Cormorant and Auk (now extinct) were eaten and exploited as a source of meat, eggs, and oil. Limpets, mussels, and periwinkles were eaten and used as bait, eels and beached whales were another source of food. There was no deep sea fishing.[6]

Household Utensils

Pumice washed ashore from Icelandic volcanoes and was used as an abrasive. The bones of slaughtered livestock were fashioned into decorated tools such as scoops, knife handles, spatulas, scrapers, awls, pins, needles, combs, bobbins, and spindle whorls. Whale bones were used to make weaving combs to beat down the weft. Walrus bones were used as boat ribs and the skins were used as boat coverings. Parts of musical instruments such as tuning pegs were also made of bone.[7]

Deer and Reindeer (possibly brought in from northern areas by trade) antlers provided combs, handles, and picks. Copper alloy was a precious commodity left over from the Romano-British era and was used for personal decoration. Penannular brooches and dress pins were imported from the South or manufactured.

Most metal objects were made from iron - for example nails, washers, knife blades, and Roman-style tweezers. Local clay was used to make pottery, both coil ware and wheel thrown pots were used for storage, cooking and to hold liquids. Most of the pottery was purely functional with little or no decoration other than a slip finish.[8]

Art and Culture

The crowning glories of early Scottish art and culture were the distinctively carved symbol stones of the Picts that appeared in greatest numbers in the seventh and eighth centuries CE. Certain symbols appear in a standardized style, all over Pictland such as double disks, serpent, crescents, crescent and v-rod, circles with central dots, double discs, z-rods, and highly stylized animals such as salmon, deer, wolf, boar, and bull.

Sometimes these stones were deliberately laid face down, implying that the magical power of the symbols was directed at the Earth and the ancestors, or at Otherworldly beings under the soil.[9]

The earliest dateable Pictish carved stone is from the mid sixth century but it is possible that the symbols appeared earlier on wood, bone, cloth or other objects that have not survived. Some of the stones appear to be road signs or advertisements. They may also have been territorial markers or memorials to the dead. The symbols may allude to personal or tribal names, or be magically protective devices. On some stones *Ogham* characters (an ancient pre-Latin, Celtic alphabet) appear alongside the symbols.[10]

6. *Ibid., P. 19*
7. *Ibid., P. 22*
8. *Ibid., P. 22*
9. *Ibid., P. 32*
10. Fraser, Iain and J.N.G. Ritchie, *Royal Commission on the Ancient and Historical Monuments*

How Scotland Got Her Name

Irish settlers to Scotland came from what would later be County Antrim, Northern Ireland, in about 500 BCE, and moved into Pictish areas on Islay, Lorn and Kintyre. They called their settlement *Ard-gael* (*Argyll*, The Eastern Irish). In the sixth century, the Picts regained control of Argyll when Aidan mac *Gabhrán* (king of *Dál Riata* from 574-608) harassed both the Picts and the High King of *Éire*. Aidan eventually settled for maritime tribute.[11]

In 603 CE, Aidan's army was destroyed by the Germanic Angles who had penetrated the East coast after Roman Britannia fell. In 637 CE, the *Uí Néill* (O'Neills) defeated Aidan's grandson Domnall Brecc and the *Dálriadans* regained control of Argyll.[12]

The Western *Dál Riata* allied themselves most strongly with the Irish while the Eastern *Dál Riata* became allies of the Caledonians. While the *Dál Riata* termed themselves *"Gaels"*, to others in Caledonia they were known as *"Scotti"*, which was the Roman name for Irish immigrants, i.e. Scots.[13]

Anglo Culture Arrives

Another group to populate Scotland was the Angles, whose most Northern colony was Northumbria. In the 630's, Edwin, king of Northumbria, occupied Dun Eidyn (Edinburgh), capitol of the Gododdin. The Goddodin then fled to Celtic Western Britain, leaving South East Caledonia (the Borders) in Germanic (Anglian) hands. The advancing Northumbrians had split British Caledonia in two. The Highlands and Lowlands were ever after separated both ethnically and culturally.

The Battle of Nechtansmere

By the late 8th century, various areas of Scotland had submitted to Gaelic (Celtic), Northumbrian and Pictish powers and then to Germanic, Anglian settlers.[14] The native Picts had been continually at war with Dalriada, British Strathclyde and Northumbria. The Picts eventually conquered Strathclyde and at the Battle of Nechtansmere (in 685 CE) crushed the Northumbrians and stopped the Anglian expansion.

The Battle of Dunnichen or Nechtansmere was fought on May 20th, 685 CE. The Northumbrians, under their king *Ecgfrith*, had decided to invade Pictavia because the Picts had been slow to pay tribute after losing a battle to the Northumbrians in 672 CE. At the Battle of Nechtansmere, the Picts were led by King *Bruide*, son of *Bili*. This battle was a crucial win for the Picts because it decisively stopped the Northumbrian expansion into Scotland. However, Dun Eidyn (Edinburgh) and the Lothian area remained in Northumbrian control for a few more centuries after the battle.

---

of Scotland, P. 5
11. Davies., PP. 182-183
12. Ibid., P. 183
13. Ibid, P. 184
14. Ibid, P. 184

A Nation is Born

One force that finally unified these warring factions was the Irish missionaries who brought with them a uniform Gaelic language and tradition which they taught and applied in all areas. This helped to set the stage for the peaceful unification of the kingdoms under Kenneth MacAlpine (*Cináed mac Ailpín*), 34th King of Dalriada. In 843 CE he unified Scotland by inheriting Pictland from his mother and Dalriada from his father.[15]

15. *Ibid., P. 190*

The Druids

*T*he Druids are the earliest historical magical and religious group in Scotland for whom we have literary evidence. The Picts and earlier inhabitants must have had their own magical and spiritual traditions but these remain speculative.

According to Caesar, there were two classes of person who had status amongst the Celts: warriors and Druids. Rulers were drawn from the warrior class and ritually elevated to kingship status.

Historians such as Dumézil theorize that Celtic society had only three classes: rulers and Druids, warriors, and producers. In my opinion, there were actually four strata to Celtic society: rulers and Druids (the sacred class), warriors, farmers and producers, and slaves. This more closely parallels the caste system of other Indo-European peoples with whom the Celts share ancestral roots, such as the proto-Vedic societies.

We know that the Druids were the equivalent of Hindu Brahmins. They were a sacred class of intellectuals, both male and female, who served the rulers and the nobility. According to Kelly, the Druid was "a priest, prophet, astrologer, and teacher of the sons of nobles".[1]

Druids were responsible for overseeing both public and private sacrifices and divinations. They carried the ancient tribal laws in their heads and were responsible for resolving disputes, passing judgment on crimes, settling boundary issues, and issuing fines and penalties. They also performed battle magic on behalf of their kingdoms.

The Druids were hierarchical, and bestowed grades based upon learning and accomplishment, and had a Chief Druid who was their chosen leader. They

---

1. *Kelly, Fergus, A Guide to Early Irish Law, P. 60*

taught the doctrine of reincarnation, and held that the Otherworld of the dead existed in the same location as the world of the living, with souls and Spirits moving between the two realms.[2]

The major focus of their public rites were the great agrarian Fire Festivals of Samhuinn (the end of the harvest when the herds were brought down from the hills), *Oimelc* (the festival for the lactation of the ewes and of the first plowing), *Bealltan* (when the cows were led out to their summer pastures in the hills) and *An Lúnasdal* (the celebration of the first fruits of the harvest).

Druids studied the stars, and calculated the size of the earth and the universe.[3] Evidence of their astronomical knowledge is found in the Coligny Calendar of the Gaulish Celts. It is worth noting that Druids from all Celtic areas met in Britain, most probably in Wales, to receive training which must have made their knowledge and practices somewhat uniform in all Celtic areas.

The Coligny Calendar was found in Coligny, France, in 1897. It was created in about 50 AD and is a now fragmented bronze tablet that shows a five year cycle of sixty two lunar months. Each month was divided into two halves, a dark half and a light half, starting with the New Moon, and each day of the month is designated as "lucky" or "unlucky". There was a thirteenth intercalary month inserted every two and a half years so that the lunar cycle and solar cycle would remain synchronized.

There is a festival that may have corresponded to Samhuinn marked on the calendar that took place over a three night interval. *Bealltan* and *Lúnasdal* are also marked by special symbols. The calendar is Lunisolar, and the year varies from 354 to 355 days.[4]

Druid physicians used herbs, surgery, magical chants and incantations to do healing. Druid lawyers and judges memorized and passed down tribal law orally. The content of the laws is still seen in the remaining *"Brehon Law"* texts, although these are admixed with later Christian overlays put in by the seventh century Christian monks who wrote them down.

Every tribe and kingdom had to have its Druid because the king or queen could not function without one at their side. The Druid was the one who had memorized the laws and precedents, while the king was an expert warrior. In ancient times the king and his Druid were known as *"two kidneys"* of a kingdom.

Tribal Druids told sacred stories at important events such as marriages, elopements, battles, births, deaths, and feasts, and held the ruler's genealogy in their heads. Druids supervised at rituals where auguries were made and where the entire community partook of the Spirit of a sacrificed animal by consuming it.[5]

The three major grades of Pagan clergy and wise ones were the *Bards* (singers, poets, and musicians), *Seers* or *Ovates* (diviners) and *Druids* (priests, philosophers, administrators of justice). Druids spent twenty years learning their craft and practicing their rituals in groves of trees, or on high hill tops.

2. McNeill, F. Marian, *The Silver Bough Vol. I, P. 22*

3. McNeill, P. 21

4. Doutré, Martin, *The Calendar of Coligny* http://www.celticnz.co.nz/Coligny/ColignyPart1.htm

5. McNeill, F. Marian, *The Silver Bough Vol. I, P. 23*

Tradition holds that Abaris, an Arch-Druid who visited Athens in 350 CE may have been a teacher of Pythagoras. There is evidence that he worshiped at Callanish, on the Isle of Lewis.

The island of Iona (*Innis nan Druidneach*) was a sacred Druid isle before the arrival of Columba. Columba met with Broichan, Arch-Druid of king Brude's court, in 565 CE.[6]

Respect for Druidic traditions continued well into the modern era. In the seventeenth century, the Church of Scotland persecuted several persons for lighting sacred fires and for refusing to plow "Druidical Fields", places given over to the Fairies where charms and spells were made and *"Gudeman's Crofts"*, small corners of gardens and fields that were kept wild for the Fairies exclusive use. Bulls were still being sacrificed in the Highlands in the seventeenth century and milk offerings were still being poured on tombs and Fairy Hills in Orkney and elsewhere. Bonfires on Druidical Holy Days were forbidden by the church.

Today, these customs are being enthusiastically revived in Scotland and other Celtic countries, and all over the Celtic Diaspora.[7]

The Bards continued as royal heralds into the middle of the eighteenth century. Today, the Lord Lyon perpetuates the ancient office of Chief Sennachie of Scotland's royal line. As keeper of the family records and of the royal pedigree, he continues the ancient Druidic function of genealogist for the tribe. The Lord Lyon's courts are held May 6 and November 6, a vestige of the ancient *Bealltan* and *Samhuinn* customs.[8]

Modern Druids are still creating sacred spaces in the landscape, and actively working to revive ancient ones. A Druidical sacred grove is called a *"Neimheadh"* (pronounced nevay). Such a site usually features a stone altar or shrine, a sacred tree or well, and a Fairy mound or cairn. The Fire Altar is a ritual focus for such sites, where offerings of thanks and praise are made to the Gods.

---

6. *McNeill, PP. 24-26*
7. *Ibid., PP. 28, 29*
8. *Ibid., P. 28*

The Old Gods

*C*ontinuing with our exploration of the ancient roots of magic, religion and lore in Scotland, it is helpful to have an understanding of the original, pre-Christian Gods and Goddesses. Scottish deities were Celtic and Romano-Celtic, Pictish and Norse, depending on the time period or geographic region (Orkney and Shetland for example still have strong Scandinavian cultural ties).

Those who are drawn to practice the old Scottish religion will want to establish a relationship with a divine Patron and Patroness. Followers of the Old Gods and Goddesses develop a family relationship with them by honoring them with poetry and praise at the Fire Festivals, and by setting a place for them at the table or on the altar at feasts and Holy Days. In essence, the best way to honor the Old Gods is to strive to be just like them, in courage, skill, and accomplishment.

Oaths are sworn to the Gods by raising a cup at the feasting table in front of witnesses, or in the presence of a Druid. You can also swear an oath to the Gods by standing on or touching a stone, being ever mindful that a stone is an ancient Spirit and a powerful ancestral force on the earth. This is one reason why coronations are performed in the presence of a stone such as the Stone of Scone (Stone of Destiny).

The Celts were true polytheists, honoring the Gods and Goddesses appropriate to their crafts and professions. Each God or Goddess was seen as a distinct personality and there was no one Great Goddess or God. There was also no Maiden-Mother-Crone triplicity. Triple deities were three deities of the same age, *Brigid* for example, or the *Matres* (triple mothers). The most popular pan-Celtic deities were, and are, *Brighde* and *Lugh*. Brigantia was the face of *Brighde* in Southern Britain. In Scotland, the *Cailleach*, who is the "*Ancient veiled woman*" and the winter face of *Brighde* or *Bride*, was especially revered.

Goddesses connected to springs and rivers were also connected to cows which provided life sustaining milk. War goddesses were often associated with carrion birds such as crows or ravens. Horse Goddesses were associated with motherhood and fertility of the crops. Gods with antlers were concerned with hunting while Gods with ram horns were connected to battle and served as sacred warrior protector deities for the tribes. Horned Gods bestowed fertility and health to both wild and domestic herds.

Some of the deities are obscure to us and all we have left of them may be a single inscription. Roman reporters equated some of the native deities with the gods of their own pantheons, an aid to our understanding of their essential natures. As you read through this list, allow your subconscious mind to play with the names and notice any feelings they evoke. Ancestral memories run strong and one or more of the Gods or Goddesses may call to you.

Airmidh, Airmidh ~ The daughter of *Dian Cécht* and Patroness of Herbal Healers (see *Dian Cécht* below).

Alator ~ *"The Nourisher"*, a warrior God. In ancient times sacred warrior Gods were associated with healing and protection for the tribes.

Andraste, Andrasta ~ *"The Invincible one"*, Warrior Goddess and Patroness of the *Iceni* tribe.

Antenociticus ~ Worshiped near Hadrian's Wall, portrayed as a youthful God with stag horns and a torc (a round neck ring symbolizing nobility) around His neck. Horned deities were especially popular in areas near Hadrian's Wall.

Anu or Ana ~ One name for the great Land Goddess and Divine Mother who nurtures the land. Landscape features such as hills were equated with her body.

Arecurius ~ *"The One Who Stands Before the Tribe"*, a solar deity equated with *Apollo* in the Romano-Celtic period, worshipped in Northern Britain.

Barrex or Barrecis ~ *"The High God"* linked with *Mars* in the Romano-Celtic era.

Belatucadros ~ *"Fair Shining One"*, a ram horned God of war worshiped by soldiers in the vicinity of Hadrian's Wall.

Belinus / Belenos ~ *"Shining One"*, a Gaulish Sun deity associated with the *Bealltan* fires (Fires of Bel). The Patron God of sheep and cattle.

Bríghde ~ *Brighid, Brigantia, Bride.* The most popular pan-Celtic Goddess. She was a triple Fire Goddess of crafts: poetry, healing, motherhood, and smith craft. Honored at *Oimelc*, the Romans compared Her to *Athena/Minerva*, a Goddess of wisdom and crafts, and with *Hera/Juno*, Mother Goddess of the Hearth. In Scotland, she was the summer face of the *Cailleach*, the great Goddess of Winter. As *Brigantia* *"High One"* *"Exalted One"* *"Queen"*, She was the Goddess of Sovereignty and divine ancestress of the Brigantes associated with the Roman Goddess Victoria *"Victory"* and with the Roman Goddess *Caelestis*. She became *Caelestis Brigantia* during the Roman occupation, a Celtic *"Magna Mater"* (Great Mother) who stood above all other local Gods and Goddesses. Mother of the Gods, She was associated with sacred wells and streams whose waters often marked tribal boundaries, illuminating Her role as a territorial Goddess. As *Brighde*, She was associated with the flocks and with cattle. Daughter of The *Daghda*, She was raised on the milk of an Otherworldly cow which was white with red ears.

Braciaca ~ *"Drunk on Malt"* From the Welsh *"brag/ brac"* or malt, possibly the God of malt induced intoxication; He was equated with *Mars* by the Romans. For the ancients, drunkenness was regarded as a virtue in warriors, who were often given alcohol as they set off to do battle, a method of instilling courage.

Branwen ~ *"White Raven"*, a daughter of the Sea with many amorous entanglements who was compared by the Romans to *Aphrodite/ Venus*.

The Cailleach ~ The ancient and mysterious veiled woman who was creatrix of the land in both Scotland and Ireland. It was said that the Western Islands of Scotland were "dropped from her apron", as were stone cairns such as *Sliabh na Caillighe* near Kells in Ireland. Loch Awe and Loch Ness were created by Her when she left magical wells uncovered. Often associated with hills and Holy Wells, She was the personification of winter, the winter face of *Bride*. She transformed herself in the Well of Youth at *Oimelc*, becoming the Summer Goddess of green fertility until She was reborn once more at *Samhuinn*. The *Cailleach* and *Bride* were the pre-eminent female deities of Scottish tradition. The *Cailleach* was honored in many locations, as a single or triple Goddess (being one of triplets implied divine status). She was known as *The Cailleach Bheara* (the oldest of all creatures) from the southern Irish coast, who had two sisters: *The Cailleach Bheur* (the blue faced Old Woman of the Highlands, the Goddess of Winter) and *Corca Duidhna* (*The Cailleach* of the area around the Dingle Peninsula in Ireland). Other *Cailleachs* included *The Cailleach Bronach* (*Cailleach* of Sorrow, from the Cliffs of Moher in Western Ireland), *The Cailleach Mal* (from Hag's Head at the Southern end of the Cliff's of Moher), *The Cailleach Uragaig* of Colonsay, Argyllshire, *The Cailleach Beinne Bric* (Guardian of the Deer), *The Cailleach Mor* (The Great One, the mother of giants), *The Cailleach Groarnagh* (Manx, Old Woman of Spells), *The Cailleach of Clibhrich*, *The Cailleach of Slyne Head*, *The Three Hebridean Cailleachs of Raasay, Rona* and *Sligachan*, and *The Muilearteach* (Cailleachs of the sea). She was also sometimes known as *Nicnevin* (Bone Mother) when she flew through the air at *Samhuinn*.

Camulos ~ Also known as *Teutates* (Gaelic, Neith) was a *Belgic* God of War who was compared by the Romans to *Aries/ Mars*. He was brought north to the area of the Antonine Wall where His carved stone altar featured a tree on each side and an Oak wreath. He was a ram-horned deity.

Cernunnos ~ His name is known from an incomplete inscription from Paris "-*ernunnos*" and from two other plaques that were found in the territory of the Celtic *Treveri* tribe in Luxembourg which were inscribed: *"Deo Ceruninco"* (to the God Cerunincos). A Gaulish inscription found in Monatgnac reads: *"Carnonos"*. A Gallo-Roman variant of His name is *Cernennus*. He was a horned God who appeared on the *Gundestrup* Cauldron (a metal cauldron of Celtic provenance, thought to date from the La Tène Period of the 2nd or 1st century BCE, which was discovered in a Danish peat bog in 1891), sitting in a half-lotus (seated with both knees bent and flat against the ground) Yogic posture, holding a ram-headed serpent. Elsewhere on the Cauldron, He was shown holding a wheel which may symbolize the turning of the seasons. Some statues of Him had removable antlers hinting at a ritual where He would lose his horns in the same way as the deer drop their antlers at certain times of year. On the *Gundestrup* Cauldron, He wore a torc (a metal neck ring), symbolic of His noble status, and wielded a second torc in one of His hands. He was surrounded by animals such as deer, serpents, lions, bear and wolves. In Gaul, He was depicted as the Patron of merchants, shown pouring gold coins from his purse, or as a nurturer of serpents who fed ram-headed snakes from His lap. Serpents in ancient thinking were akin to dragons that functioned as guardians of treasure, making Him the God who brought prosperity by increasing wild and domestic herds and prospering other mercantile efforts.

Cocidius ~ *"Red God" "Red Lord"* West of Hadrian's Wall He was worshiped as a God of soldiers, in the East as a God of wild animals, a hunter God, a God of the people, and a native warrior God.

Coventina ~ Patroness of the Sacred Well. A shrine to Her was discovered in the Carrawburgh area, near Hadrian's Wall where She was depicted as three nymphs or as a single Goddess, resting on water weeds and holding an urn from which water flowed. She was a Goddess of Fertility, Maternity and Healing.

An Daghda ~ (*Brythonic Don*) A father God from ancient Ireland who was Patron of the Druids. He had an inexhaustible Cauldron of Plenty from which He fed the people, and a magical staff that would heal or kill, depending on which end he applied. He was a Father Nature figure: nature can kill or heal depending on how wisely it is approached. He was compared by the Romans to *Zeus/*

Jupiter and to *Odin/ Wodin* (See *Eochaid Ollathair* and *Ruad Rothéssa* below). Another name for *An Daghda* was *"Aedh"* (fire), a fitting name for the father of the great Fire Goddess, *Bríghde*.

Dian Cécht ~ A God of medicine. When *Nuada*, leader of the *Tuatha Dé Danann* (tribe or people of the Goddess *Danu*) lost a hand at the First Battle of Moytura, the physician God *Dian Cécht* replaced the severed hand with a silver one, but by law, no blemished or maimed person could rule, so *Nuada* was deposed. When *Nuada* developed an infection, *Miach* and *Airmidh*, the children of *Dian Cécht*, cured him. *Miach* had the severed hand dug up and chanted the famous verse over it: *"Sinew to sinew, nerve to nerve, vein to vein, bone to bone..."* and in three days the hand was completely restored.

Dian Cécht was livid with envy at *Miach's* skill and attacked *Miach* several times, finally cleaving His skull in two. Then, three hundred and sixty five healing herbs grew out of *Miach's* grave (possibly a reference to a now lost calendrical system), each herb appearing from the body part that the herb was useful for. *Airmidh* arranged the herbs on Her cloak according to their corresponding body parts, hinting at a now lost herbal classification system. Ever jealous, *Dian Cécht* shook the cloak and the art of curing every ill was lost. *Airmidh* remains the Patroness of Herbalists and of the Herbal Arts.

Balder ~ The Norse God of light, joy, purity, beauty, innocence, and reconciliation. Son of *Odin* and *Frigg*, he was loved by both Gods and men and was considered to be the best of the Gods. A solar deity, He was responsible for the custom of kissing under the mistletoe (see Yule below).

Divine Smith ~ A native smith God equated with *Vulcan* by the Romans.

Eastre ~ The Anglo Saxon Goddess of spring whose symbols were the hare and the egg. She is still remembered in modern times when Easter baskets, bunnies and eggs are given to children.

Ériu ~ The great Land Goddess of *Eire* whose worship was brought to Scotland by the immigrant Gaels. A triple Goddess, Her other names were *Banba* and *Fodla*. She sometimes appeared as a grey-white crow.

Elen ~ (Elen of the Ways) The Green Woman, a horned, antlered Goddess who appeared dressed in green leaves with a dog at Her side, and amber around Her neck.

Eochaid Ollathair ~ "Great Horse Father" is another title of *An Daghda*, the great all-purpose Father God; war leader, bestower of fertility, law giver, patron of the Druids, and sacred warrior tribal protector.

Epona ~ "Divine Horse" She was worshiped near the Antonine Wall, Protectress of Horses, She was adopted by the Roman cavalry, and was often depicted as a woman sitting on a horse with a sheaf of grain in Her lap, a dish of grain in one hand, and a serpent in the other. The combination of serpent and grain marked Her as a Goddess who protected the fertility and prosperity of both grain and horses, of fields and herds. In Gaul, She was personified as a woman riding a goose (perhaps the original Mother Goose).

Flidais ~ The Goddess of wild animals, owner of Otherworldly cattle and mistress of stags who traveled in a chariot pulled by deer. She was the lover of *Fergus Son of Roech* (Fergus, son of Great Horse) a king of *Uster* whom only she could satisfy sexually, even though he normally needed seven women to meet his needs.

Freya ~ (or *Frayja*) The Norse Goddess of love, beauty, fertility, war, and wealth who traveled in a chariot drawn by cats.

Genii Cucullati ~ A trio of hooded cloaked figures known from stone carvings. It is unclear if they were male or female figures. They were associated with fertility, agriculture and water.

Grannos ~ A God equated with *Apollo* who was originally from Gaul.

God with a Wheel Symbol ~ Possibly *Taranis* (*Tanarus*), a thunder deity and Sky God.

God with Radiating Hair ~ Possibly *Maponos*, who was equated with *Apollo*. His hair appeared to stand out from his head in stiff spikes.

Goibniu (Ireland) / **Govannon** (Wales) ~ a divine smith who fashioned magical Otherworldly weapons for the Gods.

The Native Hercules ~ A powerful God with a large club who wore a torc (a neck ring), the symbol of nobility.

The Horned God ~ A *"genius loci"* (Spirit of place) associated with *Mars, Mercury* and *Silvanus* who was shown with antlers.

The Horned Goddess ~ Possibly *Modron* and associated with *Diana* by the Romans, She was worshiped near Hadrian's Wall. Possibly a Goddess of the hunt and of wild animals (see *Flidais*)

Latis ~ "Goddess of the Pool", "Goddess of Beer", a Goddess of pools and healing springs into which coins were tossed to petition the Goddess for good health.

Lenus ~ A God of Gaul and Britain depicted with a goose or swan. Both birds are fierce defenders of their families and were therefore associated with warriors.

Llyr ~ (Lir) A Sea God who was compared to *Poseidon/Neptune* by the Romans. Father of *Manannán*.

Lludd ~ (Nudd) **Nuada** (Gaelic) Ruler of the Otherworld under the Sea who was compared to *Pluto* by the Romans.

Lug ~ (*Lugh*) Associated with the *Lúnasdal* festival, which He founded in honor of His foster-mother *Tailtiu*, who died of exhaustion after clearing the *Wood of Cuan* in Ireland, in order to prepare the land for plowing. Similar festivals were held in Scotland, in honor of the local divine Mother Goddess of the land. He was Master of every Art. In the Christian period, many sacred sites associated with *Lug* were rededicated to Saint Michael.

Macha ~ One of the three aspects of the *The Morrígan* in which guise She is a Goddess of War. In other stories she is a Mother Goddess of Fertility and a Goddess of Horses.

Manawyddan Ap Llyr (Wales) (*Manannán Mac Lir*) ~ A God of Sea and Wind who traveled on a magical horse called *Enbarr* of the Flowing Mane, who was swift as the wind on land or sea. He was a messenger God who guided the dead to the Otherworld across the waves. Possessor of the Crane Bag of many powers, He also had a magical cloak with the power of invisibility and shape changing. He was associated with liminal spaces between water and land, symbolic of His ability to travel between one world and the next, from life to death and back. He rode over the Sea, herding fish as His flocks.

Maponos ~ "Divine Youth", "Divine Son", who was worshiped in the Border area and equated with *Apollo* by the Romans. He was a God of poetry, music, and hunting and son of *Modron*, the "Divine Mother". His name in Welsh is (*M)ap Ollo* (Son of the Highest), said to have come from the Hyperborean Isles, from beyond the North Wind.

The Matres ~ "The Triple Mothers" who may be *Brigantia* Herself in triple form. She was shown as three women, each holding a cornucopia, fruits, a baby, or bread. Sometimes shown as *Matrona*, a single, seated Mother Goddess, Her spheres were fertility and maternity.

Matunus ~ "Divine Bear" "Spirit of the Bear", a bear God.

Miach ~ Son of *Dian Cécht* and a Patron God of Herbalists (see *Dian Cécht* above)

Mither O' ~ The Sea Goddess invoked by fishermen for protection, she was the personification of summer who warmed the Ocean, calmed storms, and filled the Sea with fish. (See *Teran* below)

Modron ~ "Divine Mother", "Great Mother" The mother of *Maponos* or *Mabon* "Divine Youth" (*Mabon vab Modron*, "Son of Mother") who had no father. Equated with the Irish *Danu*, and possibly the counterpart to the Gaulish *Matrona*, she was Goddess of the Marne River.

Mogons ~ "The Great One". He was possibly a triple deity (because inscriptions referred to Him in both the singular and in plural) who was worshipped in Gaul and North of Hadrian's Wall.

The Morrígan ~ "Great Queen", "Phantom Queen" a triple Goddess personified as three battle crows or ravens who influenced the outcome of battles with Her magic. By striking terror into the hearts of warriors, she deprived them of the will to win. At times, She appeared as three Hags or as three beautiful young women. She could shape-shift into an eel, a wolf, or a heifer in order to attack any man who refused Her sexual advances. She appeared as "the washer at the ford", washing blood off of the weapons and armor of one who was about to die.

Nantosuelta ~ (Winding River). A Gaulish Raven Goddess who appeared as a raven in Her warrior context, and as a dove in the context of motherhood, hearth, and home.

Nodons ~ A Romano-Celtic God of Healing associated with dogs. He had a temple on the river Severn in Gloucestershire where the sick would come to be healed.

Ocelus ~ A God associated with the swan or goose and with *Mars*. Possibly a tribal God of the *Silures* brought North in the first century CE by those fleeing the Roman invasions.

Oengus Og ~ *Angus Og* A young god of love who was compared to *Cupid/Eros* by the Romans. He played a golden harp and aided young lovers.

Odin ~ **Odínn** (Old Norse) The chief divinity of the Norse pantheon, *Odin* was a son of *Bor* and *Bestla*. He was called *Alfadir*, Allfather, and Father of the Gods. With *Frigg* he was the father of *Balder*.

Ogma ~ A God of eloquence and fair speech, credited with inventing the *Ogham* alphabet. Called "Sun-Faced", it was said that His Bardic followers were bound to Him by a golden chain attached to His tongue. He was a God of music, spells, and the arts.

Rata or Ratis ~ "Goddess of the Fortress", Protectress of gates, entrances, and boundaries.

Rigisamus ~ "Most Kingly". A warrior God of Gaul and Britain equated with *Mars*. He was an example of the sacred warrior as a noble, kingly leader.

Ruad Rofhéssa ~ The Red One of great wisdom. The "Good God", titles of *The Daghda*.

Saitada ~ "The Sad One" possibly a Goddess of grief associated with funerals.

Setlocenia ~ "Goddess of Long Life", "The Long lived One". She was native to Cumberland.

Sequanna ~ Gaulish Goddess of the river Seine.

Silvanus ~ A horned God associated with hunting who was shown naked except for a cloak. He was worshipped on the Eastern side of Hadrian's Wall.

Sucellos ~ A Gaulish and British Sky God who was usually depicted with a mallet (possibly a symbol of thunder and lightning) and a libation plate. Called "The Good Striker" His consort was *Nantosuelta*, a personification of the Land Goddess. He was equated with *Zeus* by the Romans.

Teran ~ The Spirit of Winter who did battle with *Mither O' the Sea* at the Spring Equinox for mastery of the Oceans. *Teran's* voice was heard in the gales of March and His anger was seen in the stormy waves. At the last, *Mither* bound Him at the bottom of the Sea as Her gentle Summer reign began. At the Autumn Equinox the battle raged once more and fierce waves and wind showed that *Mither* was banished until she rose triumphant again in the Spring.

Verbeia ~ A River Goddess and Goddess of Sacred Springs. One of Her titles was "She of the Cattle". She was shown holding Serpents, powerful symbols of healing, protection, wisdom and transformation.

Vinotonus ~ "God of the Vines" equated with *Silvanus*, a God of hunting and wild animals.

Vitris ~ "Mighty Wise One" who was shown as a single or triple deity, accompanied by a serpent and or a boar.

The Gods in Place Names

Scottish place names reveal the locations where some of the above deities were worshiped. Darnaway (*Taranaich*) is derived from *Taran* or *Tarnach* (thunder), a place where the thunder deity *Taranis* may have been worshipped. Angus received its name from the God *Aengus* or *Oengus*. Annan in Dumfriesshire was named for *Anu* or *Ana*, the great Land Goddess.

In areas where Irish Gaels settled, the Goddess *Ériu* was honored. Strathearn, Perthshire is from *Strath Eireann* and Lochearn from *Loch Eireann*. Auldearn, Moray, is from *Allt Eireann* (burn of *Ériu*). Atholl is from *Ath Fodhla* (New Ireland) in honor of *Fodla* while Banff and Bamff both honor *Banba*.[1]

Sources for the list of Gods and Goddesses

Beith, Mary, Healing Threads

Bendis, Cailleach Bera, The Blue Roebuck,
    http://www.blueroebuck.com/cailleach_bera.htm

Hopman, Ellen Evert, A Druids Herbal – For the Sacred Earth Year.

Marwick, Ernest, The Folklore of Orkney and Shetland.

McNeill, F. Marian, The Silver Bough Vol. I.

Niafer, Flidas, The Cailleach: Hag of Samhain, AncientWorlds LLC, Celtia,
    http://www.ancientworlds.net/aw/HomesiteRoom/10548

Ross, Anne, Pagan Celtic Britain.

---

1. *McNeill, F. Marian, The Silver Bough Vol. I., PP. 36-37*

Lore of the Elements

A core principle in understanding the ancient Scottish approach to ritual is the profound respect given to the Sun and Moon. When approaching a sacred site such as a Holy Well, a ritual circle, a cairn, or a bonfire on one of the Fire Festivals, when blessing a new house or a boat, when setting out to Sea, etc., it is traditional to move in a "sunwise" direction or *deiseil*. Pregnant women walk three times deiseil around a sacred site to ensure safe labor; fire is carried deiseil three times around a child to protect it from being abducted by Fairies. At a hand-fasting the celebrants process three times deiseil around the house before entering. Fishing boats move in three deiseil circles before setting out to Sea. Coffins are circled three times deiseil before being carried to their place of interment.

Some believe that the practice of moving deiseil may be a reference to the movement of the Ursa Major (Great Bear, The Plow) constellation whose tail points East in the Spring, South in the Summer, West in the Fall and North in the Winter.[1] Traditionally it is very important to move *"with the flow"* of nature, or in harmony with all of creation, in order to ensure luck. To go in the opposite direction, i.e. *tuaithiuil* or *"wrang-gaites"* (counter-clockwise, *widdershins*) is considered very unlucky and implies that some kind of evil is afoot.

Only Witches deliberately dance *tuaithiuil* (some Witches have told me they do this because they are circling "Earthwise" to send energy down into the Earth). In ancient times invading armies that were bent on destruction approached their targets in this manner. One way of determining if an approaching force was an enemy or friend was to observe in which direction

---

1. *McNeill, F. Marian, The Silver Bough Vol. I, P. 53*

they circled towards their objective.[2] The number three is a sacred number in Indo-European tradition which refers to the Three Worlds of Land, Sea and Sky, or Middle Earth (the realm of humans and Nature Spirits), Underworld (the realm of the Fairies and ancestors), and Sky World (the realm of the Gods and Goddesses), and to triple deities. Celtic rituals often involve the honoring of the Three Worlds by offering gifts to fire, water and trees.

Offering a gift to a sacred fire (such as whisky, butter or dried herbs), causes the fire to send your intention skyward, to the realm of the Gods and Goddesses. Offering a gift to sacred water (such as fruit, fresh flowers, or silver) sends your intention to the Underworld of the Fairies, and to the ancestors. Offering a gift to a tree (such as honey, herbs, fertilizer, or milk) sends your intention skywards through the branches and to the underworld of the Fairies and ancestors through the roots.

Honoring the Sun and Moon

In the nineteenth century, men of the Hebrides still took off their hats to honor the Sun and women still bowed to the New Moon. As they did so, they gave thanks for the warmth and light provided so generously.[3] A *peighinn pisich* (lucky penny or silver coin) that was kept in a pocket especially for this purpose was turned three times at the first sight of the New Moon.

The ancients left us evidence of their regard for the Moon as well. Pictish standing stones were often carved with a symbol of two crescents back to back depicting the last quarter and the first quarter of the Moon.[4]

Hymns to the Moon and Sun

New Moon

When I see the new moon,
It becomes me to lift mine eye,
It becomes me to bend my knee,
It becomes me to bow my head.
Giving thee praise, thou moon of guidance,
That I have seen thee again,
That I have seen the new moon,
The lovely leader of the way.
Many a one has passed beyond
In the time between the two moons,
Though I am still enjoying the earth,
Thou moon of moons and blessings!

(Traditional –Carmina Gadelica 306)

---

2. McNeil, P. 53
3. Ibid P. 29
4. McNeill, P. 58

Queen of the Night

Hail to thee,
Jewel of the night!
Beauty of the heavens,
Jewel of the night!
Mother of the stars,
Jewel of the night!
Fosterling of the sun,
Jewel of the night!
Majesty of the stars,
Jewel of the night!

(Traditional, Carmina Gadelica 312)

The Sun

Hail to thee, thou sun of the seasons,
As thou traversest the skies aloft;
Thy steps are strong on the wing of the heavens,
Thou art the glorious mother of the stars.
Thou liest down in the destructive ocean
Without impairment and without fear;
Thou risest up on the peaceful wave-crest
Like a queenly maiden in bloom.

(Traditional, Carmina Gadelica 316)[5]

Farming by the Moon

Modern Druids and Scottish Pagans are reviving the old practices of honoring the Moon, and planting by the Moon. Each month (or *Moonth*) is divided into two halves: the *"waxing"* phase from the Dark of the Moon to the Full Moon, and the *"waning"* phase from the Full Moon to the dark of the Moon. The waxing phase is the time to harvest plants where the upper parts are what you want, such as stems, barks, seeds, flowers, leaves and berries. At this time the sap will be rising and the essence of the plant will be in the upper parts.

By tradition, the Waxing Moon is considered a good time to plant leafy and above ground crops because the Moon draws the juices skyward. Farmers and gardeners should plant, graft and pollinate above ground crops for food and medicine during this Moon phase.

Animals are slaughtered in the Waxing Moon to ensure that the flesh is moist and flavorful. Willow and Hazel rods are cut for baskets in the Full or Waxing Moon to ensure that the rods are supple and filled with sap. Pine is cut to make a boat in the Waxing or Full Moon. The Waxing Moon is considered a good time to start a journey or a new marriage.[6]

---

5. *Carmichael, Alexander, Carmina Gadelica, PP. 286, 289, 292*
6. *McNeill, F. Marian, The Silver Bough Vol. I, PP. 57-58*

From the Full Moon to the Dark of the Moon is the waning phase when the plant's energy travels downwards, sinking into roots, tubers, rhizomes and bulbs, which should be harvested at that time. When cutting wood for building, furniture making, firewood, etc, it is always wise to do it in the waning phase or the Dark of the Moon. That will ensure that the sap of the tree is concentrated in the roots, and not so much of it will be in the wood.

One reason the ancient Romans were able to move their armies across Europe so easily, was that they would wait for the Dark of the Moon to cut trees. The wood would dry very quickly and they would then use it to make bridges and roads.

The Waning Moon is beneficial for root crops (and kale). Farmers and gardeners should plant below-ground crops, transplant and weed, prune to discourage growth, and perform pest control activities during the Waning Moon.

The Waning Moon is also the proper time for plowing, reaping, and cutting peat because there will be less moisture. Eggs laid in the Waning Moon are left to hatch. The Waning moon is a good time to geld animals because there will be less flow of blood. Harvest below-ground crops for food and medicine during a waning Moon.[7]

Any animal with horns is sacred to the Moon, and in ancient times might be sacrificed to the Moon for help, for example a cow might have been sacrificed to ward off cattle disease. Symbols of horns were once buried with the dead, and horned animals were used to carry the bones of the dead to their graves.[8]

Here is a concise guide to Lunar gardening:

First Quarter (*Waxing Moon*)

> The moon pulls liquids upwards in the Waxing phase, just as it draws the tides. Plant leafy things with shallow roots like asparagus, broccoli, brussels sprouts, cabbage, lettuce, parsley, spinach, cauliflower, celery, cress, endive, kohlrabi and annual flowers. Begin new projects.

Second Quarter (*Waxing Moon*)

> Plant things with seeds inside their fruits like beans, eggplant, melons, peas, pumpkins, peppers, squash, and tomatoes. Nurture the garden and tend to new growth.

Third Quarter (*Waning Moon*)

> This is the time when the Moon's energy decreases and the best time to plant root oriented plants such as biennials, perennials, bulbs, trees, shrubs, berries, beets, carrots, onions, parsnips, peanuts, potatoes, radishes, rhubarb, rutabaga, strawberries, turnips, winter wheat.

Fourth Quarter (*Waning Moon to Dark of the Moon*)

> This is the time to cultivate the soil, pull weeds, and destroy pests. This is also the best time to begin a compost pile or a worm farm.[9]

---

7. *McNeill, P. 58*

8. *Ibid., P. 59*

9. *An invaluable reference for gardening by the moon is the Old Farmer's Almanac, founded by Robert B. Thomas in 1792.*

The Winds and Directions (The Airts)

In Scottish tradition, the winds are understood to be living Spirits. *Gentle Annis* is the Wind Spirit of Cromarty Firth whose presence is felt when the South-West wind picks up without warning. *The Cailleach Bheur* is the blue-faced Old Woman of the Highlands who controls the winter winds and Robin Hood is said to travel by horse back on the winds.[10] Leaves whirling in a circle are evidence of *Fairies* and whistling can be used to raise up a storm.[11]

The Twelve Winds

The best way to understand the winds is to actively work with them. Consult the winds on a daily basis or before setting out on a journey or any other important engagement – notice from which direction the wind is coming to determine the outcome of the day's activity. You will also want to check the prevailing wind at the stroke of midnight on New Year's Eve to see what energies the New Year will bring.

By tradition, the winds have the following qualities:

East Wind *(gaoth an ear)*
Its color is purple *(corcur)*, a color that implies nobility (because only nobles were allowed to wear the color purple) and art.

East South East Wind *(gaoth an ear ear-dheas)*
Its color is yellow *(buidhe)*, and it is a good wind for fruit, fish and corn.

South South East Wind *(gaoth a deas ear-dheas)*
Its color is red *(dearg)*, and it is a good Wind for fishing, luck and prosperity.

South Wind *(gaoth a deas)*
Its color is white *(geal)*, and it brings a rich harvest.

South South West Wind *(gaoth a deas iar-dheas)*
Its color is pallid *(glas)* or grey-green. It brings blight, battle and poor harvests.

West South West Wind *(gaoth an iar iar-dheas)*
Its color is green, and it brings healing. It is the Wind of the Mothers.

West Wind (gaoth an iar)
Its color is dun (pale) *(odhar)*, and it brings the death of a king, bloodshed, and justice.

West North West Wind *(gaoth an iar iar-thuath)*
Its color is grey *(liath)*, and it brings death, slaughter, and the fall of blossoms.

North North West Wind *(gaoth an iar-thuath)*
Its color is dusky, swarthy, sable, gloomy *(ciar)* and it brings grumbling, quarrels and sternness but also strength and vindication. It can sweep away disease.

North Wind *(gaoth a tuath)*
Its color is black *(dubh)*, and it brings battle magic and drought.

10. Lamb, Gregor, *Carnival of the Animals*, P. 116
11. Livingstone, Sheila, *Scottish Customs*, P. 110

North North East Wind *(gaoth a tuath ear-thuath)*
Its color is dark grey *(teimheil)*, and it brings sickness and battle venom.

East North East Wind *(gaoth an ear ear-thuath)*
Its color is speckled *(aladh)*, and it brings enchantments and magic.[12,13]

Water Magic

There is a rich Scottish tradition of making petitions at Holy Wells, that long pre-dates Christianity. Ancient Holy Wells are often associated with overhanging trees, with their branches that reached to the Sky World. The Well's water was understood to be a pathway to the Underworld, a water gateway to the ancestors and the Land of Fairy, thus the humans who petitioned the Well stood between two worlds.

As one example, offerings were once left at a tree that stood near Tobar Bial na Buaidh (the Well of the Virtuous Water and Tree) near Benderloch. Christian missionaries deliberately built churches near wells such as this one and re-dedicated them to Saints.[14]

A classic well ritual is to *"Silver the water"* (toss a small silver coin into the Well), take a drink, and then walk three times around the well deiseil and finally leave an offering such as a small stone, rag, pin, colored thread, or coins nearby. At *"Clootie Wells"*, small strips of one's personal clothing are torn and then hung on a tree over-hanging the well. Sometimes written requests for help, rings and jewelry are left at these places, entreating the Spirit of the Waters to help remove a sickness or other obstacles. These objects are never touched by others, because to do so might transfer the bad luck to a new person. Clootie Wells are always approached from the East on the Southern side.[15]

Offerings of cheese, barley cakes or other foods may be left for the Spirits after a well ritual. If the food disappears by the next day the illness will go with it, but if the Fairies ignore the food offerings it is a sign that someone will soon die. A coin might be hammered or pushed into a nearby Oak tree as an offering.[16]

Water from a Holy Well on *Bealltan* can be used to wash your face and increase your beauty. Wells are also consulted for good luck, protection, long life, safe travel and favorable winds for fishing. The water can be used to treat cattle plague *(connoch)* and other animal diseases.[17]

Holy Wells are visited at sunrise, or just before setting out on a journey. Water from a Holy Well can be collected to be baked into a bannock for a special occasion. The healing power of a Well is said to be strongest at the end of the first quarter of the Moon.

---

12. See this list of Winds in the Early Christian text 'Saltair na Rann', Canto 1, quatrains 12 to 24.

13. Wright-Popescul, Jean "The Twelve Winds of the Ancient Gaelic World", Canso-Chesapeake Heritage Publishing, 1997

14. Miller, Joyce, Magic and Witchcraft in Scotland, P. 43

15. Livingstone, Sheila, Scottish Customs, P. 118

16. Livingstone, P. 118

17. Miller, Joyce, Magic and Witchcraft in Scotland, P. 43

Stones are often associated with Holy Wells. Going to the *"Clachan"* (stones) was once as sacred a ritual as going to church. The correct procedure was to bow to the Well, and then walk around it three times while praying. Then you washed your hands and feet in the water and tied a *cloot* (cloth) to a nearby tree or bush. After that, you bowed to a natural stone and walked around it, praying. If there was a Fairy Mound nearby you would also process around that three times.[18]

Wells are honored at *"Well Dressing"* ceremonies on *Bealltan* (May 1) (or May 12 old style, the difference is due to the change caused by the shift from the Julian to the Gregorian calendar), *Lúnasdal* (August 1) (or August 12 old style), *Oimelc* (February 1), *Samhuinn* (November 1) (or November 11 old style) and *Summer Solstice* (June 21). Typically, the celebrants rise before dawn, drink from the well, greet their neighbors, tie a *"cloot"* on a nearby tree, drop a coin in the well, and make a wish.

Games such as ball playing, gambling, dancing, and beer drinking are part of the celebration and buns, cakes and other special foods are eaten. The Well is decorated with flowers and greenery and flowers are placed on nearby bushes, stones, and on the grass near the Well. Mistletoe is used to decorate a Holy Well on New Years Day. Young couples drink sugared Well water to announce their intention to marry. Sweetened water is given to children after they circumambulate the Well.[19]

The most powerful times to approach a Well are Sunrise and Sunset, when the first rays hit the water. It is an old magical axiom that where fire and water come together, there is the highest potential for magic.

Water drunk from a Well is ideally sipped from a human skull (obtained legally from a scientific supply house, of course) or from the horn of a living cow, or from a spoon made of the horn of a living cow.[20] Special tools such as a soldering iron or hacksaw are required to remove the horns of a living cow, and only trained farm hands should attempt this! Basically, you remove the horn, leaving about three inches of stump for it to heal over. Horns are made of keratin: a lot like finger nails, but also contain blood vessels and other tissues.

Sometimes, horns are removed from an adult cow, but generally it is best done when the cow is seven months old, or younger, and if you remove one horn, you also have to remove the other. Please don't do this unless you are very well trained.

Healing Wells

Certain Wells have developed a reputation for healing specific diseases or body parts. When approaching such a Well for a cure, there are certain basic practices that must be observed to show respect. Approach the Well barefoot and *deiseil* (sunwise, with the sun). Take a drink of the water, and then bathe the afflicted body parts. Hang a strip of cloth on a nearby tree and drop an offering of thanks into the water. Nearby stones and trees are then circumambulated with reverence.[21]

---

18. *Bord, Colin and Janet, Sacred Waters, P. 30*
19. *Bord, PP. 73-78*
20. *Ibid., P. 31*
21. *Ibid., P. 79*

Sometimes, three heaps of stones are placed near the Well. In that case, approach the Well barefoot, and wash your feet in the water, then, walk three times *deiseil* around each stone heap, taking a stone from the bottom of the pile and moving it to the top. One special healing stone will be set to one side. Take the special stone and pass it around your body and/or touch any afflicted part with it, then tear a bit of cloth (originally a bit was taken from your own clothing), and hang it on a nearby tree or leave it on nearby rocks.[22]

Healing Lakes

A *loch* (lake) is also an entrance to the Fairy realm and a gateway to the ancestors. To effect a cure from a loch, walk around it three times deiseil, then enter the loch in complete silence.[23] Another method, is to walk into the loch backwards, immersing yourself fully, then leave a coin and return to shore without looking back.

Offerings of butter are made to lochs at *Lúnasdal.* This practice is said to protect the cattle, and the poor can collect the butter (although in general it is bad luck to eat gifts that are meant for the Fairies).[24] Bread can be left as a gift for the Spirits and a rag can be tied to a sacred tree such as a Rowan.

Cursing Wells

Not all Wells have positive energies or associations. There are Cursing Wells where the name of a victim is written on paper and hidden near the Well. The name can also be carved into a rock or written on a parchment and dropped into the Well.

The person making the curse must drink some of the Well water, and then have some of the water thrown on them three times, as they declare out loud the expected outcome. A wax effigy of their target can be made and stuck with pins or thorns from a Hawthorn tree.

To undo the curse, the victim must walk three times around the same Well, retrieve the rock or parchment upon which the curse has been inscribed and drink the Well water.

Of course, no one with any sense will engage in this kind of baneful magic. No wise person will send out this kind of negative energy, knowing that it will only reverberate back on the sender.[25]

Well Magic

There are many magical practices specifically associated with Holy Wells and with water. There were once over six hundred Holy Wells in Scotland. Every spring, river, and loch was understood to have its own indwelling Spirit or patron deity. Sometimes the Spirit appeared as a trout or other fish called a *Iasg Sianta* (holy fish) on certain holy days.[26]

22. *Ibid., P. 79*
23. *Ibid., P. 82*
24. *Ibid., P. 31*
25. *Ibid., PP. 84-85*
26. *McNeill, F. Marian, The Silver Bough Vol. I, P. 66*

In modern times it may be necessary to consecrate a new Holy Well, especially if you live in the Celtic Diaspora of the United States, Australia, New Zealand, Canada, etc. (persons living in Europe and other places where Holy Wells are still common, should revive and energize the ancient Wells of their home territories).

To consecrate a new Well for magical or Spiritual use, carry stones to the Well to mark it out as a special place, then do a ritual there, invoking a specific Patron or Patroness as Guardian of the Well. Then take a candle in hand and process deiseil around the Well three times. Such a Well may be a natural spring in the ground, a stone-lined pool with steps, or even be inside a building. Ideally it should be situated near a sacred tree such as an Ash, Yew, Rowan, Oak, Hawthorn, or Holly.

Here is an Old Irish invocation to *Bríghde (Bride, Brighid)* that I recite at the Clootie Well on the land where I live. The Well that I and my Druid Grove have used for two decades, is a clear stream in the forest with a dug out pool lined with stones. A Birch tree has its roots right in the Well and there are Oaks all around it. One tree was selected to bear the cloots. We drop silver coins into the pool before we do any ritual, and in summer, we place fresh flowers and fruits in, and around, the lip of the Well.

Invocation of Bríghde by Ellen Evert Hopman
(Old Irish Translation by Alexei Kondratiev)

A Brigit, a ban-dé beannachtach
Tair isna huisciu noiba,
A ben inna téora tented tréna,
Isin cherdchai,
'Isin choiriu,
Ocus isin chiunn,
No-don-cossain,
Cossain inna túatha.
O Brighid, blessed Goddess
Come into the sacred waters
O woman of the three strong fires,
In the forge,
In the cauldron,
In the head.
Protect us.
Protect the people.

*it is perfectly appropriate to use this kind of blessing in a Scottish context because
the West Coast of Scotland was settled by the "Scoti" or Irish of Northern Ireland.*

Insults to Wells

After a Well has been consecrated, the water must never be used for mundane purposes such as cooking, and the Well should be honored with offerings at each of the Fire Festivals *(Bealltan, Lúnasdal, Samhuinn,* and *Oimelc)* to keep its powers strong.[27]

---

27. *McNeill, P. 67*

Wells can be insulted by certain acts and the power of the Well will move on, necessitating a new ritual of consecration. Insults to Wells include throwing trash into a Well, washing clothes in it, washing animals in it, cutting down the tree associated with the Well or if the tree falls down, or moving a hollow stone or statue associated with the Well.[28]

Offerings to Wells

Appropriate offerings to Holy Wells include: pins, rags, pine cones, coins, keys, bread, cheese, stones, pebbles (especially white quartz), buttons, beads, buckles, pipes, fish hooks, jewelry, religious objects, fruits and flowers. Votives can be made and nailed or tied to a nearby tree, or left near the Well in thanks for healings that have occurred. Small tin or clay objects resembling body parts can be attached to a tree, the crutches of a healed person can be left near the Well, etc.

A statue or other image of a deity, which can be situated nearby in a niche, should be washed with the Well water yearly, and then carried in procession as a way of honoring the Spirit or God/dess of the Well.[29]

Fertility Rituals at Wells and Sacred Springs

Once a Well has been consecrated for use and honored with offerings of prayers and gifts, certain magical practices can be undertaken. One Well ritual is designed to increase fertility in women desiring to conceive. In this rite, three women who are having difficulty with conception are led by an older woman to a Holy Well or spring. The three younger women take off their shoes and stockings and roll up their skirts until their genitals are exposed to the Sun, and then walk deiseil around the Well as the Crone sprinkles water on their private parts each time they pass by, three times. Then the younger women bare their breasts to the Sun as the Crone sprinkles water on their breasts three times. Finally the women rise, cover themselves with their shawls, and return home. Everything must be done in complete silence.[30]

Transporting Sacred Water to Those in Need

Water from a Holy Well can be carried in a basin to a sick person's home, and the basin must never touch the ground.

A wooden dish is set to float upon the water. If the dish turns Sunways upon the water, the person will recover. If it turns *Widdershins*, they won't.[31]

Consulting Water Spirits

A victim of theft can drop a piece of bread into the Well water, while saying out loud the name of suspects, and the bread will sink when the guilty party is named.

An item of clothing from a sick person can be thrown into a Well. If it floats they will recover, if it sinks they won't.[32]

Water can be called upon as a sacred witness to an oath or a bargain, and a South running stream is especially lucky.

28. Bord, Colin and Janet, *Sacred Waters*, P. 100
29. Bord, PP. 90, 96
30. McNeill, F. Marian, *The Silver Bough Vol. I*, P. 69
31. Bord, Colin and Janet, *Sacred Waters*, P. 87
32. Bord, P. 87

Lover's vows are made by each standing on the opposite bank of a stream, wetting their hands, and then clasping hands over the stream as they repeat their promises. In the absence of a stream, the lovers can lick their right thumbs and press them together (which is why Farmers spit once on their hands before shaking them to seal a bargain).[33]

Water and the Evil Eye

To counteract the Evil Eye (basically jealousy from a neighbor), gather water from under a bridge where both the dead and the living pass (a place where coffins are carried over water to a burial ground) and carry the water home in complete silence, never allowing the vessel to touch the Earth.

Dip a wooden ladle with a piece of silver in it into the water and give the afflicted person three sips from the dipper. The remaining water is sprinkled on the victim.[34]

Honoring Rivers at Lúnasdal

Every river is under the protective care of a particular Goddess. Offerings of flowers, fruits, silver, and other items should be given in thanks to the local River Goddess of your bio-region, yearly (usually at *Lúnasdal*). The herb Saint John's Wort (*Hypericum perforatum*) is considered to be a perfect balance of fire and water and a sacred talisman of protection and defense for the home and barn.

When my Grove honors our local mother River Goddess, we sometimes make tiny 'boats' out of wood, and place a lit candle on top of each boat along with a sprig of Saint John's Wort, and sail them down the Connecticut River, in thanks for Her blessings all year.

Watery Places of Power

A place where two streams meet is filled with natural power and the water at these intersections has strong inherent magic.

The power of Fairy can be broken by crossing a running stream, and a child can be cured of disease by passing it back and forth over the waters for one hour.[35]

The great Mother Ocean has powerful magic of Her own. To ensure plentiful butter, a Skeely Woman (a skilled woman, a charmer) takes a bucket to the sea and puts three *gowpens* (as much water as two hands can hold) into her pail. This water is then put into the churn along with the milk (nicely salting the milk in the process).[36]

Certain activities should always be done at the incoming tide such as cutting turf for the thatch, pulling deep rooted weeds such as Dock, and churning. Fish bite more readily at this time. Rabbits should be hunted at the incoming tide, because by ebb they will go underground. Bringing a cow to the bull at the rising tide will result in a larger calf.[37]

33. McNeill, F. Marian, *The Silver Bough Vol. I*, P. 73
34. McNeill, P. 73
35. Livingstone, Sheila, *Scottish Customs*, P. 124
36. McNeill, F. Marian, *The Silver Bough Vol. I*, P. 73
37. Marwick, Ernest, *The Folklore of Orkney and Shetland*, P. 78

The Power of Dew

The most sacred form of water is dew, especially when gathered on *Bealltan* morn when it is used to wash the face as a magical way to ensure beauty.[38] It can also be sprinkled on cattle and farm implements to ensure fertility and a rich milk yield.

Rub the limbs of sick children with *Bealltan* dew and apply it to weak eyes, goiters, and to the chest as a healing agent. Bottle it and add it to healing lotions and ointments (adding a tiny amount of alcohol such as Vodka or Gin will preserve the water nicely for later use).

This practice closely resembles the creation of "Flower Essences" as invented by the Renaissance Swiss physician Paracelsus, and later developed into a spiritual counseling and medical healing technique by the Welsh physician Dr. Edward Bach. Paracelsus collected the dew from plants and stored it in glass vials. Bach created a method of exposing flowers to sunlight for four full hours in a crystal bowl, adding brandy as a preservative, and then bottling the water to treat medical and emotional conditions.

Fairy Pools

Fairy Pools are wild pools that are not touched by humans (similar to the Gudeman's Crofts that are left to grow wild at the corner of a field). A Fairy Pool should be left alone for the Fairies' use, however, at *Midsummer*, children may come and dress it with flowers and white stones.[39]

Fire Magic

In the ritual context, sacred fire is the vehicle by which offerings are sent to the Sky World of the Gods. The highest holy days are all celebrated with large bonfires designed to send messages of hope and thanksgiving to the deities. Offerings of sacred woods, fragrant herbs, butter, and oils are made to the flames, as petitions are spoken and prayers recited.

The hearth fire is the mystical center of the home which acts as an anchor for sacred activities such as prayer and story telling, and the central altar of the home which protects it from evil Spirits.

The hearth fire should always be kept lit (modern Druids may have to make do with a pilot light in an oven or a candle). Traditionally the peat fire was banked and kept smoldering all night (wood was generally too expensive to use as fuel), so that coals and embers always remained. Smooring the fire was the sacred duty of the woman of the house. Here is a traditional blessing from the Carmina Gadelica:

---

38. McNeill, F. Marian, *The Silver Bough Vol. I*, P. 74
39. Livingstone, Sheila, *Scottish Customs*, P. 123

Smáladh an Teine (Smooring the Fire)
The sacred Three
To save,
To shield,
To surround
The hearth,
The house,
The household,
This eve,
This night,
Oh! This eve,
This night,
And every night,
And every night,
Each single night,
Till white day shall come to the embers.
Traditional, Carmina Gadelica 84 and 85 (adapted)[40]

When a child is born, a fresh fire should be lit in the hearth or elsewhere. When a cow has calved, a lit peat should be brought into the barn and waved over the cow's back several times while saying: *"May the fire protect thee, may good be about thee".*[41]

Tein-eigin (The Need-Fire)

One of the most powerful fire rituals undertaken by a community is the Tein-eigin or "Need-fire", a sacred fire that must be made by friction. Such a fire is made to light sacred bonfires at the Fire Festivals and to perform community-wide healing magic.

To start the fire, a stick is drilled into a piece of dry wood with a hole in it. As the stick is turned, tinder such as straw is used to catch the spark, then tiny bits of Agaric, fungi that grow on Birch trees, are slowly added. The men who make the fire should be married men, and they should remove all jewelry and metal from their bodies as they work. Certain woods are considered sacred and appropriate to build a Need-fire:

The nine sacred woods:

"Choose the Willow of the streams,
Choose the Hazel of the rocks,
Choose the Alder of the marshes,
Choose the Birch of the waterfalls,
Choose the Ash of the shade,
Choose the Yew of resilience,
Choose the Elm of the brae,
Choose the Oak of the Sun".

(Traditional)[42]

---

40. Carmichael, Alexander, Carmina Gadelica – Hymns and Incantations, PP. 94-95
41. Marwick, Ernest, The Folklore of Orkney and Shetland, P. 78
42. McNeill, F. Marian, The Silver Bough Vol. I, P. 84

For the ninth wood, Apple or Pine is appropriate. Alternatively, the fire can be made entirely of Oak.

When a serious human or cattle disease afflicts the community, nine times nine men are employed to make a huge fire by friction. Every house in the area must put out their hearth fire and then re-kindle their home fire with the sacred flames. If the Need-fire fails to catch, the assumption is that someone in the village has failed to dowse their home fire, or that one of the eighty one men assigned to build the Need-fire is guilty of some hidden crime.

Once everyone has the new fire in their home, they should take water from a sacred spring or a Holy Well and put it to boil on the new fire (this must be the first thing heated on the new fire). When the water has come to a boil, it may be taken from the flames and sprinkled on affected people and animals to heal them.[43]

Saining

Crops, fields, herds, fishing boats, homes, ritual circles, newborn babies, etc., are *sained* (blessed or purified) by carrying a lit torch in a Sunwise circle around them.

Beannachadh na Cuairte (The Blessing of the Circle)

In this rite, an iron hoop is wound with straw that has been soaked in oil and melted bees wax, and then set on fire (be careful to leave a bare space on each side, so that the hoop can be held using fire proof gloves or mitts).

Two women hold the flaming circle while a third woman passes a sick child through the hoop as she prays.[44]

To Bless a Newborn Child

Every newborn child should be passed three times across the flames. The *bairn* can also be placed in a basket on top of cheese and bread that has been carefully wrapped with linen. The oldest woman present carries the basket around the flames three times and then briefly holds the basket over the fire. Afterwards, the food is shared with everyone assembled.

If no sacred fire is available, the Midwife can put a lit peat in a shovel and carry it three times around the new born and its mother.[45]

Earth Magic

Earthen mounds, whether natural or made by the ancestors, are seen as the homes of the *Fairies*. These are places to do ritual, declare laws, and mete out punishments. *The Brehons* (ancient law keepers of the tribes) once held court on the side of a hill while seated on the earth.[46] It is irreverent and even dangerous to remove earth or wood from a Fairy Hill.[47]

---

43. McNeill, PP. 63-64

44. Ibid, P. 65

45. Livingstone, Sheila, Scottish Customs, P. 9

46. McNeill, F. Marian, The Silver Bough Vol. I, P.60

47. McNeill, P. 105

The Gudeman's Croft

Also known as *"Halyman's Rig"*, *"Cloutie's Croft"* and *"The Black Faulie"*, it is a piece of land left wild for the exclusive use of the Earth Spirits and the Fairies. It must remain untouched by human tools. The Gudeman's Croft can be a corner of a field that is dedicated to the Fairies after a promise to leave it wild, or it can be a section of garden that is enclosed by a wall. [48]

Making Oaths on Sacred Ground

Every inch of ground is sacred because it holds the bones and blood of the ancestors, be they animal, vegetable, mineral, or human. Hallow an oath by lifting a clod of earth and swearing on it. When swearing, take care to remove your shoes and socks so as to be in close contact with the earth.

Earth to Earth and Dust to Dust

Earth and salt are placed on a dish and laid on a dead person's chest when the departed is laid out for viewing. Earth represents the physical body of the deceased, and salt represents the Spirit, reminding everyone that the one who has passed over is more than just a physical shell. [49]

---

48. *Ibid., P. 62*
49. *Ibid., P. 62*

Stones, Bones, and Talismans

Minerals, Crystals and Fairy Stones

Salt

Scatter salt or salt water around a new house for luck, before moving any furniture into it. When the herds are moved to a new pasture they are sained with fire, water, and salt.[1]

A particularly powerful way to obtain salt for saining is to take it from the ninth wave of the sea.

Silver

Silver is a metal particularly associated with the Moon, and with sacred water. A silver coin can be dedicated to the Moon and used as a charm.[2] Turn the silver coin in your pocket at the first sight of the New Moon. Place a bit of silver near, or on, the bairn to protect it from sorcery or Fairy abduction.

Silver bullets are a must when seeking to kill Vampires, Demons, and the Undead.[3] Scrofula (tubercular swelling of the glands) can be treated by wearing a silver coin around the neck.[4]

Gold

Gold is a mineral with strong associations to the Sun and with sacred fire. Golden earrings are helpful to those with sore eyes, or simply rub the ears with jewelry of pure gold. Rub sties and ringworm with golden rings or jewelry.[5]

---

1. *McNeill, F. Marian, The Silver Bough Vol. I, P. 75*
2. *McNeill, P. 72*
3. *Miller, Joyce, Magic and Witchcraft in Scotland, P. 58*
4. *Beith, Mary, Healing Threads, P. 159*
5. *Beith, P. 159*

A golden wedding ring or engagement ring carries luck all its own. Rub a wedding ring over a sty to heal it. Place the ring in a ladle or glass, pour water over it, and drink the water for luck.[6] At a party, the ring can be dropped into a bowl of water and all unmarried females in the house compete to fish it out. The first to secure the ring will be next to marry.

It is very good luck to take a friend's wedding or engagement ring and put it on your left hand, turning it three times towards the heart, while making a wish. To increase milk yield in your cow, milk her through a golden wedding band. To improve bad vision wear golden earrings.[7]

Iron

Iron is a metal abhorrent to the Fairies and with protective power against ill-intentioned Witches (as everyone knows there are Witches who bless and heal, and others who are more interested in power struggles). A particularly potent talisman is an iron horseshoe or nail that is made by a smith, because smiths by tradition have mystical powers, conferred by the smith-God *Goibniu* and by the Goddess *Brighde* in her aspect of patroness of smiths.

Horseshoes and nails made by a smith are placed in the bedroom during labor, to protect the mother and child during this vulnerable time. Iron placed on the threshold, or above the door, prevents evil from entering.

Iron can cure disease when the affected part is touched with it. Afterwards, the iron object is nailed to a tree (to transfer the disease). Nails are left on the chest of a corpse or on a gravestone, to prevent the dead from rising to haunt the living. Place a red-hot iron poker into the butter churn to prevent a sorcerer from spoiling the milk (this process probably sterilizes the milk, conveniently preventing it from going bad!).[8]

Lead

Molten lead is held briefly over a sick person, and then poured into cold water, to diagnose which organ is affected (the lead will form a shape that the healer interprets). The sufferer then wears the piece of lead as an amulet over their heart to ward off misfortune.[9]

Amber

Amber beads (or *Lammer*) are strung on red thread and worn as protection against eye diseases, sorcery, and bad dreams.[10] Clutching a piece of Amber helps a woman in labor to relieve the pain.

Amber is a perfect balance of male and female, fire and water. It is hard and yellow-orange meaning it has an affinity for the Sun and sacred fire, yet it derives from molten tree sap, which is a watery substance.

---

6. *Miller, Joyce, Magic and Witchcraft in Scotland, P. 57*

7. *Livingstone, Sheila, Scottish Customs, PP. 32, 95*

8. *Miller, Joyce, Magic and Witchcraft in Scotland, PP. 59-60*

9. *Miller, P. 60*

10. *Ibid., P. 60*

Molluka Beans, Bonduc Beans

Molluka beans (*Guildandia bonduc*) (Gaelic – *Cnó Mhoire* – Mary's Nut) are seeds from the West Indies that wash up on the beaches of the Western Isles of Scotland, via the Gulf Stream. They are especially powerful if a cross naturally appears on the shell. (For Pagans the Solar Cross is a powerful symbol that pre-dates Christianity).

Mounted in silver, the white ones are reputed to turn black if the wearer is threatened by sorcery. The seeds help with childbirth when a woman in labor holds one in her right hand.

If a cow gives blood streaked milk, the suspicion is that a Witch has "stolen" the milk. To counteract the spell, a bean is placed in the milk pail and left there, until the blood streaked milk turns the bean brown. At the next milking the same bean is put into the pail again.[11]

Serpent Stones and Serpent Beads

Serpent Stones (*Adder-Stanes* in Scots or *Clach Nathrach* in Gaelic) are prehistoric spindle-whorls. Serpent Beads or Serpent Glass (*Glaine Nathrach* in Gaelic), are Iron Age glass beads. These stones are used as charms to heal "snake-bitten" cattle, humans, or sheep. "Snake-bitten" refers to any disease where there is peeling or flaking of the skin.

The stones are suspended by a red woolen thread and dipped into water which is given to the sufferer. The patient can also be bathed in the water.[12]

Other Healing Stones

When using a stone for healing work, it is best to begin by "clearing" it, and then "charging" it. The stone should first be buried in the earth for three days, then exposed to the sun and Moon for three days, and then placed in a tree (to charge it with healing energy) for three days. A stone can also be placed in running water (such as a stream) for three days to clear it.

Snail-Stones (*Cnaipein Seilcheig*) are hollow, cylindrical glass beads used to heal sore eyes. Cock's Knee Stones (*Clachan-glúin a' choilich*) are small fossils used for healing. Frog or Toad-Stones (*Clachan nan Gilleadha Cráigein*) are fossilized fish teeth used to stop bleeding and remove poison.[13] Pictish "Cold Stones" are small white quartz pebbles onto which Pictish symbols have been inscribed. These can be dipped into water which is then given to a sick person or animal to drink. If the quartz dries swiftly the illness will heal swiftly. Fever Stones are white or rose quartz which is boiled in water. When the water cools, it is drunk for a fever or rubbed onto rheumatic limbs.[14]

The White Stone of the Fairies is a stone found on a Fairy Hill (after making a suitable offering) which can be rubbed on a painful part. In general, all white stones are said to belong to the Fairies.

---

11. *Ibid., PP. 60-61*
12. *Beith, Mary, Healing Threads, P.157*
13. *Beith, PP. 157-158*
14. *Ibid., PP. 154, 147*

The Brahan Seer had a stone that he received as a child, when he fell asleep upon a Fairy Mound. On waking, he found a small, smooth white stone on his chest that had a hole in it. By looking through the hole, he was able to see the future as well as people's true motives and intentions.

Fairy Arrows (also known as Elf Shot) are tiny, ancient flint arrowheads or spear heads which can be mounted in silver and worn to protect against, or to cure the effects of, "Elf Shot". Fairies and Elves are known to make the arrows which they will shoot at a person or a cow to cause sickness or even death. If a sick cow is suspected of being "Elf-shot", the cow's body must be examined for a lesion. Once the lesion is found, the "Elf-shot wound" will disappear.[15]

Green pebbles from the South Beach of Iona are reputed to be a charm to protect a person from drowning.[16] A blue stone found on the Isle of Skye once cured *Briochan* the Druid. The stone was steeped in water which was drunk, or used in a bath, to cure stitch in the side. A similar stone was found on the Isle of Troda. Fishermen would wash the stone to bring a helpful wind.[17]

Crystals

Quartz stones and crystals can be soaked in water, which is then given to a sick person or animal to drink. Rock crystal balls (Gaelic- *Léigheagan* – healing objects) are carried by a Clan Chief and dipped into a bowl of water taken from a Fairy Spring. The water is used to cure both humans and animals.[18]

Silver mounted crystals are dipped into a Holy Well and asked to heal all sick and suffering creatures. The stone is kept in a woolen cloth and kept hidden from sight until needed. To use such a stone, draw it deiseil around a bowl of water, and then dip it in three times. The water is then given to people or animals to drink, or be bathed or washed in. The animal or person may also be rubbed with the stone. The stone should never be far from its guardian, and water treated by it may be bottled for distance healing.[19]

Charm stones are often egg shaped crystals set in silver, but they may also be carnelian, garnet, or flint. The stone can be touched and a wish made.

The Campbells owned a large crystal called the *Clach Bhuaidh* (the Bright Stone) and the *Ballochyle Brooch*, which was a crystal set in silver. Both were dipped into water which was sprinkled on sick animals and humans. The *Clach Dearg* (The Red Stone of *Ardvorlich*) is also a crystal set in silver that was rubbed on affected parts or dipped in water (these stones are now at the National Museum of Scotland).

The MacDonnells had the *Keppoch* stone, which was dipped into Saint Brigid's Well in Lochaber as prayers were recited.

15. *Ibid., P. 154*
16. *McNeill, F. Marian, The Silver Bough Vol. I, P.94*
17. *Beith, Mary, Healing Threads, P. 156*
18. *Livingstone, Sheila, Scottish Customs, P.81*
19. *Beith, Mary, Healing Threads, P. 154*

The Lockharts have a red stone set in silver called the *Lee Penny*. When a healing was called for, the stone was dipped in water three times, and then swirled deiseil.[20]

The Mackintoshes and MacDonalds used the *Ball Mo-Luidhe* or *Molingus Globe*, a green stone the size of a goose egg. It was placed by the bedside of a sick person in hopes that the illness would be absorbed by the stone. (If the case was hopeless, the stone would remove itself). The stone was held by those who were swearing an oath, and carried into battle to cause opponents to flee.[21]

Healing Threads and Knots

Knots and threads are widely used in Scottish magic. Red is the most magical color of all, which is why red coral beads and red Rowan Berry necklaces were once worn for protection. Rowan twigs were bound with red thread to make tiny, equal-armed, Solar crosses which were sewn into clothing, hung above the door, or hidden in the home as a potent charm against evil sorcery. Amber beads (*Lammer*) were strung on red thread as a form of magical protection.[22]

Red threads are tied around a child's wrist as a protection from sorcery, and red silk can be tied around a body part to ward off rheumatism. A red thread is tied around the neck to expel evil from the head. Green threads are also wrapped around an injury.[23]

Blue thread is worn by a woman who is subject to fevers while nursing. These protective blue threads are handed down from mother to daughter. A black thread spun from black wool, with nine knots tied into it, is tied around a sprain or any other injury to a limb,[24] while chanting the following:

> *Joint to joint,*
> *Vein to vein,*
> *Sinew to sinew*
> *Hide to hide,*
> *Marrow to marrow,*
> *Bone to bone,*
> *In the name of the three.*

(Traditional and slightly re-Paganized)

Two black threads are tied around the body to help cure Scrofula (tuberculosis of the cervical lymph nodes).[25] When applying the threads, a spoken charm is always recited, and the threads are left on until they rot, or fall, off.

---

20. Miller, Joyce, *Magic and Witchcraft in Scotland*, P. 71
21. McNeill, F. Marian, *The Silver Bough Vol. I*, P.74
22. Miller, Joyce, *Magic and Witchcraft in Scotland*, P. 73
23. Miller, Joyce, *Magic and Witchcraft in Scotland*, PP. 61-64
24. McNeill, F. Marian, *The Silver Bough Vol. I*, P.75
25. McNeill, F. Marian, *The Silver Bough Vol. I*, P.75

The Charm of the Thread (Eólas an t-snáithein)

Three threads colored red, white and black (or blue) are wound around an affected part while a prayer is recited. Here is an old Gaelic charm:

> *I put my trust in the remedy*
> *Which Dian Cécht left with his people,*
> *In order that whatever it goes upon may be healed.*
>
> (Traditional)[26]

Knots

When a woman is in labor, her hair should be combed loose, and all knots in her shoes, clothing, etc., should be untied (windows and locks in the birthing area should also be unlocked and unbolted).

A Sorceress can cause impotence in a man, by tying a knot in a handkerchief. To cure warts, rub a length of string over them, and then tie as many knots in the string as there are warts to be healed. Bury the string in the ground, and as it dissolves, so will the warts.[27]

A Wise Woman can tie three knots in a thread and give it to a fisherman heading out to sea. If a light wind is needed, one knot is untied, the second knot is untied to fetch a stronger breeze, and if the third knot is untied it will raise a storm.[28]

Wearing Healing Charms

Sometimes prayers and invocations for healing are written on parchment and sealed in wax, to be worn on a thread by a person needing help. The recipient of the written charm must never open it, or its power will be lost. The charm is worn until it rots, or falls, off.[29]

Bone Magic

Bones for Healing

In old Scotland, a criminal was hung on the gallows tree (called the "greetin tree") and left there until only bones remained, no doubt as a salutary warning to would-be criminals. Bones taken from the skeleton were said to have healing powers.

The ancient Celts used skulls as drinking cups at healing wells. The Well of the Head in Wester Ross preserved this tradition until the twentieth century. The skull of a woman who had been buried on the moor gradually worked its way above ground, and eventually was found and preserved in a silver box. A *Dewar* (guardian, Wise Man) used it to cure epileptics.

The patient and their family would go to the house of the guardian, then the guardian and the patient would climb to a Well on a hill, between sunset and dawn, in complete silence. The skull was removed from its box as the patient

---

26. Beith, Mary, *Healing Threads, P. 195*
27. Miller, Joyce, *Magic and Witchcraft in Scotland, PP. 64-65*
28. Livingstone, Sheila, *Scottish Customs, P. 88*
29. Beith, Mary, *Healing Threads, P.195*

walked three times deiseil around the Well. Then the guardian filled the skull with water, and gave it to the sufferer to drink three times. *Geasa* (prohibitions, taboos) were laid on the patient, which were never to be revealed.

Severed heads were sometimes carried around a village to bring good weather. Water could be poured from a cleaned skull and bottled for healing work.[30] *Caution:* **do not** use any human bones unless they are legally obtained from a licensed scientific supply house.

Bones for Luck and Love

To make a Love Potion: Kill a frog on the Summer Solstice and remove a crooked bone. Clean it, dry it over a fire of Rowan wood, and then powder it with a mortar and pestle. Sprinkle the powder on the food of your intended, or use it to end a lover's quarrel.[31] *Caution:* It is very bad karma to use love magic on an unwilling or unsuspecting object of desire. Remember that all magic returns to the sender. Frogs are now an endangered species, and if you need a bone from one, get it from a market that sells frogs for food. (Buy it, or barter for it, on the day of the Summer Solstice).

The big toe of an old man can be touched for luck (after politely asking permission of course). Two persons can pull the wish bone of a fowl. The one who gets the larger half should make their wish in silence.

Cursing Bones

Cursing bones are made from the hollow bones of a deer. Witches bent on sorcery once visited the hen house of their victim in the dark, killed a chicken by strangulation, and poured its blood through the bone while laying a curse on the dwelling.[32] *Caution:* As all magic returns to the sender, no intelligent person will carry out this kind of vengeful malice.

Stones of Power

Stones, especially large ones, carry potent magic, perhaps because they endure through the generations, linking the living with those long gone. When cut and polished, stones capture light and shine like the Sun, Moon, and Stars. In the old Fairy Tradition, it is held that there is a Star inside every stone. Our own planet has a blazing Sun in its center, known as "The Emerald Heart of the Earth", which can be linked to mentally, or called upon spiritually, for strength.

Healing Stones

For thousands of years, natural clefts and hollows in rocks that collected water, querns (stones to grind grain) left outside to collect rainwater, and old baptismal fonts have been regarded as repositories of sacred water suitable for healing. Coins are left in thanks at such places, for the Spirits who sanctify the water.

Stones and wood are carved to resemble body parts: breasts, limbs, the head, the heart, etc., and offered to the waters of a Sacred Spring in hopes of a cure. The

30. *Livingstone, Sheila, Scottish Customs, PP. 87, 89*
31. *Livingstone, P. 88*
32. *Ibid, P. 88*

source of a river has always been a place of sanctity for Celts, and such votives may be offered there. Lakes, the Sea, or any body of living water carries its own magic and may be called upon for healing help by placing stone or wood votives into the waters.

One method of healing is to wash a votive in a waterfall, and then rub it on to the afflicted body part before drying off. In this case the stone should be rubbed three times deiseil, and then three times *tuaithiuil*, around the afflicted area. Lastly, the stone is rubbed over the whole body, while a healing incantation is recited. This rite is especially effective if there is a large sacred tree nearby.[33]

Healing stones should be ritually purified at least once a year by pouring milk and honey, or water and wine, over them. Keep healing stones on your altar for use when someone is in need. (Large standing stones in a ritual circle should also be ritually washed at least once a year using liquids such as milk and honey, milk and whisky, or milk, water and wine).

To cure wasting diseases and nervous conditions, go to the seashore and remove your pants. Straddle a stone that is half submerged in shallow water every day, until your strength returns.[34]

Protective Stones

At Glen Lyon in Perthshire (an ancient Pictish stronghold), gateposts are often topped by river stones that have been shaped by the action of the water. These stones are said to be protective.

Glen Lyon stretches from Fortingall to Loch Lyon, and by tradition, it was once the hunting ground of the greatest warrior of the *Fianna, Fionn MacCumhail.* The oldest tree in Europe is the Fortingall Yew (1000 BCE) which was a sacred tree and Pagan shrine for the district long before the Christian missionaries arrived. The missionaries built a church right next to the Yew, but were careful to put two stones well worn by the waters of the river Lyon on top of the gateposts, as a form of magical protection.[35]

In the Upper Glen, a stone shrine with a thatched roof known as *Tigh na Cailliche* (the house of the ancient Land Goddess), contains three stones within it that are worn and shaped by water. The largest is called the *Cailleach* (the Hag Stone), the second largest is the *Bodach* (Her consort), and the smallest stone is called *Nighean* (Her daughter).

Regarding these stones, the following tale is told. Many years ago, a huge man and woman appeared in a snow storm, walking down the mountain of the Upper Glen. They were strangers and they asked for, and received, hospitality. Eventually the local folk gave them a thatched house to live in, and there, the woman gave birth to a baby girl.

As long as the family lived in the Glen, the weather was kind and the crops and herds flourished, but one day, the family announced that they had to go. They said that as long as they were remembered and their house preserved, they would ensure that peace, prosperity, and good weather stayed with the people.

33. Beith, Mary, *Healing Threads*, PP. 149-150
34. Beith, P. 147
35. Ross, Anne, *Folklore of the Scottish Highlands*, P. 110

Every *Bealltan*, the three stones were taken out of the house and positioned to face the Glen while the house was re-thatched. The stones were put back every *Samhuinn*. A local shepherd ensured that the ritual continued, but unfortunately the last such caretaker recently passed over.[36]

Stone Magic

To utilize a stone for magical work, visit it at the Full Moon for nine months (*Moonths*) in a row. At each visit, circle the stone nine times on your knees, then make your wish.[37]

Stone Circles

When setting a stone circle for magical and ritual use, first select your site, and stand within it with a circle of friends while holding hands, then let go of your hands, and slowly walk backwards until the size of the circle reveals itself. Place a wooden stake in the center of the space, and for one year, rise before dawn on each Holy day (Quarter Days and Cross Quarters) and tie a rope to the stake, pulling it taut to the exact direction the Sun rises. Mark the position of each Sunrise with a wooden stake. This is how you will know where to plant your stones.

When you are ready to raise the stones, dig a deep hole and shape the earth into a steep slope on one side. Lay a stone on the slope, and see-saw it, until it slides into the hole. Bring the stone to vertical, and pack it in with rocks, gravel, and dirt.

A Moon Circle can be made in the same way by observing the direction of the Full Moon for a year. Some of the so called "recumbent" stone circles in Scotland feature a stone altar at the position of the southernmost Moonrise of the Year. That direction is marked by a recumbent stone in a circle of otherwise upright monoliths. Of course the Moon's position in the sky changes over its twenty nine year cycle so the very southernmost Full Moon happens only once every twenty nine years.

Other circles are aligned to the southernmost setting of Venus, or to the Midwinter or Midsummer sunrise.

Recumbent stone circles are most abundant in northeast Scotland. Prominent examples include Midmar Kirk and Sunhoney Farm in Aberdeenshire. Tomnaverie, also in Aberdeenshire, is located on a hill top with an amazing three hundred and sixty degree view of the surrounding mountains. These Bronze Age circles date to approximately 2000 BCE.

There are two famous circles in Orkney called the Ring of Brodgar (The Temple of the Sun, 2800 BCE) and The Ring of Stenness (The Temple of the Moon, 3200 BCE). At the Ring of Stenness, a woman would kneel before her lover and pray to Woden, asking for help to keep the promises she was making to her lover. Then the couple would go to the nearby Ring of Brodgar, where the man kneeled and prayed in a similar fashion before the woman.[38]

Most of these types of stone circles and landscape temples were built during the Neolithic and Bronze Ages, yet they still have power today. The Clava Cairns

36. Ross, P. 113
37. Marwick, Ernest, *The Folklore of Orkney and Shetland*, P. 59
38. Marwick, P. 60

near Inverness, Callanish on Lewis, Machrie Moor on Arran, and the Hill o' Many Stanes in Caithness are but some examples of stones of power.

Some of these circles are oriented to the Midwinter Sunset or Sunrise, others to the positions of the Moon. Burial cairns are often found nearby and also collections of sheep and cattle bones, indicating that these circles were places for feasting, ritual, and honoring of the dead.[39]

Each of these circular stone temples has its own unique characteristic. Callanish is oriented to the pole Star, and was once used for Druid rituals. The Ring of Stenness points directly to the large burial mound of Maes Howe (2,900 BCE), which is oriented to the Winter Solstice sunset. There is a Holy Well (Bigswell) situated near the Ring of Brodgar. The Clava Cairns (2000 BCE) are surrounded by rings of stones and a thick forest of Rowan trees.

Standing Stones, Dolmens and Barrows

Other types of stone constructions can be found or constructed. A *Menhir* is a large, single upright stone. A *Dolmen* consists of three or four uprights with a flat slab on top. This construction usually features a burial in the center. Chambered Tombs or *Tumuli* are a later type of construction for the bones of the dead, consisting of a long stone hall that is divided into separate "rooms" and roofed with stone. *Cromlechs* are stone circles surrounding a *Dolmen* or a Barrow.[40]

Gruagach Stones

These are solitary standing stones to which offerings of milk are brought to honor the Fairies.[41]

Stones and Sympathetic Magic

Stones shaped like a tooth can help with toothache. Women needing help with childbirth or fertility can sit on a stone shaped like a chair called a *Clach-bhan* (wife stone). A single woman may sit on the stone to attract a mate, while a woman near her due date may sit on it to ensure easy labor. For fertility, a woman should sit on the stone during the Waxing Moon.[42]

I visited such a chair in County Tyrone at Altanadevan, Augher, Northern Ireland, a place thick with Scots heritage. The chair, called "The Druid's Chair" by the locals, is carved out of a single boulder. It rests on top of a hill in the midst of a dense Larch forest.

Near the chair there is a stone with a small depression in it that collects rain water, an ancient Holy Well dedicated to *Brighde*. Folk still come there to tie their cloots and make their prayer requests. Supposedly Saint Patrick sat on the chair to hear confessions, but the chair long pre-dates Christianity. Locals gathered on the hill until the 1960's to celebrate "Bilberry Sunday" by picking ripe berries, drinking and picnicking on the hillsides. Today, modern Druids are reviving the ancient customs.

39. *Miller, Joyce, Magic and Witchcraft in Scotland, P. 66*
40. *McNeill, F. Marian, The Silver Bough Vol. I, PP. 84-86*
41. *McNeill, P. 86*
42. *Miller, Joyce, Magic and Witchcraft in Scotland, P. 67*

Holed Stones

Small holed stones ("Holey Stones") are collected and worn around the neck. *Coinneach Odhar*, the famous Brahan Seer, was able to see the Otherworld through such a stone.

Large stones with natural holes in them can be used to cure asthma, consumption, and other lung conditions. A couple may clasp hands through a holed stone to be hand-fasted, in the ritual they vow to stay together for a year and a day with no hard feelings if they part due to incompatibility. Women crawl through holed stones to aid pregnancy and childbirth. Offerings of bread and cheese are often left at these stones.

Children may be brought to a holed stone for a cure. First, a fire is built, and then the child removes its clothing, and is passed through the hole. Baked cakes are left on the rock in thanks, and if the cakes are gone the next morning the child will recover, but if the cakes are still there, the child could die.[43]

Likewise, to determine if a child or other patient will recover, water is taken in silence from under a bridge without spilling any of it, and poured on the corner of a stone building while uttering the name of a patient, to see if the stone cracks or splits. If so, the sickness will be fatal.

Children can be healed of rickets or mumps by passing them under a "rocking stone", a large stone that can be easily rocked on its fulcrum by simple hand pressure. Rocking stones are particularly plentiful in Ayrshire, where some have been associated with the ancient Druids.

Passing through a cleft in a rock is said to heal wounds.[44]

Stones for Luck

Fishermen and newlyweds may walk around a stone deiseil seven times to seal their good luck.

Clach na h-Iobairte (Stone of Offering)

Making an offering to a stone brings good fortune to the giver. Leave a gift of milk for the *Gruagach* of the area, or leave a gift of milk at a Brownie Stone for the Brownies.[45]

Oath Stones

An Oath can be sworn while resting the hand or foot on a stone. Clan Chattan on Arran once had such a stone, with a footprint incised into its surface. When a new Clan Chief was inaugurated, he stood on the stone and swore to uphold the ways of his ancestors. He was then given a wand (usually of Yew, an old Druidic tradition), a sword, and a white robe of faithfulness, handed down from the previous chief.[46]

Boundary Stones

Boundary stones have special powers because all boundaries are liminal places. In Celtic tradition, any liminal space such as the shore of the Sea, the

43. McNeill, F. Marian, *The Silver Bough Vol. I*, PP. 90-91
44. Livingstone, Sheila, *Scottish Customs*, P. 81
45. Miller, Joyce, *Magic and Witchcraft in Scotland*, P. 67
46. Livingstone, Sheila, *Scottish Customs*, P. 80

edge of a lake, a hill between land and sky, the times of dusk and dawn, and at the crossing point between one season and the next, was a magical interval or space between the Worlds, where Spirits and humans could more easily interact. In ancient times, offerings such as butter (and sometimes bodies) were buried in a bog at the place where one territory ended and another began.

Judgments and contracts were made in the vicinity of a boundary stone. Chiefs went to the stone to settle disputes, and any clansman who wandered past the boundary stone could no longer expect protection. Troops assembled at such a stone and the burial cairns of noble warriors were placed near them. The gallows tree was often in the vicinity of a boundary stone.[47]

When marking a boundary, the ancient technique was to lay down wood ash (probably from a ritual fire), and put a large stone on top. If in the future anyone questioned the boundary line the stone was lifted to see if there was ash beneath it.[48]

Elf Cups

Stones into which water has naturally bored a hole are called Elf Cups. These are strung in groups of three on a horsehair rope and hung in the byre on *Bealltan* to prevent Fairy mischief.[49]

Magic Cups

A 'Magic Cup' is any hollow in a stone that fills with water. Such water brings luck and healing.[50]

The Knocking Stone

A lump of rock shaped like a bowl in which grain is ground using a thick stick. Kept in the barn, it holds the luck of the home. It is carried from house to house as the family moves.[51]

Sanctuary Stones

Stones and stone circles once had the same kind of power that was later given to churches. Criminals and those in debt could claim sanctuary in the vicinity of refuge stones.[52]

Keel-Stane

A cairn or ring of stones, about five feet long and shaped like a boat. It marks the grave of someone who was drowned.[53]

The Stone of Destiny or Stone of Scone

By tradition, this stone was Jacob's pillow at *Bethel* which was carried to Ireland by *Scota*, daughter of an Egyptian Pharaoh, in 900 BCE. It became the *Lia Faill* at *Tara* (the stone that cried out when touched by the true king).

---

47. Livingstone, P. 80
48. Ross, Anne, *Folklore of the Scottish Highlands*, PP. 108-109
49. Livingstone, Sheila, *Scottish Customs*, P. 84
50. Ibid., P. 85
51. McNeill, F. Marian, *The Silver Bough Vol. I*, P. 92
52. Livingstone, Sheila, *Scottish Customs*, P. 78
53. Marwick, Ernest, *The Folklore of Orkney and Shetland*, P. 61

Migrating Irishmen brought it to Scotland (named for the *"Scotti"* or Irish), where it served as the coronation stone of the *Dál Riatan* kings. Kenneth MacAlpine, whose reign united the Scots and Picts, took the stone to Scone, the capitol of Southern Pictland.

The last Scottish king to be crowned using the stone was Alexander III in 1249. In 1297, the stone was supposedly carried to London by Edward I of England, to be sat upon by English kings.[54] However, local tradition states that when the monks of Scone were alerted to Edward's advance they hid the true stone and put a piece of local sandstone in its place, handing the real stone to the Knights Templar and that on March 25, 1306, Robert the Bruce was crowned while seated on the true stone.

The true stone is said to be black and polished, while the current "Stone of Scone" is red sandstone, proven to be local. On his deathbed, Robert the Bruce is said to have sent the true stone to the Hebrides for safekeeping.

In 1950, four Scottish students removed the stone that was resident in Westminster Abbey, breaking it into two pieces. It was repaired by a stonemason and then deposited on the altar of Arbroath Abbey. Police were alerted and the stone was returned to Westminster. In 1996, a decision was made by the English that the stone should be re-patriated to Scotland, to be used by the English only for coronations. It now resides at Edinburgh Castle, the regimental headquarters of the Scots Dragoon Guards.[55]

54. McNeill, F. Marian, *The Silver Bough Vol. I, PP. 88-89*

55. McAlister, Neil Harding, *The Stone of Destiny,* Brigadoonery Canada http://www.durham. net/~neilmac/stone.htm

Holy Days and Holidays

The Fire Festivals

*I*n Celtic thinking, the year proper began with the festival of *Samhuinn*. For the ancients, a day began at dusk, not at dawn, as we now suppose. Similarly, the year was divided into two halves: the dark half and the light half. The dark half of the year was "winter" which lasted from *Samhuinn* to *Bealltan*, and the light half of the year was "summer" which lasted from *Bealltan* to *Samhuinn*. The year began in the dark half.

Given that the Celtic seasonal round of festivals and feasts was largely based on the agricultural calendar, it is not difficult to follow this reasoning. A seed begins its life cycle in the dark of the soil, and an animal or person starts its life journey in the dark of the womb.

The ancient Fire Festivals of *Samhuinn, Oimelc, Bealltan* and *Lúnasdal* are the most potent times to do magic. The very best time for spell casting is at dawn or at twilight on one of these festival days (because these are liminal times between day and night). Need-fires may be ritually built to protect the community from disease and misfortune at these times, and crops, fields, herds, boats and buildings are sained. Wells are visited and dressed with flowers, stones are washed, and divinations made.

The Fire Festivals are always an auspicious time to start a journey, or any new project, but certain prohibitions apply.[1] It is very bad luck to give fire out of the house on a Fire Festival, because your luck might go with your neighbor. If fire is given out for some dire reason, a burning coal or chunk of peat must be dropped into water as soon as the neighbor leaves, to counter any misfortune. Similarly, rennet should not be given away lest milk products lose

---

1. McNeill, F. Marian, *The Silver Bough Vol. I*, PP 54-55

their luck, nor should a loan be made on such a day (because your luck might disappear along with the money). The same cautions and prohibitions apply on the first Monday of each Quarter.[2]

It is traditional to bake a *bannock* or cake at each of the Fire Festivals. At *Oimelc*, the cake is called a *Bonnach Bríghde*, in honor of *Bride*. At Bealltan, it is called a *Bonnach Bealltan*, at Lúnasdal, it is a *Bonnach Lunastain* and at Samhuinn, it is a *Bonnach Samthain*.

Several cakes are baked, and every clan member goes out to the fields, eating the cakes and tossing small bits over each shoulder, while invoking any malevolent Spirit or entity that could hurt the farm. A piece of bread is tossed out for the wolf that it might spare the lambs, and another piece for the fox that it spare the ducks and chickens. Other pieces are tossed to appease ravens, eagles, crows, and any other force of blight or disaster for the farm.[3]

Here are some traditional recipes for festival breads and cakes. It is very easy to make your own fresh butter to go with these breads. Just place whole heavy cream (not low fat) in a jar with a tight lid, and shake vigorously for about twenty minutes.

Bannock Bread (Oatmeal Bannock)

225g (8 oz) fine oatmeal
55g (about 2 oz) plain flour
1 tsp salt
1 tsp bicarbonate of soda
1 pint of buttermilk

Preheat your gridle. It is hot enough to cook on when flour sprinkled on it takes a few seconds to brown.

Put the oatmeal, flour and salt into a large bowl and mix well.

Put the buttermilk into a small bowl, add the teaspoon of bicarbonate of soda and mix briskly.

Add the buttermilk mixture to the dry ingredients and bring together into a soft dough. Be careful not to overwork the mixture. Work quickly, as the bicarbonate of soda will be kicked into action by the buttermilk.

Roll the mixture out on a lightly floured surface, to a depth of about ½ inch. Cut into a round (cut around a suitable size plate).

Dust the gridle with a small amount of flour, and put on the round of dough to cook. Turn the bannock over when the underside starts to brown. (It will be a large, flat oat cake).[4]

---

2. *McNeill, P. 55*

3. *Ibid., P. 57*

4. *http://bakingforbritain.blogspot.com/2006/06/oatmeal*

Scottish Oatcakes

2 cups oatmeal**
1 Pinch sea salt
1 Pinch bicarbonate of soda
½ oz beef drippings (or lard, butter)
8 oz hot water

(**use old fashioned oats, not the quick cooking variety)
Mix the oatmeal, salt and soda.
Make a well in the center of the bowl and pour in the melted drippings, and then add the water until a pie dough consistency is achieved.
Cover your hands with oats and knead into a ball, then roll out on a floured pastry board to ½ inch thickness.
Sprinkle some oatmeal on top and cut into squares.
Cook the squares on a hot griddle until the edges curl and toast slightly.[5]

The Year in Scotland

The Festival of Samhuinn – October 31 - November 1

Samhuinn marks the official end of the harvest and the time when the cattle must be brought down from the hills, into the safety of the barnyard. Animals for which there is not enough fodder are slaughtered at this time, the official end of summer, and the start of winter and the dark half of the year.

The oldest extant name for this festival is *Trinouxtion Samonii* (three nights at the end of summer) from the Coligny Calendar of the Gaulish Celts (a bronze calendar found in Coligny, Ain, France, near Lyon in 1897 which is believed to be of Romano-Celtic provenance and which was possibly made by Druids).

This festival marks a time of feasting and plenty when fresh meat, sausages, bacon, milk, butter, fresh breads, fresh fruits and nuts are available. Rents were once paid in the form of cows, pigs and sheep in time for the feasting. The bounty was shared with dead relatives by setting a place for them at the table and games were played at the celebration, especially ones involving apples and water (apples being mystically connected to Avalon or Abhalloch, the Otherworldly Island of Apples, and water the gateway to the realm of the ancestors).

The Christian church adapted this ancient Celtic festival to its own ends, naming it "All Saints Day" and "The Day of the Dead".

Samhuinn is a liminal time when the walls between the worlds are thin, a portal between the seasons of light and dark. It is a time for divinations and the time when Spirits can more easily make contact with this world. It is a wise idea to travel in disguise, to fool any irate discorporate entities at this time. Children dress as guisers, and go from house to house, wrecking property and indulging in mischief, imitating the chaotic forces abroad in the land.

5. *Smith-Twiddy, Helen, Celtic Cookbook, P. 34*

Large fires are lit to strengthen ties with The Fires of Life, and to regenerate the Earth. Householders douse their own hearths, and relight them from torches brought by runners from the ritual fires.

A *samhnag* (bonfire) is lit for every house: youths collect wood for months to make it memorable. Wood shavings and tar barrels are added to the pyre by the adults who supervise the proceedings carefully. Once the fire is lit, everyone holds hands and dances around it deiseil and tuaithiuil.[6] Those who are able, take turns leaping the fire (the elderly and infirm can demurely step over the coals as the flames die down).

Youths carry burning torches around the fields to sain them from Fairy influence. They toss the burning brands high into the air and then leave them on the ground where they dance over them.

Divinations at Samhuinn

The old date for the festival was November 11, though in modern times "Halloween" is usually celebrated on October 31. At Samhuinn the world is open and exposed to the Otherworld and so it is a good time to take omens and make predictions. One method of divining a future spouse or lover is to take two Hazelnuts and assign each of them a name. Place both in the fire and see which pops towards you.

Egg whites are dropped into boiling water and a divination made, based on the shapes that appear. Hot wax from a candle can be dripped into a cold pond or stream and the hardened patterns examined. Another traditional divination is to place six plates on the floor with a different object or symbol on each plate. Young women and girls are blindfolded and led to the plates, and the one they touch reveals their future fate.[7]

Horse Racing at Samhuinn

Until 1866, there was a traditional horse race that was held on *Michaelmas*, but which was originally held at *Samhuinn*. On the eve of the race a large bannock called a *"struan"* was baked from the new grain by the oldest female child of the house. In the morning, the struans were taken to a local church to be blessed and then the family returned home to eat them along with a ritually slaughtered male lamb. The remaining struan were distributed to the poor.

Afterwards, the riders went to the church again, more prayers were recited, and everyone circumambulated the church and graveyard deiseil, led by the priest on a white horse with the entire congregation, all on horseback and singing. The chief piper then picked a place for a ceilidh (party).

The Sunday before the race was called *"Carrot Sunday"*. Women and girls harvested the roots while singing songs to *Bríghde* and Michael (a thinly disguised version of the God *Lugh*) and to harvest a forked carrot was considered particularly lucky. The carrots were deposited into a bag called a *crioslachan* (little girdle) that hung from a girls waist, tied into bunches with red string (a very magical color) and given to men as gifts. The fertility aspects of this ritual are obvious.[8]

---

6. Ross, Anne, *Folklore of the Scottish Highlands, P. 148*
7. *Ross, P. 149*
8. *Ibid., P.145*

By tradition, anyone could steal a horse the night before, to ride in the race, and suffer no legal consequences (so long as at least one old nag was left for each man of the house), so men carefully guarded their horses on that night.

The actual race had strong fertility connotations: a boy and a girl rode bareback on each horse, with no bridle. When the race was over, the girl presented the boy with a bouquet of the freshly harvested carrots.[9]

The Goddess at Samhuinn

The Goddess most closely tied to *Samhuinn* in Scotland is the *Cailleach*, the "Hooded One" or "Veiled One" who is the great Hag of Winter. She is said to live on the high mountain tops from whence she rides with her eight sister Hags to hammer frost into the ground.

She is the only creator deity known from Celtic tradition. It is said that She dropped stones from Her apron to form the islands of Scotland. She is an old woman at the start of winter when she carries a magic wand called a *"slachdan"* with which she controls the weather and it is said that when the first snow falls it means She has arrived.

She grows gradually younger as the winter ebbs, until *Oimelc* when She washes Her face in the Well of Youth and transforms into *Bríghde*, throwing Her *slachdan* into the roots of an old Holly or Gorse bush. Her power remains stored there, safely hidden until the next winter.

All Souls Day – November 2

Christians adopted the ancient Samhuinn custom of honoring the dead and renamed it "All Souls Day". It is appropriate to make a donation to the poor on All Souls Day in the memory of those who have passed over.

Martinmas, Hallowmass Foy November 11-12
(also called Old Samhuinn)

This is the last legal "Quarter Day" when rents and contracts were once due. Since cattle and sheep were often killed at this date, it was the traditional time to make Haggis out of minced livers, hearts and lungs. The offal was mixed with oatmeal and suet and seasoned with salt and pepper. It was then stuffed into a sheep's stomach and boiled. Black Pudding was also made with sheep's blood.

To Make a Haggis: Lady Login's Receipt, 1856

> 1 cleaned sheep or lamb's stomach bag
> 2 lb. dry oatmeal
> 1 lb chopped mutton suet
> 1 lb lamb's or deer's liver, boiled and minced
> 1 pint (2 cups) stock
> The heart and lungs of the sheep, boiled and minced
> 1 large chopped onion
> ½ tsp. each: cayenne pepper,
> Salt and black pepper

---

9. Lamb, Gregor, *Carnival of the Animals, P. 97*

Toast the oatmeal slowly until it is crisp, then mix all the ingredients (except the stomach bag) together, and add the stock.

Fill the bag just over half full, press out the air and sew up securely.

Have ready a large pot of boiling water, prick the haggis all over with a large needle so it does not burst and boil slowly for 4 to 5 hours.

Serves 12.[10]

Black Pudding (Marag Dubh)

1 lb suet
1 lb oatmeal
2 onions
Fresh sheep's blood
Salt and pepper to taste

Chop the suet and the onions finely.

Mix the dry ingredients then add the blood.

Stuff into a casing and tie.

Put into a large pan and boil in water gently for three hours.

Remove and cool.

Cut into slices and fry in hot fat.

A classic side dish with fried bacon and eggs.

Serves 4.

If you slaughter your own animals, use fresh blood, or get fresh blood from an abattoir (ask your local butcher shop where you can purchase sausage casings).[11]

A banquet is held after a day of fasting. A wether (a male castrated ram) is sacrificed. Guizers enter from the kitchen, hobbling and dancing in pairs. They are dressed in white with petticoats beneath their robes and tall, woven straw caps, making noises like human grunts and bird calls and rapping on the floor with a staff. One of them plays a fiddle and another has a straw basket on his back. They beg for money and food and are given coins, butter, mutton, and cakes.

Cattle are given their feast of an entire sheaf of grain each. Turnip lanterns (the original Jack O'Lanterns) are lit.

Guy Fawkes – November 5

An English festival that commemorates Guy Fawkes' attempt to blow up the Houses of Parliament in 1605, Fawkes was a Catholic and the event took place shortly after James VI of Scotland became king of England and Wales. James was the son of Mary Queen of Scots, and born a Catholic but he was educated as a Protestant and had strong Protestant sympathies.

Saint Andrew's Day – November 30

This festival originally commemorated a Pictish battle in 747 AD.

---

10. *Kreitzberg, Tom, Haggis Recipes, http://www.smart.net/~tak/haggis.html#four*
11. *Black Pudding, FoodDownUnder, http://fooddownunder.com/cgi-bin/recipe.cgi?r=28464*

Sowans Nicht – Christmas Eve – December 24

Named for *"sowans"* a dish made from oat husks and fine meal that have been steeped in water for about a week. After straining, the solid matter at the bottom is the sowans which is eaten like porridge. The poured off liquid is called *"swats"* which may be made into a fermented drink.[12]

Branches of Rowan are burned on Christmas Eve to purge any bad feelings between friends or relatives at Yule.

Yule (Christmas) – December 25

This festival was originally celebrated at the Winter Solstice when the Norse God Odin was the gift-bringer who traveled the sky in a chariot drawn by horses or goats. Yule is the time of the "Wild Hunt", a phantom horse race that occurs during stormy weather in winter and especially during the twelve days of Yule. When the Wild Hunt passes overhead, celestial riders can be seen, accompanied by black hounds, riding black steeds and black he-goats, and blowing their horns.

The Yule Log burns in the hearth, keeping the Fires of Life alive during the magical twelve day interval of the darkest time of year. Before lighting the log prayers, wishes and petitions for luck can be tied onto it using natural twine. As the string burns the prayers and hopes are sent to the Gods via the smoke.

There is kissing under the mistletoe in honor of Balder, the Norse God of innocence, beauty, joy, purity, and peace who is Odin's second son.

The home is decorated with Holly, Pine, and other evergreens as a reminder that life is eternal despite the cold, and to provide a safe haven for any Nature Spirits seeking shelter at this dangerous time. Solar wreaths of evergreen are hung on the door and trees are illuminated with candles and lights to honor the strengthening sun.

The Yule festival actually lasts for about a month starting on December 12. From that day on neither carding nor spinning should be undertaken in a home with sheep. Knitters, shoemakers and dress makers may work until Yule Eve but should not work again after that until the feast is over, either the twelfth day after Yule or the twenty fourth day after Yule.

On Yule Eve, the kitchen is cleared of furniture, husks are strewn on the floor, and a fiddler brought in for the celebration. Costumed revelers dance all night as potent spirits are shared by all.

In some areas, straw images that represent the Grain Goddess, the bitch, the wolf, the goat, or the horse, are brought out and paraded through the village, bringing the fertility and luck of the last year's solar cycle to all. These images embody the female Spirit that inhabits the grain and nurtures the people. This Spirit stays with the last sheaf which must be ritually cut and preserved.

According to tradition, Robin Hood bled to death on Yule Eve and reappeared as a hobby horse. Until the nineteenth century all over Britain, Austria, and other Celtic areas, horses were bled that evening to make them healthy (possibly a remnant of an ancient horse sacrifice ritual).

---

12. *Porridge, Carrbridge Community Council, http://www.goldenspurtle.com/porridge.htm*

Men disguised as animals, often in straw masks, appeared at the door to bless the house with their presence. Offerings were made to them of food, drink, and coin, in gratitude to the nurturing animal Spirits who protected the house and farm.

On Yule Day, precautions were taken to foil the Trows (Trows are the mischievous sprites and Fairies of Shetland, Orkney, and other culturally Norse areas). The person who fed the cows had to appear at the barn before dawn, carrying a cow's skull with a candle inserted in its eye socket.

The Yule breakfast consisted of boiled mutton, pork, scones, ale and spirits. The Yule supper included Flummery.

Flummery
1/3 cup almonds (sliced)
2 ounces oatmeal
1 cup heavy cream
4 tablespoons honey
cup whisky
2 teaspoons lemon juice
1-2 cup berries

Toast the almonds and oatmeal in a pan until slightly browned.
Set aside.
Whip the cream until it is smooth, but not stiff.
Warm the honey VERY slightly, so that it will run easily.
Fold the honey, whisky, half of the toasted almonds and oatmeal, and half of the berries plus the lemon juice into the cream.
Mix thoroughly but lightly, and spoon into tall individual glasses.
Sprinkle the remaining almonds, oatmeal and berries on top.
Chill and Serve.
Serves 4-6.

A green Yule is bad luck because "A green Yule means a full graveyard". Hard frosts are always needed to ensure that pestilences are killed off.

Tug of war games are played at Yule. A tree is stolen without permission from someone's land and taken to the town center. Ropes are attached and teams vie to pull the tree to their side of the goal line. Football (soccer) games are played where the object is to kick the ball to fantastic heights and spectacular distances.[13]

Boxing Day – December 26
Gifts in boxes are exchanged.

Hogmanay – New Years Eve – December 31
The name of this festival may derive from the Norse *"Hoggunott"*, the night when animals were killed for the midwinter feast. For Scots this is actually a more important festival than Yule. The house must be thoroughly cleaned (including

13. Marwick, Ernest, *The Folklore of Orkney and Shetland*, PP. 118-120

a thorough cleansing of the hearth) in preparation for the visits of friends and relatives who arrive in the wee hours of the morning on January 1.

"First footing" is an old custom: ideally the first visitor should be a tall, handsome man with dark hair (a woman is less lucky and a red head the worst of all!). He should bring with him symbolic gifts of coal (that the house be always warm), bread or shortbread (that there always be good food to eat), salt (a symbol of purification), black bun (a spiced cake), and whisky.

A band of men or boys may appear at the door in *guizing* masks to *wassail* the house and demand butter, bacon, ale, cakes, scones, and money. Once admitted, they dance around the living room or around the fire. Here is a collection of traditional songs and chants used by guizers:

> *Hogmanay, Trollolay,*
> *Give us of your white bread, and none of your gray*

These are even more demanding:

> *Get up, goodwife, and shake your feathers,*
> *An dinna think that we are beggars;*
> *For we are bairns come out to play,*
> *Get up and gie's our hogmanay!* (give us)

and

> *My feet's cauld, my shoon's thin;* (shoes)
> *Gie's my cakes, and let me in!*

This one attempts to use moral pressure:

> *Get up, goodwife, and dinna sweir,*
> *And deal your bread to them that 's here;*
> *For the time will come when ye'll be dead,*
> *And then ye'll need neither ale nor bread.*

This one may be about the Virgin Mary or a Queen named Mary:

> *This night it is grid New'r E'en's night,* (New Year's night)
> *We're a' here Queen Mary's men;* (soldiers of Queen Mary)
> *And we're come here to crave our right,* (claim our right)
> *And that's before our Lady.*
> *The very first thing which we do crave,*
> *We're a' here Queen Mary's men;*
> *A bonny white candle we must have,*
> *And that's before our Lady.*
> *Goodwife, gae to your butter-ark,*
> *(a slate bottom table upon which butter is cut)*
> *And weigh us here ten mark.* (ten pounds' worth)
> *Ten mark, ten pund,* (a mark is the same value as a pound)
> *Look that ye grip weel to the grund.*
> *(get to the bottom of the container)*
> *Goodwife, gae to your geelin vat,*
> *(a vat where cheese and curds are made)*

> *And fetch us here a skeel o' that.* (a wooden scoop with a handle)
> *Gang to your awmrie, gin ye please,* (cupboard)
> *And bring frae there a yow-milk cheese.* (a ewe-milk cheese)
> *And syne bring here a sharping-stane,* (a stone for sharpening knives)
> *We'll sharp our whittles ilka ane.* (a sheath-knife or dirk)
> *Ye'll cut the cheese, and eke the round,* (supplement, enlarge)
> *But aye take care ye cutna your thoom.*
> *(take care not to cut your thumb)*
> *Gae fill the three-pint cog o' ale,* (a three pint wooden vessel)
> *The maut maun be aboon the meal.* (serve it with the meal)
> *We houp your ale is stark and stout,* (strong and powerful, healthy)
> *For men to drink the auld year out.*
> *Ye ken the weather's snaw and sleet,* (snow and sleet)
> *Stir up the fire to warm our feet.*
> *Our shoon's made o' mare's skin,* (shoes)
> *Come open the door, and let's in.*
> (Traditional, from Deerness, in Orkney)

In order for the New Year to begin correctly, short bursts of thrifty activity are symbolically undertaken. Men may fish for an hour, women begin one new knitting or weaving project, a straw rope might be started, one turf turned, a stone moved or set up, a coin saved, the barn cleaned, fishing and hunting gear repaired, a garment mended or a new one started.[14]

On New Year's Day in Kirkwall, Orkney, the men of the two original wards of the town fight for the possession of a ball (which may have originally been the head of a decapitated enemy or of a ritually slaughtered animal). These contests are also featured at weddings (the groom must provide the ball), at summer and winter solstice, at *Samhuinn* and at *Bealltan*. The game symbolizes the struggle of transition during a liminal time of passage: from one reality to the next, the old year to the new, summer to winter and vice versa, and from bachelorhood to marriage.[15]

Here are some traditional toasts for Hogmanay:

> *Here's tae us, wha's like us*
> *Damn few and they're a' deid.* (they're all dead)
> *Lang may yir lum reek!* (long may your chimney smoke!)
> *May the best yer've ever seen be the worst yer'll ever see,*
> *May a moose ne'er leave yer girnal' wi' a tear drop in its e'e,*
> *(mouse, grain store)*
> *May yer lum keep blithely reekin' until the day yer dee,*
> *(chimney, smoking, dead)*
> *And may yer a' be as happy as I'd like yer a' tae be.*
> (Traditional toast from Canisbay, a small village near John O'Groats)

14. Marwick, P. 105
15. Lamb, Gregor, *Carnival of the Animals*, P. 102

Here's tae them that wish us weel, (well)
And for the rest...ye ken yersel! (You know who you are)
(Traditional toast from the Island of Stroma near Orkney)

Robert Burns (1759-1796)

A Guid New-year I wish thee, Maggie!
Hae, there's a ripp to thy auld baggie;
(a handful of grain for your belly)
Tho thou's howe-backet now, an knaggie, (sway backed)
I've seen the day,
Thou could hae gaen like only staggie
Out owre the lay.
(a lull between waves during which a horse may cross the surf)
(The Auld Farmer's New-Year Morning Salutation To His Auld Mare,
Maggie, on giving her the accustomed Ripp of Corn to Handsel
(a good luck gift) in the New Year, 1786)[16]

Mannies an Horses

8 oz flour
½ tsp. bicarbonate of soda
1 tsp. ground ginger
3 oz lard
5 tbsp golden syrup
Warm water as needed

Preheat the oven to 350 degrees.
Mix the lard and syrup together.
Mix the dry ingredients and combine the two mixtures.
Shape into mannies (men) and horses.
Bake until golden brown.[17]

Handsel Monday – First Monday of the New Year

The day when employers give a gift to their employees, it was once the only holiday workers had other than the day of the local fair. Families would get together, couples marry, and servants and employees received gifts of cash.

Burning of the Clavie – January 11 Eve (Old Hogmanay)

This is an ancient festival with Pictish, Celtic, or Viking roots that takes place at Burghead, Moray. A half barrel is filled with wood shavings and tar or creosote (originally a herring barrel but in modern times a whisky barrel). The barrel is nailed to a post (the same nails are re-used each year) and placed on the shoulders of a local resident.

The Clavie (from Gaelic *cliabh*, a basket used to hold kindling) is lit with peat from the hearth of a local Povost and then carried by the chosen *Clavie*

16. Wilkie, George Scott, *Understanding Robert Burns*, Electricscotland.com, www.electricscot-land.com/burns/

17. *Mannies an Horses*, Electricscotland.com, http://www.electricscotland.com/newsletter/070105

King. Ten or more men (traditionally fishermen) take turns with the *Clavie*, carrying it deiseil around the town, stopping to give a burning faggot from the *Clavie* to chosen citizens to bring good luck to the house in the New Year.

The procession ends up at an old stone altar on Doorie Hill, reputedly a place where Druids used to light their ritual fire. The *Clavie* is put down and fuel is added to make a large bonfire. Those in attendance take a faggot home to re-kindle their own New Year's fire or to send to distant friends and relatives for luck.

This practice was once common all over North-East Scotland until it was condemned by the Presbyterian church as *"superstitious, idolatrous and sinfule, an abominable heathenish practice".*[18]

Up-Helly-Aa – last Tuesday of January

Also called Yule's End, this festival from Viking times is now celebrated in Lerwick in the Shetland Islands. A fully equipped Viking ship, complete with oars and shields is pulled to the beach by a torch bearing crowd of fully dressed Viking warriors. Three cheers and a bugle call and the ship is set ablaze by 800 burning torches.[19]

In this ancient Fire Festival blazing barrels are dragged through the streets, accompanied by *Guizers* carrying torches which are piled together at midnight to form a huge fire. At the stroke of midnight all house doors are opened and using brooms, mops, and other devices, evil spirits and hunger demons are magically "swept' out of the house.

Dances are held where *Guizers* show off their costumes, sing songs, and perform comedy routines.

Burns Nicht – January 25

A celebration of the birthday of the poet Robert Burns in 1759 which features toasts, music, praising of Burns, recitation of Burns' poetry and of course the "piping in" of the Haggis. The piper leads a procession consisting of the chef who bears the Haggis on a silver platter, the person who recites the "Address to A Haggis", and a third person who carries whisky so that each person in the procession can properly toast the Haggis.

The Haggis is ritually slaughtered by *"trenching its gushing entrails"* with dramatic flourish.[20] (I can personally attest that the very best way to eat Haggis is a after a wee drap o' Single Malt).

The Festival of Oimelc – February 1-2

Renamed "Candlemas" by the Christian church, this Fire Festival is an ancient Celtic observance in honor of the goddess *Bríghde (Bride)*. It is a legal Scottish quarter day when rents and other contracts were once due.

---

18. *Clavie Burning, Hopeman F.C., www.hopemanfc.com/clavie_burning.htm*

19. *Traditional Scottish Festivals, Up-Helly-aa, Rampantscotland.com, http://www.rampantscot-land.com/features/festivals.htm*

20. *Article by "Mac", The Burns Supper, The World Burns Club, The Robert Burns World Federation, http://www.worldburnsclub.com/supper/burns*

> *If Candlemas Day be bright and Fair*
> *Half the winter is to come and mair* (more)
> *If Candlemas Day be dark and foul*
> *Half the winter was over at Yowl* (Yule)
> (Traditional)

Girls and women decorate a straw doll made from the last sheaf of the harvest with flowers and shells. Dressed in white, they carry the *Brideag* (Bride Doll) around town from door to door, finally putting her to rest in a bed of rushes by a hearth.

A stick of birch (a *"slachdan"*) is placed in the Doll's hands, symbolic of Her magical power to soften the weather. The next morning the ashes of the hearth are examined to see if *Bride* has left a footprint. If no mark is found an offering has to be made in *Brighde's* honor (such as a chicken) which is buried at a place where three streams meet. [21]

A party is held at Oimelc for all girls of the village that features music, food, and dancing until dawn.

Oimelc is the milk festival that celebrates the lactation of the ewes. In a time before supermarkets it was impossible to purchase or obtain milk until the herd animals were pregnant and lactating (which happens just before the ewes give birth). The availability of new milk was a cause for rejoicing, the first sign of the return of the Fires of Life and of the renewal of the seasonal cycle of farm activity. To celebrate the first sparks of spring, candles were placed on the windowsills.

Oimelc was also the time of first plowings. The plow and other agricultural tools were ritually blessed with Whisky before the first furrow was cut and the fields were sained with a burning brand to ward off bad luck.

Winter stores of food such as vegetables, grain, and meats, were low so milk dishes were cooked for the feast. Butter was made from the new milk and the churn was dressed to look like the Goddess *Brighde*. Omens were read in the weather – good weather at Oimelc meant that winter would continue, but if a hedgehog or snake emerged from its den on Oimelc it meant that winter was on the wane (this is the origin of the American celebration called 'Ground Hog Day'). Rain at the time of Oimelc meant a good summer for the crops.

The Goddess at Oimelc

The Goddess associated with this festival is *Brighde (Bride)*. She is the daughter of *The Daghda, Deagh Dia* (The Good God) and of *Boann*, the Cow Goddess of the Boyne. She is Patroness of the Druids and Bards and a triple Fire Goddess whose spheres are poetry, healing, and smith craft. She is also the Goddess of Motherhood appealed to by women in labor. When a woman is giving birth, the midwife stands in the doorway with her hands on the doorjambs and welcomes Bride in:

> *Bride! Bride! Come in,*
> *Thy welcome is truly made,*
> *Give thou relief to the woman*
> *And give the conception to the sacred three.*
> (Traditional and slightly re-Paganized)

---

21. Nicholson, Francine, et al., *Land Sea and Sky* http://homepage.eircom.net/~shae/ Chapters 14-15

The midwife places three drops of water on the child's brow when it is born, in remembrance of *Bríghde* and of the sacred three.[22]

Equal-armed Solar Crosses, *Bríghde's* own special symbol, are woven from rushes and hung in the house and barn as protective talismans on the night of the festival. The rushes are spread under the table on the night of the feast and woven after the family dinner. Left over rushes are used to make *Bríghde's* bed by the fire, and scattered around the barn for luck.

In the Highlands these Solar Crosses are also made before weddings and tucked under the mattress to ensure fertility.[23]

A Bride's Girdle (*Crios Bríghde*) is made of a straw rope that is about nine feet long. The rope is tied to make a circle through which the family passes (men generally step through it and women usually pull it down over their heads). Three tiny Solar Crosses are tied to the rope.

An image of the Goddess is made and drawn around the edges of the fields in a cart, followed by singing and dancing townsfolk and clergy. Highland women make a figurine out of the butter churn and carry it from house to house, bringing the blessings of Bride to every door. They collect cakes, bread, and butter as they go, to be eaten with the men later at a village dance. Holy Wells are visited on this day. [24]

It is very good luck to recite *The Descent of Brigit* at Oimelc. Here is a slightly re-Paganized version:

Praises of Brigit
Brigit daughter of Dugall the Brown
Son of Aodh son of Art son of Conn
Son of Criara son of Caibre son of Cas
Son of Cormac son of Cartach son of Conn
Brigit of the mantles,
Brigit of the peat-heap,
Brigit of the twining hair,
Brigit of the augury.
Brigit of the white feet,
Brigit of the calmness,
Brigit of the white palms,
Brigit of the kine.
Brigit, woman-comrade,
Brigit of the peat-heap,

---

22. Ross, Anne, *Folklore of the Scottish Highlands*, P. 131
23. Nicholson, Francine, et al., *Land Sea and Sky* http://homepage.eircom.net/~shae/ Chapters 14-15
24. Nicholson, Francine, et al.,

> *Brigit, woman-helper,*
> *Brigit, woman mild.*
> *Each day and each night*
> *That I say the Descent of Brigit,*
> *I shall not be slain,*
> *I shall not be wounded,*
> *I shall not be put in cell,*
> *I shall not be gashed,*
> *I shall not be torn in sunder,*
> *I shall not be despoiled,*
> *I shall not be down-trodden,*
> *I shall not be made naked,*
> *I shall not be rent.*
> *Nor sun shall burn me,*
> *Nor fire shall burn me,*
> *Nor beam shall burn me,*
> *Nor moon shall burn me.*
> *Nor river shall drown me,*
> *Nor brine shall drown me,*
> *Nor flood shall drown me,*
> *Nor water shall drown me.*
> *Nightmare shall not lie on me,*
> *Black-sleep shall not lie on me,*
> *Spell-sleep shall not lie on me,*
> *Luaths-luis* shall not lie on me.*
> *I am under the keeping of Brigit,*
> *My companion, my beloved.*

(Traditional and slightly adapted, from Carmina Gadelica 263) [25]
(*Luis means Rowan and luaith means ashes
so this may refer to a spell that uses burned Rowan wood)

Candles are placed in the windows to honor the rekindling of the fires of spring and to welcome the Goddess. A dish of water or salt, healing threads, ribbons, cloths, or a cloak are left out all night to receive Bríghde's blessing, which are later used for healing throughout the year.

The early Christian church recognized that the people would not give up their beloved Goddess so they morphed Her and many of Her stories and traditions into Saint Brighid of Kildare.

Bannock Night

Also known as *Beef Brose, Shriften E'en, Fastern's E'en*, it takes place on the first Tuesday of the New Moon after Oimelc

Small boys take torches and seek out older boys who are dressed as old women wearing masks. The "old women" chase the younger boys with flailing ropes until the younger boys finally get away. The "old women" represent troll-women.

---

25. Carmichael, Alexander, Carmina Gadelica – Hymns and Incantations, P. 236

It is also celebrated as a carnival and feast on the last Tuesday before Lent, to use up the meat, butter and fat. Rowdy ball games are played.

Valentines Day – February 14

Names are written on bits of paper and placed in a hat. Everyone takes a paper and if someone draws the same name three times a marriage is destined.

Whuppity Scoorie – March 1

A boy's festival from Lanark where pennies are tossed and boys compete to gather them up. Wadded up balls of paper tied with a string are used by the contestants to strike each other. The object is to make a lot of noise and to frighten away evil Spirits.

Spring Equinox - March 21-22

At this time a *"Kern Doll"*, made from the last sheaf of the previous year's harvest, is taken outside and ritually burned in the barnyard (this activity can also be done at the Fall Equinox). Curses are laid on any person or power that might interfere with the new Kern Doll from the next harvest.[26]

In Orkney, a small patch of ground is plowed and sewn with grain. The success or failure of the plot predicts luck or disaster for the farm in the coming year. Grain harvested from that plot is for ritual use only, to be ground and baked into cakes which are offered to the Harvest Goddess. It is very lucky to be the first farmer to get your seed into the ground.

In Shetland, a hen's egg is placed in the store of grain to bless it with fertility. Only those with a proven "green thumb" or with a "growin' hand" should be allowed to handle or sow the grain.[27]

Spring Equinox marks the start of battles between *Teran* and the *Mither O' the Sea*. *Mither* eventually wins, bringing calm summer seas.

Easter

A Pagan festival named for the Saxon Goddess of spring, *Eastre*, whose symbols are the hare and the egg. This festival was adopted by Christians as a counterpart to Jewish Passover. The date is based on the phases of the Moon.

Hot cross Buns are baked, with Solar crosses on them. Colored hard boiled eggs are rolled down hills on Easter Monday.

Hot Cross Buns

1 cup milk	½ tsp. nutmeg
2 tablespoons yeast	4 eggs
½ cup sugar	5 cups flour
2 tsp. salt	1 1/3 cup currants or raisins
1/3 cup butter, melted and cooled	1 egg white
1 tsp. cinnamon	

---

26. Lamb, Gregor, *Carnival of the Animals*, P. 140
27. Marwick, Ernest, *The Folklore of Orkney and Shetland*, P. 69

Glaze

| 1 1/3 cup confectioner's sugar | ½ tsp. lemon extract |
| 1 ½ tsp. finely chopped lemon zest | 1- 2 tablespoons milk |

In a saucepan, heat the milk to very warm, but not hot (110°F).

Pour the warm milk into a bowl and sprinkle in the yeast. Mix to dissolve and let sit for 5 minutes.

Add the sugar, salt, butter, cinnamon, nutmeg and eggs and gradually add in the flour. The dough will be wet and sticky. Continue mixing until smooth.

Cover with plastic wrap or a clean cloth and let the dough "rest" for 30-45 minutes.

Knead again until smooth and elastic.

Add currants or raisins and knead until well mixed. At this point, the dough will still be fairly wet and sticky.

Shape the dough into a ball, place in a buttered dish, cover with plastic wrap and let rise overnight in the refrigerator. Excess moisture will be absorbed by the morning.

Let the dough sit at room temperature for about a half-hour.

Line a large baking pan (or pans) with parchment paper (you could also lightly grease a baking pan, but parchment works better).

Divide the dough into 24 equal pieces (in half, half again, etc.).

Shape each portion into a ball and place it on the baking sheet, about ½ inch apart. Cover with a clean kitchen towel and let rise in a warm, draft-free place until doubled in size, about 1½ hours.

Pre-heat the oven to 400° F.

When the buns have risen, take a sharp or serrated knife and carefully slash the buns with a Solar (equal armed) cross.

Brush the buns with egg white and place in the oven. Bake for 10 minutes, and then reduce the heat to 350° F. Bake until golden brown, about 15 minutes more.

Transfer to a wire rack for cooling. Whisk together glaze ingredients, and spoon over the buns in a Solar cross pattern. Serve warm, makes 2 dozen.[28]

Hunt The Gowk – April 1

A *"gowk"* is a fool, from the Old Norse: *"gaukr"*. This is a day to play tricks, tell lies, and send people on foolish errands, but the jokes must stop by noon.[29]

Tailie Day or Preen-Tail Day – April 2

The day after Hunt the Gowk, paper tails are attached to a person's backside as a joke. In past times, butchers would save pig's tails for the boys. Pierced with hooked pins, the tails were attached without anyone noticing.

---

28. *Recipe For Cooking Hot Cross Buns, Fabulous Foods, http://www.fabulousfoods.com:80/recipes/breads/yeast/hotcrossbun.html*

29. *Traditional Scottish Festivals, Hunt the Gowk – 1st April, Rampantscotland.com, http://www.rampantscotland.com/features/festivals.htm*

Borrowing Day – April 3

Anything borrowed on this day becomes the possession of the holder.

Whitsunday – Seventh Sunday after Easter

Another Scottish legal quarter day when rents were once due.

Bealltan – May 1

In the times before radio, television, and the internet, the date of this Fire Festival was calculated in different ways. One was the blooming of the Hawthorn tree, the signal that summer was indeed upon the land. It was the task of the local Druid to keep an eye on the Hawthorns to announce the first blossoms and the inauguration of the *Bealltan* feast.

The second method for divining the date was the observation of the skies. *Bealltan* marks the day when the Pleiades "disappear into the sun", that is, the Pleiades are no longer visible after sunset. If we are to take into account the movements of the stars in the last two thousand years this would place the *Bealltan* festival on April 26 or 27 of the current Gregorian calendar.

At Bealltan, great bonfires are lit on the hilltops in the sun's honor. All hearth fires are extinguished to be re-kindled with sacred flames from the ritual pyres. A large bannock is baked and divided into as many pieces as there are celebrants. One piece is blackened with charcoal and all the pieces are placed into a hat. Whoever draws the blackened piece must jump the flames six times.[30]

Sacrifices were once offered at this time to preserve the health of the cattle as the *áiridhean* or *"Shielings"* (summer grazing) began. Women and children drove the cattle, sheep and goats out to their summer pastures and lived in bothies (small huts or cabins), while tending to the herds, milking, butter-making and cheese-making.

Men left the fields and came to the hills for a visit every once in a while whereupon singing, story telling and courting ensued. A male lamb was sacrificed and eaten in celebration when the men came to visit.[31]

At the official start of summer, the weather was warm but the crops were not yet in, and so it was a time of hunger. Fertility of the herds and crops was a major concern and rituals were done to ensure success. The Maypole with its strong phallic symbolism is an English custom that found its way into the Lowlands of Scotland.

In modern times, young women still wash their faces in dew collected in the morning, a magical beauty aid which can be collected and bottled for later use. A large festival happens every year on Calton Hill in Edinburgh. "Year and a day" trial marriages (hand fastings) end so that couples are free to pursue other partners. Large bonfires are lit and everyone dances around them as men and boys jump the fire.

Animals born at Bealltan are not expected to thrive. Kittens and chickens born the first week of May are destined to be scrawny.

30. Ross, Anne, *Folklore of the Scottish Highlands*, P. 137
31. Ross, P. 135

Bealltan Magic

Remove a piece of turf (to be replaced afterwards) and build a fire of nine sacred woods. Place each bit of wood with care, uttering a prayer of blessing as each stick is laid down. Make a caudle of eggs, oatmeal, butter and milk and cook it over the fire. First offer some to the Fairies by spilling it on the ground, then eat or drink it (depending upon the recipe).

Caudle

1 pt milk
2 tbsp oatmeal
¼ tsp salt
2 tsp honey
¼ tsp nutmeg
whiskey or heather ale to taste

Heat the milk in a pan with the oatmeal and salt.
Stir well and bring to the boil.
Leave to stand for 10 minutes and then press the mixture through a sieve into a clean saucepan.
Add the honey and nutmeg and bring the mixture to a simmer.
Stir well to make sure the mixture doesn't burn or stick to the pan.
Remove from the pan and add in the whiskey or heather ale.[32]
Serve immediately.

Bake a bannock with nine raised bumps dedicated to forces such as blight, drought, or animals that could harm the herds and crops. Break off the pieces one at a time, and throw them behind you saying: *"This is for you, crow, preserve my corn. This is for you, fox, preserve my hens"* and so on.

Break a bannock into as many pieces as there are celebrants and blacken one piece. Put the pieces in a jar. Whoever draws the black piece must jump the fire three times.

Pass small animals through a hoop of rowan to protect them from sorcery. Make large animals walk over a rowan branch. Make a bannock and toast it to a fire of rowan (any left over flour should be carefully sprinkled on the animals). Make a charm of rowan such as an equal armed Solar Cross bound with red thread and sew it into your clothing where it can't be seen.

As at Samhuinn, the gates between the Worlds are thin at this liminal time between the dark and light halves of the year. Otherworldly Spirits are about, so Bealltan is a good time to take omens.

The "Fairy Rade" (Fairy Ride) occurs when the Fairies ride out on May Eve. The tinkling of their horses bits and bridles and the sound of their singing keeps country folk awake.

Couples are encouraged to pair off and mate in secluded, wild places lending fertile energy to the landscape (but marriage at this time is very unlucky).

---

32. *Caudle recipe http://theskirmish.com/seren/?page_id=53*

A feast is held, to ensure prosperity by sympathetic magic, where oatmeal porridge, bread, soft cheeses, new greens and roots are the main fare. Sprouts of young herbs such as wood sorrel, dandelion, and silverweed are eaten and a male lamb is sacrificed for the meal.[33]

The Crescent Moon nearest Bealltan is a good time to sacrifice an extra bull. Offer parts to the Gods by placing them in the fire. Distribute the rest to your clan.

A man dressed in women's clothing, or a butter churn and pitchfork dressed as a "man and wife" are paraded through the town. Carts filled with burning mugwort are dragged around the edges of the fields to sain them, as drums are beaten to drive away evil Spirits that might harm the farm.

Symbolic battles are staged, between the Oak King (king of summer) and the Holly King (king of winter) and between the forces of the Queen of Summer and the King of Winter. The Summer Lord or Summer Queen must always win and the Lord of Winter must be driven away to the West, the direction of death and sunset.

Temporary marriages (hand-fastings) end at Bealltan so that couples are freed to find new mates. Families "beat the bounds" or "ride the marches" by walking the borders of their lands, honoring the Spirits and leaving offerings for protection and blessing (this activity helps to fix the borders of the land in people's minds). The rite is followed by horse racing, games, and a feast.[34]

Robin Hood Games

May Day games or Robin Hood Games are so called because participants donate to their place of worship in their own name and in the name of their family. The money is used to maintain the place of worship, and also to help the poor, in effect "robbing the rich to give to the poor".

In one such game, a band of "grenadiers" goes into the forest in search of an "outlaw", who wears a straw mask and a necklace of old, rock-hard biscuits around his neck. When caught, the "outlaw" is led out of the forest accompanied by a hobby horse and a fool, and sitting backwards on a donkey. The backwards riding posture is a position seen in Otherworldly riders.

The "outlaw" is then "shot" by the "grenadiers" and "dies", but is soon revived by the fool. The "outlaw" is none other than Robin Hood.[35]

The sun shining on water at this time is considered potent magic, and well or spring water is collected as the first rays hit, to be sprinkled on people, animals and objects for healing and protection. Butter churned on Bealltan morning is called "May Butter". Salt water and dew gathered at dawn on May Day are added to it and it is used afterwards to cure fevers (see more about the magical uses of dew in the Water Magic chapter above).

The first water taken from a well or spring on Bealltan is especially lucky, but if someone else gets there first they might steal your luck. (Holy Wells are exempt from this because their luck does not diminish with use).

---

33. *Nicholson, Francine, et al., Land Sea and Sky http://homepage.eircom.net/~shae/ Chapters 14-15*
34. *Bord, Colin and Janet, Sacred Waters, P. 98*
35. *Lamb, Gregor, Carnival of the Animals, P. 120*

Purification by Fire

The name of this festival probably derives from *"Belinus"*, the patron God of the Bealltan Fires. It is a time of ritual purification by sacred fire, when the herds are sained by driving them between two fires on their way to their summer grazing in the hills (the fires are supposed to be close enough that the hair of a white heifer will be singed brown). At the start of the light half of the year, warriors and raiders set out to serve their chieftain.[36]

The Shieling Feast

At Bealltan, when the cows have arrived safely in their summer pastures, make a feast of lamb and ale to celebrate.

Victoria Day – May 24

Fans of Queen Victoria celebrate her birthday.

Guid Nychburris – Mid June

"Good Neighbor Day" is a weeklong festival that originally took place when court was in session to resolve disputes between neighbors. Crown a *"Queen of the South"* and perform a neighborly deed by doing an errand or favor for your neighbor. Leave a surprise gift of flowers, or a coupon good for a service on your neighbor's doorstep.

Selkirk Common Riding – June 18

Riding the Marches (boundaries) or Beating the Bounds is done in many areas. The object is to refresh everyone's memory as to where boundary lines are drawn.

Summer Solstice (Midsummer) – June 21

Locals go to a hill top before dawn to watch the Midsummer sunrise. When the Sun appears, hands are raised to catch the first rays, and held up to the Sun until the Sun clears the horizon. Then everyone kisses, sings and dances, and attends a breakfast feast.

Older boys and girls have gathered materials for a bonfire by pulling heather and tying it into bundles, carrying peat, and collecting twigs and branches. The peat is placed at the center of the fire, heather on top, and finally the wood. Adults supervise the lighting of the fire (that is ideally lit by friction) which should be respected as a "Fire Altar", and is not to be used for mundane purposes such as trash burning, cooking, etc.

Everyone dances around the fire, making offerings to it (such as dried herbs, butter, oil, and whisky) and then the young pull out flaming torches which they carry to the fields, barns, and hills. The fields, horses and cattle are sained with the burning brands which are carried in a Sun-wise circle around the boundaries and animals.

The sick and those making petitions walk around the bonfire deiseil. Sick animals are led around the fire. Old bones are gathered and burned in the fire, and those who are able take turns jumping the flames (because the grain will grow as high as they can leap).

36. *Nicholson, Francine, et al., Land Sea and Sky http://homepage.eircom.net/~shae/ Chapters 14-15*

Unmarried women carry home a partially burned peat, extinguishing it in the vat of stale urine kept for the conditioning of wool cloth (traditionally a barrel was kept out of doors for the gentlemen to pee in just for this purpose – over time the urine becomes ammonia). Then, the peat is placed over the door lintel.

The next day, the peat is broken open and the color of the fibers inside will reveal the hair color of their future husband.

Sailors and fishermen throw silver coins into the sea as they set out for the summer fishing, for luck and a calm sea. *Selkies* drop their skins on this night, to come to shore and join the humans in their dancing.[37]

Glasgow Fair – last two weeks of July

This fair goes back to William the Lion in 1190.[38]

Lúnasdal – August 1

This Fire Festival is another legal Quarter Day when rents were once due. In some areas it marks the celebration of the "first fruits" of the harvest and the ritual cutting of the first sheaf of new grain. Christians adopted this festival and re-named it *"Loafmass"*. Loaves were baked from the new grain and placed on the altar to be blessed.

Grain from the first sheaf of the harvest is dried and ground, and the head of the clan should be the first to taste the new flour. If the harvest is poor, a more genial member of the tribe is chosen to taste the first grinding, because the disposition of the "first taster" predicts the harmony of the family in the coming year.

A small triangle shaped corner of the last field to be harvested is left untouched for the Fairies.

Part of the final sheaf to be cut is saved to be fed to the work mare and her foal on New Year's morning, thus transferring the luck of the harvest to the next year. In northern areas such as Orkney a *"bikko"* (bitch) or straw dog is also made from the last sheaf and hung from a farm building for luck. Some of the grain is fashioned into a Kern Doll and a bannock is baked from some of the grain of the last sheaf, as a way of ingesting the Spirit of the corn and the luck that is in it.

The last person to bring in grain is forced to eat a piece of buttered bread before they are allowed into the farmyard (to cancel bad luck).

Harvest knots are made from plaited grain and exchanged by lovers. If someone manages to secretly place one in your shoe you must provide all the harvesters on the farm with whisky.

The Lammas Fair

This is a traditional gathering that takes place at this time, in many Celtic areas. To protect yourself against hucksters, place a four leafed clover in your shoe, as this will give you the ability to see through any deception. Four leafed clover is luckiest of all plant talismans and a powerful charm against sorcery, and has the strongest power if found accidentally.

To advertise that you are looking for work, put a spray of oats in your buttonhole.

---

37. *Marwick, Ernest, The Folklore of Orkney and Shetland, PP. 111-113*

38. *Traditional Scottish Festivals, Glasgow Fair, Rampantscotland.com, http://www.rampantscotland.com/features/festivals.htm*

Lammas "Brother and Sister"

At the Lammas Fair a couple may decide to be lovers for the duration of the fair, during which time they may enjoy all the pleasures of love.

Fishing Ends

Old Lammas (12 or 13 August) marks the official end of the fishing season. Fishermen hold a feast and celebrate with good food, story-telling, cup-reading (divinations), and many toasts.

Harvest Suppers

"Cuttin' Butter" is a simple feast given for those who helped with the harvest, once it is done. *"Herding bannocks"* are large bannocks made specifically to celebrate the end of the harvest. Made of the new grain they are so large that they provide breakfast for several days. *"Harvest-home"* is a large feast that often features a ram, culled from the flock.

In Ireland, the festival is called *Lughnasad* and is celebrated for a three week period beginning August 1. In Scotland, perhaps because it is more northerly and thus the "first fruits" of the harvest come in later, the same festivities take place as in Ireland, but on September 29, or on the feast of Saint Michael (see Michaelmas below).[39] It is worth noting that many churches dedicated to Saint Michael were placed on hills once sacred to *Lugh*.

Lúnasdal marks a time of celebration because the first fruits of the harvest are available, but it is also a time of tension. The crops are not yet safely in and rain is still needed to ensure a healthy harvest. Rain on *Lúnasdal* is a special blessing and a very good omen.

Purification by Water

In Indo-European tradition, cows are animals associated with the Moon and sacred water because they produce milk, while horses are viewed as Solar animals. *Bealltan* is a festival of sacred fire where the cows are purified by leading them between two ritual fires, and *Lúnasdal* is a festival of sacred water, the time to ritually bathe horses in a river or pond as an act of purification. Thus we again see the magical admixture of fire and water at play.

Giving Thanks for the Harvest

The name of the festival is derived from the *násad* of *Lugh* (games of Lugh). Lugh is not a Sun God as is often supposed. He is "Master of Every Art": poet, magician, harper, swordsman, goldsmith and more. He represents the intelligence and skill that are necessary to survive the vagaries of pestilence and of weather, and to bring the harvest safely in.

The God Lugh is a son of *Cian* of the *Tuatha de Danaan*, and of *Ethlinn*, daughter of *Balor*, King of the *Fomor*, and foster son of the *Fir Bolg Queen Tailtiu*, wife of *Eochaid Garb*.

Tailtiu died of a broken heart as a result of Her labor to clear the Wood of Cuan in Ireland, to create a plain of cultivation known as *Oenach Tailten*. This site later became a place of great assemblies sponsored by the High Kings of *Ériu*.

39. Ross, Anne, *Folklore of the Scottish Highlands*, P. 139

Lugh inaugurated the festival at *Tailtiu's* request, as funeral games in *Tailtiu's* honor and the festival was transported to Scotland via the *Scoti of Dalriada.*

Another name for the festival is *Brón Trogain* (sorrow of the Earth's Travail) and *Tailtiu* can be none other than a representation of the Earth Mother, who sacrifices Herself each year at the time of the harvest. It is fitting that She should be mourned and honored at this time when we all enjoy the fruits of Her labor.

In ancient times, the month preceding the harvest was hard, with sometimes only wild foods such as nettles and old cabbages were available. The ewes were separated from their lambs in preparation for breeding which meant a scarcity of milk.[40]

The cutting of the first sheaf of new grain is a solemn occasion. The family dresses in their finest and walks out to the fields. The head of the clan removes their hat and places it on the ground while facing the sun, and using a sickle ritually cuts the first sheaf of grain. Then they twirl the sheaf three times *deiseil* around their head while turning on their heel, and singing a song in praise of the Harvest Gods. The family joins in the praising of the Gods of the Harvest who have given bread and grain, herds and meat, wool, clothing, health and strength.[41]

Berry picking (especially blueberries), horse racing and other forms of competition follow. Couples go high into the hills to picnic, gather berries, and make love.

Lúnasdal is a lucky time to marry (perhaps because the herds and fields of a potential mate can be evaluated) and to sign contracts of all kinds. The feast features fresh berries and bread made from freshly ground new grain, as well as other "first fruits" from fields and gardens. Carrots and oatcakes are traditional *Lúnasdal* fare.

Magic at Lúnasdal

The *Lúnasdal* festival is a time to climb high hills and honor the Sun. If a stone seat is available on top of a hill, it is sat upon and offerings are left for the Spirits along the way. Water is bathed in for purification, and Holy Wells are visited. Plants growing around Healing Wells have a special magical potency at this time, and ropes used to tether animals are hung near the Well to absorb its protective powers.

It is a good time to make a devotional offering to your local sacred Mother River Goddess. Float a tiny boat or wooden plank laden with Saint John's Wort or other flowers and a lit candle, out to the waters of a river or lake.

Standing stones are garlanded with flowers and grain stalks, and washed with milk and honey.

It is also a good time to take omens and do divinations. The first cut of grain is thrown with eyes closed. If it falls in one bunch it means good luck.[42]

Bardic and craft competitions are held, and stories are told of great battles such as the Battle of Moytura where the *Tuatha Dé Dannan* who were under *Lugh's* leadership bested the *Fomoire.* The *Fomorians*, who always sought to keep the harvest

---

40. Nicholson, Francine, et al., *Land Sea and Sky* http://homepage.eircom.net/~shae/ Chapters 14-15
41. Ross, Anne, *Folklore of the Scottish Highlands, P. 138*
42. Ross, P. 139

for themselves, symbolize the forces of chaos and blight that farmers must constantly strive to control. The *Fomoire* may have been an actual people at one time who were later used by the poets to symbolize the forces of blight, disease and bad weather.[43]

Mock battles are fought at *Lúnasdal* fairs. Tradition holds that the Fairies do battle at this time for the best portion of the harvest.[44]

Marymas – August 15

A bannock is baked in honor of Mary. Here is a traditional description from the Carmina Gadelica that bears undertones of having once been an ancient ritual in honor of the Grain Goddess:

The Feast Day of Mary

On the feast day of Mary the fragrant,
Mother of the shepherd of the flocks,
I cut me a handful of the new corn,
I dried it gently in the sun,
I rubbed it sharply from the husk
With mine own palms.
I ground it in a quern on Friday,
I baked it on a fan of sheepskin,
I toasted it to a fire of rowan,
And I shared it round my people.
I went sunwise round my dwelling,
In name of the Mary mother.

(Traditional, Carmina Gadelica 76)[45]

Braemar Gathering - First Saturday of September

A major Highland Games that dates back to the 11th century when king Malcolm III "Canmore" gave a prize to the winner of a race to the top of Craig Choinnich.[46]

Fall Equinox – September 21-22

When the harvest is done, the reapers run to the highest hill and *"Cry the Kern"* by yelling that the harvest is finished. Some grain from the last sheaf is kept to be mixed in with the stores of new grain that will be saved for the next year's sowing. This transfers fertility magic from one year to the next.[47]

A Doll is made from the last sheaf to be taken (see Farming, Fertility, and Harvest Customs below).

Mither O' the Sea and *Teran* do battle once again. *Teran* prevails as the harsh winter seas set in.

Michaelmas Day – September 29

This is the feast day of St. Michael, patron of the sea and of sailors. In Barra, in the West of Scotland, a bannock was baked from the new grain and shared. It

43. *Nicholson, Francine, et al., Land Sea and Sky http://homepage.eircom.net/~shae/ Chapters 14-15*
44. *Nicholson, Francine, et al*
45. *Carmichael, Alexander, Carmina Gadelica, P. 86*
46. *Traditional Scottish Festivals, Braemar Gathering, Rampantscotland.com, http://www.rampantscotland.com/features/festivals.htm*
47. *Lamb, Gregor, Carnival of the Animals, P. 142*

is a day for horse racing and in some northern areas, the celebration of the "first fruits" of the harvest (see *Lúnasdal* above). A woman gives a suggestive bunch of carrots to her lover, bound with red string.

A dance called *Cailleach an Dúdain* (Hag of the Mill-Dust) is done on St. Michael's night (September 29). A man holds a *Slachdan Druidheachd* (Druid's Wand) or *Slachdan Geasachd* (Magic Wand) over his and a woman's head, and the woman falls as if dead at the man's feet. He dances around her as if in mourning, then touches her left hand with the wand. The left hand slowly comes back to life. Then he dances his joy and touches different parts of her body as they too come back to life. Finally, he breathes into her mouth and touches her heart with the wand. She springs to her feet and both dance happily together.

Musicians accompany the dance with pipes, fiddles, or mouth music that shifts and changes with each aspect of the dance. Sword dances are also performed which have roots in pre-Roman Gaul.[48] These dances sometimes feature a mock "decapitation" of one of the dancers, symbolic of the cutting of the grain.

Winter Sunday – Third Sunday in October

The cattle are brought in from the hills and stabled in the barn. Everyone who works on the farm spends the night with their employer. Trout are seen moving from streams and lakes to the ocean and it is very bad luck to molest them in any way.

Fireworks and bonfires are lit and children beg for pennies. (This is probably a modern vestige of the old *Samhuinn* observance).

---

48. Ross, Anne, *Folklore of the Scottish Highlands*, P. 139

Life Passages

Courtship and Marriage

According to one tradition, the Goddess who oversees courtship, marriage, and childbirth is *Bríghde (Bride)* who spends each winter trapped inside *Ben Nevis* until She is rescued by *Oengus Og*, the ever-youthful patron God of young lovers who arrives on his white horse to free Her.[1] *Oengus Og* and *Bríghde* are both children of *The Daghda* or "Father Nature", with his enormous appetites, his ever-full cauldron of plenty, his vast fertility, and his wisdom.

At her marriage every woman becomes a living manifestation of the Goddess *Bride* and her groom takes on the qualities of *Oengus Og*. But before there can ever be a wedding there must first be courting. Here are some Scottish courtship customs.

Rocking

The women gather in the kitchen to spin using *distaffs* or "rocks". A *distaff* is a stick with a cleft in it through which flax is drawn for spinning by hand. The flax line is "drafted" or pulled off of the *distaff* a little bit at a time to be spun with a drop spindle or with a wheel.

Later in the evening the men join them and make a party.[2]

Waulkin O' the Fauld (Watching the Fold)

When watching the sheep to keep the weaned lambs away from their dams, a young lad and lassie have a chance to spend the night together. Afterwards, the lad puts "Lad's Love" or wormwood in his cap or lapel – to announce that he has taken a lover.[3]

1. *Livingstone, Sheila, Scottish Customs, P. 21*
2. *Livingston, P. 27*
3. *Ibid., P. 27*

Bundling

A custom that was once especially popular in Orkney. A lad and lassie are encouraged to share a bed. They must remain fully clothed and the lassie's legs are tied to the bolster, or the bolster is propped in the center of the bed between the pair. It is a nice way to pass a long winter night in conversation, with the full blessings of the clan.[4]

Marriage Divinations

Two lovers sit by the fire and place two straws which they have named for each other on a glowing peat or ember. One straw should have a knot tied in it. If it jumps towards the other straw they will be married.

On *Oimelc* morn, an unmarried lassie should chase the first crow she sees because it will fly towards her future home. But if it lands in a kirkyard she will never marry.

At Midsummer, a couple pick stalks of ribwort plantain in bloom, removing the flowers and placing the stalks on a flat stone. If more flowers open before the stalks wither they are destined to marry.

At the appearance of the first New Moon of winter, select a large earth-fast stone (a stone that is half in and half out of the ground). Run around it three times *deiseil* (sunwise) and three times *tuaithiuil* (widdershins) saying:

> New Moon, New Moon tell me true
> Whether my love be false or true
> If s/he be true, the first time I her/him see
> Her/his face to me and his/her back to the sea
> If s/he be false, the first time I her/him see
> Her/his back to me and her/his face to the sea.[5]

(traditional)

Asking for His Hand

On a Leap Year a lassie may propose. If her intended says "no" he has to buy her a dress.[6]

The Speerin' Bottle

A prospective groom comes to his lover's house and places a small bundle on the bed. He shakes hands with all family members, studiously ignoring his intended. The father of the lassie makes an excuse to go outside and the suitor follows him, to ask for the daughter's hand. If the father says "yes", they go back inside and the bundle is opened, revealing a bottle of whisky which is passed around for a toast. Then the family discusses the wedding plans.[7]

Réitach

Another way to do this, perhaps if the hopeful groom is too shy, is to host a gathering at the prospective bride's home. The couple's friends get together and pick one of their number to ask the father's permission in the groom's stead. The marriage is not directly alluded to, instead the friend makes casual

---

4. *Ibid., P. 27*

5. *Marwick, Ernest, The Folklore of Orkney and Shetland, P. 85*

6. *Livingstone, Sheila, Scottish Customs, P. 32*

7. *Livingstone, P. 31*

conversation and mentions that a lamb or a boat needs to be looked after and he would be very happy to arrange for this to happen. If the father agrees, it is settled. Then neighbors and family members contribute food and drink for a celebratory meal. Musicians appear as if by magic and everyone pretends to be pleasantly surprised.[8]

Choosing the Date

It is very bad luck to marry in the Waning Moon, in January, or at *Bealltan*. Friday is sacred to *Freya* the Norse Goddess of Love, and is the best day for a wedding. *Lúnasdal* is the most auspicious time of year for a marriage rite.[9] In all cases the Moon must be Waxing or Full.

The Tocher (dowry)

Every bride should have new sheets, blankets, table linens and bedroom furniture. The whole clan pitches in to collect these necessaries. She should also come to the union with cattle, sheep, or money.[10]

Wee Mindings

Neighbors, family and friends give the couple *"wee mindings"* or gifts of handcrafted wooden, wickerwork, or horn items. The night before the wedding, a supper is served for the bridal party and the wedding gifts are put on display.[11]

"Booking Night" or "Contract Night"

The family and close friends come together to share a feast. The engaged couple spend the night together to seal the contract.[12]

Fit-Washin'

The night before the wedding a group of unmarried women go to the bride's house. The bride's father removes her shoes and her mother takes off her stockings. Then the mother pronounces a blessing on her daughter and the bride's feet are washed in a tub filled with one half volume of salt and one half volume of water which must be exposed to the Sun for twelve hours before the rite.

Afterwards, a ring is dropped into the tub of water and the women compete to claim it. The groom's feet should be washed in the same tub by a group of men.[13]

In another version of this ritual of purification, the clan gathers to wash the feet of the bride and groom with oil or grease and then rub them with soot. Afterwards there is music and dancing.[14]

The Wedding

In an ancient ceremony that does not involve the blessings of clergy, the couple stand on opposite banks of a small stream, dip their hands in the water and then join

8. *Ibid., P. 30*
9. *Ibid., P. 32*
10. *Ibid., P. 30*
11. *Ibid., P. 33*
12. *Marwick, Ernest, The Folklore of Orkney and Shetland, P. 87*
13. *Marwick, P. 88*
14. *Livingstone, Sheila, Scottish Customs, P. 31*

hands across the water while speaking their vows. If there is no stream available they can lick the thumbs of their right hands and press them together tightly.[15]

In order to protect the couple and the house, care must be taken that no one in the bride or groom's party walks *tuaithiuil* (against the sun). In fact, to do that while carrying a dried fish will ensure that the bride will have no milk for her first bairn![16]

The Bride's Dress

A new gown is made and one stitch is left undone. The bride must not make her dress alone, and any color will do except black. A green gown is especially lucky, being the favorite color of the Fairies. Blue is also lucky because as the saying goes: *"Marry in blue, love ever true"* and *"Something old, something new, something borrowed, something blue"*. To wear a blue garter is also very lucky.

The color silver is lucky because it is associated with the Moon. Gold is also lucky and associated with the Sun and Stars.

The bride should put a silver coin in her left shoe, and put her right shoe on first, for luck. She must not look in the mirror once fully dressed, and must remain veiled until after the ceremony.

The Groom's Attire

Silver buckles are very lucky, as is an embroidered vest. It is good luck to slip salt into the groom's pocket without his knowledge. All knots must be undone before the ceremony, in both the bride and groom's clothing, as an aid to fertility (after the ceremony the knots may be re-tied).[17]

Bride's Maid and Best Man

The custom of appointing a bride's maid and best man goes back to the time when women were forced to marry against their will. They were there to make sure the bride didn't escape, or to protect the bride in case her family came to steal her back. Sometimes mock *"abductions"* were staged where the groom had to overcome difficulties, in order to claim his bride and prove his and his men friend's mettle.

On the night before the wedding, the best man would sleep in the same room with the groom and bridesmaids would sleep with the bride. The bride and groom had to be well-guarded until the first sunrise after the wedding ceremony (to prevent the Fairies from stealing the bride or groom out of envy). Shots were fired at weddings because the noise kept the Hill Folk at bay.

In modern times, the job of the bride's maid is to issue invitations to the friends of the bride and groom. The bride and groom are responsible for inviting their own family and close friends.[18]

Stag Night

The best man organizes fun activities for the groom and his friends a few nights before the wedding, such as blackening the groom with soot or cocoa, and the more mess the better. He might take off the groom's pants and tie him

---

15. Livingston, P. 27

16. Marwick, Ernest, *The Folklore of Orkney and Shetland*, P.88

17. Livingstone, Sheila, *Scottish Customs*, P. 39

18. Livingstone, P. 34

up, or get him drunk and leave him on a bus, giving the driver money to take him as far as the money will last. (These tricks should be played enough days before the wedding to give everyone a chance to recover).

The bride is also subjected to tricks such as covering her with treacle (molasses), feathers, soot, and chocolate, or forcing her to dress with her clothing inside out, or with a jacket, flowers, or towel around her head. Once the bride is dressed, she is wheeled around town in a wheel barrow or a supermarket cart, and then everyone ends up at a house or pub for a party.[19]

Hen Night

This is a women only party specifically for the bride on the night before the wedding. The name comes from the days when the women would gather to pluck hens for the wedding feast.[20]

The Burning O' The Sneud

A *"sneud"* is a ribbon used by the bride to tie back her hair before she is wed. The elder women present at the party gather in secret to burn it in the fire. As it burns, they examine its shape and divine the bride's future.[21]

Salt

The night before the wedding, the bride carries salt to her new home, and sprinkles it on the floor as an act of purification. The *tocher* (dowry goods) are taken to the home and the bed is made. Presents are set up, and care must be taken that the bride does not trip and break a dish, which would be very bad luck.[22]

Wedding Ceremonies

There are several different types of ceremonies. A *"free wedding"* is one where the bride's father pays for everything. A *"penny wedding"* is one where the guests bring food and help defray the costs for music, drink, and so forth. At a *"dinner wedding"*, friends and family attend a dinner provided by the bride's father and afterwards there is music and dancing as more guests arrive.[23]

Hand-Fasting

A trial marriage or *"hand-fasting"* takes place before witnesses at a fair or *Lúnasdal* gathering. It lasts for a year and a day, after which a permanent wedding can take place (if both parties are willing), or they may part with no obligation.

Any child of a hand-fasting must be provided for by the child's father and his clan, according to the ancient laws. The child is fully legitimate and has full inheritance rights.[24]

The Wedding Walk

The women of the wedding party meet at dawn at the bride's home while the men assemble at the groom's house. After breakfast, the men walk to the

19. *Ibid., P. 34*
20. *Ibid., P. 35*
21. *Marwick, Ernest, The Folklore of Orkney and Shetland, P. 90*
22. *Livingstone, Sheila, Scottish Customs, P. 35*
23. *Livingstone, P. 36*
24. *Ibid., PP. 37-38*

bride's house making as much noise as possible along the way (to repel evil Spirits). The men fire three shots towards the bride's door and it is flung open. The bride and her attendants emerge in all their finery, kiss the men present and process *deiseil* around the house to arrive at the opposite side of the front door.[25]

A fiddler or piper leads everyone to the ritual site (care must always be taken that the musician is well fed or whisky might affect their playing). The piper is followed first by the groom and matron of honor or best maid, then the best man and the bride, next all couples, and finally the single folk and children. Older married couples may walk before the bride and groom out of respect. The very last person in line is the *"tail-sweeper"* who clears the trail behind the procession with a heather broom. The procession must cross water two times (in order to fool any bad Spirits seeking to do mischief).

When the party arrives at the place of ceremony, the bride and groom walk deiseil three times around the building or space before entering it. After the ceremony the newly joined couple lead everyone to the place of celebration, closely followed by the matron of honor and best man.[26]

The Ring

Wedding rings are an old Pagan custom going back to at least Roman times. The same ring may be used as both an engagement ring and a wedding ring. Before the wedding it is worn on the right hand. During the ceremony it is transferred to the left hand.[27]

After the Ritual

Small gifts are loosely sewn onto the bride's gown, and as soon as the ritual is over everyone tears one off. Such gifts are filled with luck from having been in close contact with the bride. The bride's mother also passes around a basket of favors supplied by the groom.[28] It is very lucky to be the first person to kiss the newly married bride.

As they leave the ritual area, the couple should pass under an arch of items relevant to their trades: farm tools, swords, fishing poles, artist's brushes, and the like.[29] The couple is showered with rose petals, confetti or bird seed at the same time (never throw rice as it is hardly traditional to Scotland, and it swells in the body of a bird, possibly killing it!).

The bride's father throws a shoe after the bride and groom, symbolic of his transfer of responsibility[30] and the bride throws the *"marriage ba"*, a decorated ball which the men vie to capture. The groom throws coins which children scramble to collect.[31]

The Broose (from Norwegian bruse – "to rush") (Horse Wedding)

In this type of wedding, horses are borrowed from far and wide to be ridden bareback (or covered with a cloth but not a saddle) by couples to the seat of the local

25. Marwick, Ernest, *The Folklore of Orkney and Shetland*, P. 88
26. Marwick, P. 89
27. Livingstone, Sheila, *Scottish Customs*, P. 37
28. Livingstone, P. 43
29. Livingstone, P. 41
30. Ibid., P. 41
31. Livingstone, P. 39

laird. After their vows are made, everyone races back to the barn where the wedding celebrations are to be held. Guests thunder across the fields taking the shortest possible route and facing great danger, and the first couple to arrive receives a prize.[32]

Horses figure in marriage ceremonies in other ways: hobby horses processed in the wedding of Mary Queen of Scots to the French Dauphin, and it is worth recalling that the mare is a symbol of sovereignty in Celtic tradition. Ancient king making rituals involved the sacrifice of a mare where the new king had to bathe in a broth of her blood and eat of her flesh in order to become one with or *"married to the land"*.

In Le Mans, France, a hobby horse called a *"bidoche"* still appears at weddings, to bring luck. In old Scotland the hobby horse was returned to the couple if their marriage soured due to infidelity or abuse. A straw effigy of a horse and rider, meant to represent the guilty party, was paraded through the town and then burned. Or a procession led by a man holding a horse's head with clacking jaws would spend several days making noise at the house of the offender.

An offending woman might be placed in *"branks"* (bridle), an iron bridle with a bit to prevent her from speaking. She was led around the town by a rope and labeled a *"scold"*.

"Kettling" was the banging of kettles, tin pails, tongs, and bones in the vicinity of a house in order to drive away the evil Spirits that were ruining a marriage.[33]

Running the Broose

Races and competitions were once a regular feature of Scottish weddings. When more than one couple was joined in a ceremony, they all raced to see which couple would get home first. The first couple to arrive would have a happy and prosperous marriage, but the last to come home would have bad luck.[34]

In ancient weddings, the mothers of the bride and groom did not always attend the rites but rather waited at the couple's new house. This custom dates back to the time when there was danger that the bride might be abducted. Young men ran to the house right after the ritual to let the mothers know that the couple was safely wed, and the first man to arrive was awarded a bottle of whisky.[35]

The Wedding Feast

In Highland weddings, the supper consisted of cold mutton and fowl, cheese, butter, milk, scones, oatcakes, and whisky, followed by an energetic dance. The meal was pot luck and supplied by all the neighbors. Celebrations went on all night and for the next few days.[36]

A *"cog"* was passed around to all guests at frequent intervals. The bride and groom took the first sip and then the vessel began to circulate.[37] Inside the cog were hot ale, sugar, whiskey, cream, spice, and eggs. The cog was always passed

32. Lamb, Gregor, Carnival of the Animals, P. 100
33. Lamb, PP. 104,107
34. Ross, Anne, Folklore of the Scottish Highlands, P. 121
35. Livingstone, Sheila, Scottish Customs, P. 41
36. Ross, Anne, Folklore of the Scottish Highlands, P. 121
37 Marwick, Ernest, The Folklore of Orkney and Shetland, P. 90

in a sun-wise direction from guest to guest, and frequently re-filled. Everyone drank to the bride's health.[38]

If anyone attended a penny wedding and did not contribute to the feast or forgot to bring a dish they were called *"whistlebinkies"*. All was forgiven if they sang or told a good story.[39]

The Cake

The top tier of a formal wedding cake is kept for the naming ceremony of the first child. The cake is cut by the bride alone and distributed to all.

The bride's mother bakes a large bannock or shortbread and breaks it over the head of the bride. It is very good luck and signifies fertility if the bannock breaks into many small pieces. Everyone takes a bit home to put under their pillow and dream on. A thimble and a ring are hidden inside the bannock, and whoever gets the ring will soon be married, but whoever gets the thimble will remain single (at least for a while).[40]

The Bride's Garter

The best man does his best to pull the bride's garter off of her leg. She eventually drops it on the floor, preventing mayhem.[41] (The garter is an object of luck, having been in intimate contact with the bride).

Guizers

Young men in masks and costumes made of straw and ribbons enter unexpectedly and kiss the bride and all female attendants while dancing around them. The leader of the *guisers* carries a straw broom and dances around the bride and groom, raising the besom over their heads as a blessing. One of the dancers, the *"fool"*, keeps laughing.

The *guizers* do not reveal their identities and must be well provisioned with spirits. When they depart, they leave handsel-money (handsel is a gift given to someone to bless any new venture) for the bride.[42]

In Shetland, men wearing straw masks and dresses appear at a wedding led by a *"scudler"* wielding a straw broom. They dance with all the ladies present, bringing the magic and fertility of the Grain Spirit to all.[43]

The Handsel Bairn

The youngest child present is placed in the bride's arms. If it raises its left foot, her bairns will be mostly boys. If it raises the right foot, her bairns will be mostly girls.[44]

The Wedding Dance

After the wedding supper there is a dance. The bride and groom dance first, followed by the best man and matron of honor, then the bride's mother

---

38. Livingstone, Sheila, *Scottish Customs*, P. 42

39. Livingstone, P. 43

40. Marwick, Ernest, *The Folklore of Orkney and Shetland*, P. 89

41. Livingstone, Sheila, *Scottish Customs*, P. 42

42. Marwick, Ernest, *The Folklore of Orkney and Shetland*, P. 91

43. Lamb, Gregor, *Carnival of the Animals*, P. 151

44. Marwick, Ernest, *The Folklore of Orkney and Shetland*, P. 90

and the groom's father, and finally the bride's father and the groom's mother.[45] After the last dance everyone kisses their partner.

After the Feast

The evening after the wedding all who helped cook, serve, and otherwise assisted at the feast, are given a meal. The best man and male friends host a dinner and entertainment for the bride's friends called a *"back treat"*. The bride later hosts a party in her new home soon after moving in called *"the hame-fare"*.[46]

Beddin' O' the Bride

First the mothers of the bride and groom must sprinkle water on the couple's new bed to bless it. Then the groom carries the bride over the threshold to prevent her from tripping (which would be most unlucky). The mothers hand over the keys to the bride, and she is also presented with tongs with which to place a peat on the fire.[47] It is worth noting that the hearth is the ritual center for the home, making the woman of the house a priestess as she carefully *smoors* (prays over and then banks) the fire each evening.

The bride enters the bedroom with a troop of female attendants who help her undress as a group of men assist the groom to remove his clothing. The groom's men may also attempt to invade the bride's chamber and steal articles of clothing.[48]

Creeling the Groom

In the days following the wedding, every attempt is made to keep the groom humble after his incredible good fortune in snaring a life mate. He may be loaded with a basket full of rocks, held by a band around his head. Everyone adds a stone until the bride comes along and cuts the band, freeing him.

The groom is also expected to pay for a round of drinks for his workmates. If he fails in this they may retaliate by rubbing him all over with dirt, soot, and grime.[49]

Other Weddings

Owre-Boggie Wedding (Elopement)

This is a secret wedding that takes place before two witnesses. It is often performed *"over iron"*, that is, a black smith allows the rite to take place over his anvil which is a very lucky way to wed.

Weddings amongst the Fisher Folk

Among fishermen, if a member of the crew marries, their boat is draped in flags and funds are given to the crew so they may buy whisky. The youngest member of the crew takes a flag to the bride's house, wraps it around her, and receives a kiss.[50]

45. Marwick, Ernest, *The Folklore of Orkney and Shetland*, P. 90
46. Marwick, Ernest, *The Folklore of Orkney and Shetland*, P. 91
47. Livingstone, Sheila, *Scottish Customs*, P. 44
48. Marwick, Ernest, *The Folklore of Orkney and Shetland*, P. 90
49. Livingstone, Sheila, *Scottish Customs*, P. 45
50. Ibid., PP. 37-38

Conception and Childbirth

Childbirth is always a magical event, a time when the walls between the worlds are thin, because a being is visibly moving from one world into the next. But before the great magic of birth can occur, steps must be taken to ensure conception.

To ensure fertility, a branch of willow is placed under the newlywed's bed, and the chamber pot is filled with salt with a doll placed inside of it as sympathetic magic. But if a woman is still unable to conceive, there are several possibilities: someone might have tied a knot in the groom's handkerchief when they were wed, or the house where the couple are living may have been built directly on top of a Fairy track.[51]

In any case, certain rituals can be undertaken. A woman can crawl through a holed stone while chanting an invocation of Bríghde, or enhance her fertility by embracing a standing stone or a large tree. She may also walk around a Holy Well three times deiseil and then drink the water.[52]

Another form of sympathetic magic involves placing a doll in an empty cradle, and then rocking it while singing a lullaby.[53]

Once a woman has conceived, she should keep the fact a secret and show no ostentatious preparations, in case the Fairies find out about it (there is always the danger of abduction). However, if the village sees a very bright rainbow ending at a certain house it is a prophecy that a boy will be born there.[54]

To Divine the Sex of the Child

Drop a sheep bone into your lap three times saying:

> "Prophecy bone, prophecy bone,
> Will my friend have lass or boy?"

(Traditional)

If the hollow side comes up twice it will be a lassie. If the protruding side comes up twice it foretells a laddie.[55]

Thread a needle and suspend it over the mother's belly. If it moves in a circular path the bairn will be a lassie. If it moves back and forth in a straight line it will be a laddie.[56]

Birthing

> Monday's child is fair of face,
> Tuesday's child is full of grace,
> Wednesday's child is full of woe,
> Thursday's child has far to go,
> Friday's child is loving and giving,

---

51. *Livingstone, Sheila, Scottish Customs, P. 2*
52. *Livingstone, P. 2*
53. *Ibid., P. 3*
54. *Marwick, Ernest, The Folklore of Orkney and Shetland, P. 82*
55. *Marwick, P. 82*
56. *Livingstone, Sheila, Scottish Customs, P. 3*

> *Saturday's child works hard for a living,*
> *But the child that is born on a Sabbat day,*
> *Is blithe and bonny and good and gay!*
>
> *(Traditional, adapted)*

When the birth appears imminent, a black cock should be borrowed or otherwise kept near the house, because the cock will crow if Fairies or Trows are about.[57] Iron is placed in the bed to repel the Fairies.[58] Every clock in the house must be opened, bottles uncorked, animals taken out of the house, and mirrors covered.[59]

To ease the laboring mother's pain, the father of the child should walk around the house three, seven or nine times deiseil and then place his pants under the marriage bed. An arrow may be fired from East to West, leaving the quiver empty, or a gun may be fired in the same direction, and all cartridges removed from other guns in the house.

The mother can clutch a Molluca bean, a piece of coral, or amber, to help with labor pains. Rowan berries or amber strung on red thread will be very protective for the mother.[60]

To keep the Fairies from stealing the bairn, place leaves or petals of Móthan (Pinguicula vulgaris) behind the mother's right knee. An iron nail made by a blacksmith or other iron object, such as a horse shoe, may be placed under the bed and a branch of rowan hung over the bed or placed in the cradle for magical protection.[61]

The bed can be placed over a spot where a piece of furniture made of rowan wood once stood, to protect the mother from enchantment.[62]

Once the child emerges and before it is bathed, mattress material such as straw is taken from under the mother and woven into a rope. The rope is wound three times deiseil around the child's body, then cut into three parts (the three parts must never come together) and thrown into the fire as a charm against ill wishes and epilepsy.

If the child is born in winter, it should be taken outside and a mark made in the snow with its foot.

A lit peat is carried deiseil around the bed seven times, or may be carried around the house instead. The mother is given a glass of whisky and an oat cake (dark ale or stout is also a good choice, because it helps to bring down breast milk.[63]

The midwife places salt or a tiny pat of butter in the bairn's mouth to protect it from Fairies and the bairn is bathed before a fire made with rowan sticks. Gold and silver are put into the bath water to attract wealth to the child. Salt is added to the bath water which is used to bathe the mother's breasts.

57. Marwick, Ernest, *The Folklore of Orkney and Shetland*, P. 82
58. Beith, Mary, *Healing Threads*, P. 98
59. Livingstone, Sheila, *Scottish Customs*, P. 2
60. Livingstone, P. 3
61. Livingstone, Sheila, *Scottish Customs*, P.5
62. Livingstone, P. 7
63. Beith, Mary, *Healing Threads*, P. 98

A bairn born in the fall is given hazelnut milk as its first food. A dish of oatmeal is passed around and every person present at the birth takes three spoonfuls to protect the house.[64]

It is very good luck to feed the bairn a bit of warmed sugar water with a silver spoon, or a sip from a cup or spoon into which a wee bit of silver has been placed. The child should also be given a bit of silver to hold.[65] (Caution: NEVER give honey to a newborn as this could prove fatal due to bacteria).

A bairn born at the incoming tide will have an easier life than one born at the ebb tide. A bairn born during the Waxing Moon will be more prosperous than one born during the Waning Moon.[66]

A *"Lucky Bonnet"* (foetal membrane or caul) is considered to confer magical protection to anyone who possesses it. A child born with a caul, or the seventh child of a seventh child, will have the Second Sight. A child born between midnight and one AM will be able to see ghosts.[67]

Difficult Labor

Place gold and silver pieces into fresh water from a Holy Well, stir the water and give the mother three sips in the name of the Three Worlds.[68] After the birth, the child should be taken outside, dipped in a running stream to strengthen it, and immediately bundled into a warm blanket.[69]

Fire Blessing

A basket is filled half full of bread and cheese which is wrapped in clean linen. The child is laid on top of the bread and cheese, and the oldest female present carries the basket three times around the fire deiseil, and then suspends it briefly over the fire. Then the bairn is placed in the cradle, and the parents distribute the bread and cheese to all who are assembled for the birth.[70]

To Prevent Abduction by Fairies

A tub of water is set before the fire. Three glasses of whisky, three glasses of wine, three teaspoons of salt, and three swords are placed in the tub.

The child is passed hand to hand to all the assembled relatives who stand in a circle around the tub. Then the bairn is washed in the water as the officiant says:

"I name thee_____ in the presence of thy relatives. May you be protected from the evil desires of your enemies and from the evil desires of the enemies of your ancestors."

But the child must never be called the name spoken in the ritual! The purpose of this is to confuse the Fairies.[71]

64. Livingstone, Sheila, *Scottish Customs*, PP. 6, 7

65. Marwick, Ernest, *The Folklore of Orkney and Shetland*, P. 84

66. Livingstone, Sheila, *Scottish Customs*, P. 9

67. Ross, Anne, *Folklore of the Scottish Highlands*, P. 120

68. Ross, P. 119

69. Ibid., P. 120

70. Ibid., P. 120

71. Beith, Mary, *Healing Threads*, PP. 98-99

The Afterbirth

The afterbirth is buried out of doors. If a tree grows on the spot where it has been buried, and if the tree is healthy, strong, and straight, the child will also be healthy and strong.

The Umbilical Cord

The cord may be placed in a drawer. If it stays moist it is a very good omen. If it dries and shrivels it is a bad omen for the child.[72]

Celebrating the New Arrival

The Cryin' Bannock (or Cryin' Cheese and Groaning Malt)

All women who helped with the birth are treated to a party by the women of the house. The father of the new bairn must first offer them food and drink but they must refuse him. Then the women relent and eat cheese and ale, and an oatmeal bannock baked in an iron pan. Any left-overs are taken home by the women to be shared with their families.[73]

Weet the Heid O' the Bairn (Wetting the Baby's Head)

The menfolk have their own celebration. They pass around a bottle of whisky and toast the child's health.[74] Kinfolk and neighbors also drink the health of the newborn with whisky.[75]

The Blithe-Feast

The first feast held in the child's honor. Women, who are friends, neighbors, or kin, come to visit the new mother and to eat scones and ale.[76]

The Fittin' Feast

A family feast to celebrate the mother's return to her household duties.[77]

The Christening Feast

A child is generally baptized about eight days after being born. If a group of children are baptized together, the boys are baptized first, because if the girls go first they will eventually grow beards (and the boys will never grow a beard!).[78]

The Naming Ceremony

The appointed Godparent should be an unmarried woman. The mother and child, and all who are present walk three times deiseil around the ritual circle, and then three drops of water are placed on the bairn's forehead in the name of the Three Worlds.

If more than one bairn is named, there should be separate water for the males and females. Babies of the same sex who are named together are bound to be fast friends for life.

72. Livingstone, Sheila, Scottish Customs, P. 9

73. Livingstone, P. 10

74. Ibid., P. 10

75. Marwick, Ernest, The Folklore of Orkney and Shetland, P. 84

76. Marwick, P. 84

77. Ibid., P. 84

78. Ibid., P. 84

That night, the bairn is not bathed at home so that the ritual water may have longer to "work".

An old way of picking a name is to name the child after a relative. If it is a girl, *"ina"* is added to the father's name: Thomas becomes Thomasina, Joseph becomes Josephina, Edwin becomes Edwina, Paul becomes Paulina, and so forth.[79]

Birthing Luck

When a new mother comes for a visit, she must be given food to eat or to take home. Any household that denies her this will be overrun with mice. The bath water of a healthy newborn can be poured onto the barn roof to bring luck. It is bad luck to carry fire out of a house where the bairn has not yet cut its first tooth.[80]

Neighbors and friends should take turns rocking the cradle both day and night for several days after a birth, to keep the bairn from being stolen by Fairies. It is very good luck to drop a silver coin into the pram of a new bairn.

If the Bairn Dies

All of the clothes and furnishings assembled for the newborn should be burned to clean away the bad luck. On the day the mother first leaves the house, a hot peat or live coal is thrown after her to ward off evil.[81]

Death Rites

The pre-Roman natives of Scotland believed in a life after death. The evidence is the fact that graves were supplied with meat (especially pork), and with containers and implements for wine and ale drinking. Cauldrons for cooking or serving of liquids were also deposited in burials, and warriors were often interred with their weapons and chariots. Ancient funerals were celebrated and hallowed by funeral games.[82]

The Bronze Age Picts buried bodies in stone cists (square stone boxes) after allowing eagles and crows to pick the bones clean. (It takes about twenty minutes for a body to be cleaned of flesh by carrion birds. In my opinion this practice may have led to the belief in angels, winged beings responsible for helping the dead to cross over to the Otherworld).

In the Iron Age, bodies were cremated and buried in urns. In more modern times, the body lays in the home for three days before internment.[83]

In the Highlands, when a person died they were said to have gone into the *"saoghal thall"* or the *"yonder world"*. The word *"death"* was only used for animals. You could also say *"shiubhaile"* (he travelled) or *"chaochail e"* (he changed). Mourning women (*bean-tuirim*) chanted the *coranach* (lament) for the dead, telling of their heroic deeds, their hunting prowess, their generosity and nobility.[84]

79. Livingstone, Sheila, *Scottish Customs*, P. 12

80. Marwick, Ernest, *The Folklore of Orkney and Shetland*, P. 84

81. Livingstone, Sheila, *Scottish Customs*, P. 12

82. Ross, Anne, *Pagan Celtic Britain*, P. 356

83. Livingstone, Sheila, *Scottish Customs*, P. 47

84. Ross, Anne, *Folklore of the Scottish Highlands*, PP. 118-119

It is said, that at the moment of death, the soul can be seen leaving in the form of an insect such as a bee or a butterfly.[85] I myself have seen this when a young woman was struck by a car. I went to her bedroom to burn herbs of purification and a very large white moth appeared and flew out of the window. The moth was immediately swallowed by a blue jay in a nearby bush, showing that the cycle of life continues forever.

Death Omens

Before someone dies, certain signs will appear so that the clan and the person themselves can prepare for the transition. Signs of imminent death include: a mouse squeaking behind the bed, a raven flying over the house, a cock crowing at midnight, and ringing in the ears.

If a dog howls at night, or shies away from a sick person, or barks three times, or if a crow or magpie lands on the roof, it may be a death omen. The death of a child is foretold if a flock of sparrows stays near the house, or if three meadow-pipits sing near the house.

Other omens include the *"deid-drap"*, the sound as if water were dripping onto the ground, unexplained knocking sounds, or if a coffin shaped coal leaps out of the fire.[86] There are also the ticking sound of a wood-worm, the song of a quail, a rail croaking in a field, a raven or crow croaking from the roof or flying around the house.

"Deid-lights" or phosphorescent glows in the forest warn of an impending death and can also reveal the location of a murder victim. [87]

To dream of a ship sailing over dry land, or when both ends of a rainbow fall between the borders of a single township, means a death is likely. When a wife is washing her husband's trousers in a stream and they fill up with water, death is near.

To hear your spirit animal moan is a sign of death. If your *co-walker* (ghost or Fairy double), a figure that looks exactly like you, suddenly appears after noon, it means death is nigh (if your *co-walker* appears before noon it presages a long life). The *co-walker* of someone who is far away may suddenly appear just before, or at the exact time of, their death.[88]

Individual families have unique warnings that tell them when a member of the clan is about to cross over. When a *Breadalbane* is about to die, a bull will roar at night. The MacLachlans will see a small bird. Other families might hear whistling or see lights. In some cases, the air turns cold and screams and sobs are heard. A meteor may be seen shooting from the house where the death will occur to the graveyard.[89]

Some families will hear a *Benshi* (Fairy woman) cry and shriek along the processional route that the funeral is destined to take.[90]

85. Ross, P. 121
86. Livingstone, Sheila, Scottish Customs, P. 50-51
87. Marwick, Ernest, The Folklore of Orkney and Shetland, P.92
88. Marwick, P. 92
89. Ross, Anne, Folklore of the Scottish Highlands, P. 122
90. Ross, P. 116

The Straiking (Lying Out)

A bell should be rung at the exact moment of death and also at the time of interment, to frighten away evil Spirits. A Druidical tool called a *"bell-branch"* may be used for this purpose (a tree branch with nine bells attached). The body should be guarded and watched until it is buried, because the Spirit stays with it until it goes under ground.[91]

The eyes of the corpse must be closed so that the Spirit is prevented from escaping to haunt the living. For this reason coins are laid on the eyes, to keep them shut. A plate of salt and a plate of earth are placed on the chest of the deceased, who is covered with a linen shroud, with feet facing the door, and laid on a board. The earth represents the physical body and the salt represents the Spirit.

All animals are kept away from the body. If a dog or cat walks over the corpse they must be killed, according to Highland tradition.[92]

The coffin lid is left open until the funeral, and a window is left slightly open at all times so that the Spirit can escape if it wants. Crossed ash twigs or branches are placed on the body as protection and all clocks are stopped. Mirrors and pictures are covered, so the Spirit won't become confused, curtains are drawn, fires put out, and all locks opened.

If the deceased has died of cancer a pat of butter is placed on the corpse to draw out the disease and purify the body. If the person has died of a contagious disease all of their clothing is burned.[93]

Friends, family and neighbors are encouraged to touch the corpse as a way of saying farewell and of achieving closure. The coffin should have a candle lit at its head and feet for as long as the person is laid out (it is very bad luck for the person who lit the candles if one of the candles blows out).

Oak is a very good wood for a coffin, especially for a Druid. Sprays of mistletoe and oak leaves may be arranged around the body and in the coffin. Ritual tools and magical items should be placed in and around the coffin to be buried with the deceased.

In the old days, it was the first duty of a newly married woman to make and embroider a cloth shroud. These *"deid-claes"* (dead clothes) were kept clean and freshly laundered and packed away with rosemary, until needed. The cloth was natural linen or wool.[94]

The Wake

A *"Late Wake"* is held in the deceased's honor which consists of music, song and dance, wrestling, riddling, card games, and the playing of tricks. Liberal quantities of whisky are provided and everyone stops to place a hand on the deceased's forehead to utter a blessing. Some of these celebrations became so rowdy that participants left for the churchyard and forgot to bring the coffin! Children are encouraged to participate so they won't be haunted by memories.

91. Livingstone, Sheila, Scottish Customs, P. 53
92. Ross, Anne, Folklore of the Scottish Highlands, P. 116
93. Livingstone, Sheila, Scottish Customs, PP. 56, 69
94. Livingstone, P. 58

If there is a concern that the deceased may try to haunt the living, grain is placed in-between their fingers and toes, in their mouth, and on their chest. The coffin may be lined with grain as well.[95]

Young people stay up all night to guard the corpse and keep it company: drinking whisky, telling ghost stories, gossiping, playing music and dancing. These activities continue every night until the burial. Guisers, usually boys, show up at the house to beg for food or money.[96]

The family may also host a ball where people, laughing and weeping in turns, dance until dawn. They weep in sadness for their personal loss and feel happy because their kin has passed beyond the trials of this life.[97]

The coffin is usually placed on two kegs or small stools which must be kicked over as soon as the coffin is lifted. If the corpse has been lying on a bed of straw, the straw is burned as soon as the coffin leaves the house.[98]

Telling It to the Bees

If the household has bees, the hives are draped in black crepe or ribbon and the bees are told of the death because the bees are the Gods' messengers.[99]

The Funeral Procession

The procession begins in the evening and is lit by torches and led by a bell ringer or piper who ties black ribbon to their pipes. The company stops from time to time, lowering the coffin and taking refreshment such as whisky, ale, shortbread, bread, and cheese. No one should attempt to overtake or precede the coffin. It is very bad luck if a dog crosses in front of the procession and this should be prevented.[100]

Sometimes a *bean-tuirim* (keening woman), barefoot and dressed in black, follows the hearse or coffin, wailing and beating the coffin like a drum.[101] The *bean-tuirim* is often the local mid-wife who births souls into and out of this life.[102] Every township in Scotland once had its own mid-wife and mourning woman who received free grazing and fodder for her beasts in payment.[103]

If a person encounters a funeral procession unexpectedly, they should politely remove their hat and walk a short distance with the procession, help carry the coffin for a bit and then bow and continue on their way.[104] As the procession passes, houses should turn out their lights and close their doors.

Burial

All persons, whether rich, poor, laird, or simple farmer, should have a decent burial and the community should band together to cover any expenses.

95. Marwick, Ernest, *The Folklore of Orkney and Shetland*, PP. 93-94

96. Livingstone, Sheila, *Scottish Customs*, P.62

97. Ross, Anne, *Folklore of the Scottish Highlands*, P. 115

98. Marwick, Ernest, *The Folklore of Orkney and Shetland*, P. 94

99. Livingstone, Sheila, *Scottish Customs*, P. 56

100. Marwick, Ernest, *The Folklore of Orkney and Shetland*, P. 94

101. Ross, Anne, *Folklore of the Scottish Highlands*, P.116

102. Livingstone, Sheila, *Scottish Customs*, P. 56

103. Ross, Anne, *Folklore of the Scottish Highlands*, P. 123

104. Livingstone, Sheila, *Scottish Customs*, P. 52

Islands are especially good places for burials because they give protection from wolves and wild beasts, and also because they are an echo of the Isles of the Blessed, where Spirits go on their Otherworldly journey.

As the procession wends towards the gravesite, relatives and friends take turns carrying the coffin or urn to its final resting place. In coastal areas, burials should be done when the tide is going out.[105]

Cairns

Cairns, or mounds of stones, were once erected to honor dead warriors and other persons of note. To build a cairn, every member of the funeral party lays a stone on a single grave, or a stone is placed in memory of each deceased warrior in the event of a mass grave. Related to this, the cry for clan Farquharson is "Carn na cuimhne", the cairn of remembrance.

Burials at Sea

Those who die at sea are sewn into a canvas bag. A person who drowns is buried on the "black shore" (between the line of seaweed and the water) so as not to offend the Spirits of the ocean.[106] Fishermen's Spirits are sometimes so tied to their boats that old fishermen will stay alive as long as their old boat is whole and mended.[107]

After the Funeral

A party may be held in the barn or in the best room of the house, or a meal taken at a hotel or restaurant. Shortbread, oatcakes, and spirits are the traditional fare.

Money is collected to help the widow or widower, and the genealogy and virtues of the dead are recited. The door of the house is painted black or covered with black cloth, or a black wreath is hung upon it.[108] The name of the deceased is not spoken lest it call back their Spirit, instead expressions such as "him that was taken" are used.[109]

Visiting the Gravesite

Wreaths of heather and sprays of flowers should be taken to the gravesite throughout the year when visitors come to the grave to tell the departed the latest news.[110] On Samhuinn a bowl of water and a lit candle are placed by the gravesite, and a place is set at the supper table for deceased relatives. The door is left ajar so they might feel welcome to enter and join the Samhuinn feast.[111]

105. Livingstone, P. 64

106. Ibid., P. 62

107. Marwick, Ernest, *The Folklore of Orkney and Shetland*, P. 93

108. Livingstone, Sheila, *Scottish Customs*, P. 52

109. Marwick, Ernest, *The Folklore of Orkney and Shetland*, P. 93

110. Livingstone, Sheila, *Scottish Customs*, P. 69

111. Thoms, Penelope Ann, *Thin the Veil*, P.29

Divination Practices

Many divination practices have been mentioned above, associated with the Fire Festivals and other ritual observances. Here are a small assortment of divinations which involve love and marriage.

A Gentleman Desires To Know If He Will Marry

Put the man in a blindfold. Place three coggies (bowls) before him, one filled with water, one filled with soot and water, and one that is empty. Move the bowls about and then ask him to choose one. If he chooses the bowl filled with clear water, he will marry a virgin. If he chooses the sooty water, a widow. And if he chooses the empty bowl, he will never marry.

A man can walk into a newly plowed field with furrows that run north to south. Entering from the west he crosses eleven ridges and then stands on the twelfth. If he hears crying, death is approaching. If he hears music and dancing he will soon marry.

A Lady Desires to Know if She Will Marry

A woman may put a bit of mugwort root, a piece of bannock, or a bit of wedding cake under her pillow to dream of her future husband or lover. She may also dream of a future mate by putting a ring on her finger and a shoe under the bed, which must be a bed she has never slept in before, and she must get into it backwards.

Dipping the Sark

A woman may go to a south running stream and soak a shirt in the water, then take it home and dry it by the fire. The wraith of her future husband will appear.

To Divine the Behavior of Your Mate

Throw a herring fish at the wall. If it slides down in a straight line, your spouse will be upright and true. If it slides down in a crooked fashion, your spouse's behavior will be the same.

On Midsummer Eve pick stonecrop (Sedum telephium) and hold it over your head. If it bends to the right your lover is true, if it bends to the left your lover is false.

Assign the name of a man to one nut, and the name of a woman to another, and place them into the fire. If the nuts split and pop, their love will be rocky, but if they burn quietly, their love will go well.

To Divine a Future Lover

Take the first laid egg of a spring chicken, and drop the egg white into pure spring water. Take a mouthful, but do not swallow. The first name you hear will be the name of your future spouse or lover, and the remaining egg white will form into a shape in the water, and an object associated with your future mate's occupation will appear.

Sit before a mirror at midnight and cut an apple into nine sections. Then stand with your back to the mirror, and point eight of the pieces in turn to your left shoulder. Eat the pieces. Toss the ninth piece over your left shoulder, and turn your head to the left. Your future spouse will appear in the mirror. The poet Robert Burns refers to this and other divination methods in his poem "Halloween":

> *Wee Jennie to her grannie says,*
> *"Will ye go wi' me, grannie?*
> *I'll eat the apple at the glass*
> *I gat frae Uncle Johnnie:"*

Another method is to pare an apple so that the skin comes off in one piece. At the stroke of midnight swing the paring three times around your head, taking care to keep it intact. Then fling it over your left shoulder, and it will form the first letter of your future mate's name. But if the paring breaks, there will be no hand-fasting that year.

You may also set the paring above the lintel of the door. The first person to enter through that door will have the same name as your future spouse.

If someone puts shoes on the table, that means a marriage is in the offing. If you consult a Spaewife (fortune teller), her hand must be crossed with silver so that she can predict your future lover.[1]

Dá-Shealladh (Second Sight)

The ancient Romans reported that the Gaulish Celts had Seers whom they called "Vates" or prophets. The Fili were a very high grade of poet amongst the Irish Celts who were so highly trained that every utterance from their mouth was prophecy.

Taghairm is an ancient Druidic practice, that was still being undertaken in the Highlands as late as the eighteenth century, which involved sewing a Seer into an ox-hide and putting him or her into a space behind a roaring waterfall to incubate a vision. The Highland word for seer is Taibhsear and the practice of seeing is called Taibhsearachd.[2]

1. *Livingstone, Sheila, Scottish Customs, PP. 23-25*
2. *Ross, Anne, Folklore of the Scottish Highlands, PP. 43-44, 59*

In the Western Isles, an augurer is known as a frithir and a divination is called a frith. Frithirs can locate lost people and animals. The best day to do this kind of augury is on the first Monday of the quarter, before dawn.

The frithir rises before the Sun and goes fasting, bare headed and barefoot, and with eyes closed, to the door. They place one hand on each door jamb, invoke the Gods, and ask to see that which is hidden. When they open their eyes, they get their answer from the objects that appear before them.[3]

Other ways that those with The Sight can make an augury are by staring at a fire, or by looking through the blade bone of a sheep's shoulder.[4] A Seer might hear a cry out of doors that sounds like a person who is about to die. They may also have a premonition by smell such as smelling a meal that won't be cooked for months.

A Seer can describe a person who is coming to visit and give an accurate account of their appearance, even if the visitor is a total stranger. A Seer might suddenly feel themselves in the midst of a crowd, bearing a coffin. They will later be able to identify the pall bearers, but not the deceased. If a true Seer is having a vision and they touch someone near them, that person will also experience the vision.[5]

When a vision is "seen" in the early morning, it means that the event will happen in a few hours. If at noon, it will take place on the same day. If in the evening, it will take place that night.

To "see" a funeral shroud wrapped around someone means their death is coming. If the shroud is below the waist, the death won't happen for at least a year. If further up the body, the death is more imminent.[6]

If a man "sees" a woman at his left, she will be his future wife, even if he is already married. If he "sees" more than one woman, they will each be his wives in turn, starting with the woman closest to his left hand. To "see" a spark or fire fall on someone's arms or chest, means a child will soon die.[7]

Seers can sometimes see a person's Fairy double (or co-walker). If a Seer sees their own twin, then the Seer's death is imminent. If they see a relative lying in a coffin or dressed for burial, this means that their death is nigh. If they see the relative in street clothes, then the death is further off. The Seer may witness blue lights moving along the route of a future funeral procession, or around the bed, of a person about to die.[8]

A person with "the Sight" can hurl an object at a person's double, and the person will be blinded. They can also "see" a person's future spouse. They may "see" a bad event involving a boat.[9]

---

3. *Ross, P. 55*
4. *Ibid, PP. 56-57*
5. *Ibid, PP. 50-51*
6. *Ibid., P. 49*
7. *Ibid., P. 50*
8. *Ibid. P. 64*
9. *Ibid. PP. 47-50*

Dogs and horses can also have "The Sight". They will "see" the fetch of a person about to die. Dogs will howl if a family member is about to die, and horses will shy away from a haunted place, or a place where there has been a murder, or where a murder will eventually occur. Cows can also see supernatural visions, and will run away in fright. In my experience, cats have "The Sight" and will often react to unseen presences, as if receiving a message.

Famous Seers

Reverend Robert Kirk

The Reverend Robert Kirk (minister of Balquhidder 1664-1685 and of Aberfoyle, Stirlingshire, 1685-1692) was the author of "The Secret Commonwealth of Elves, Fauns, and Fairies" published in 1691. He had "The Sight" and was a seventh son of a seventh son (such children are often born with the gift of Sight). Kirk was "taken" by the Fairies in 1692.

Kirk reported that the Fairies, or the Good People, live by rule of law but are not devoted to Jesus, or to God as understood in the Christian context. They do not believe in death, but rather in cycles of creation and re-creation similar to the recurring seasonal wheel of the year and the motions of the Sun and Moon.

He also said that Fairies are intelligent beings with bodies of light that are most visible at dusk, and that they can appear and disappear at will. Those with "The Sight" can most easily see them at the start of each quarter.

According to Kirk, the Fairies labor within their mounds at tasks such as the baking of bread and smith craft. They move house at the start of each quarter, which is why it is polite to leave them a gift at this time, to help them in their travels. They wear clothing in the style of the land in which they live, and their women spin cloth from cobwebs and rainbows.[10]

Kirk reported that Fairies can steal milk from a distance as far as a bull can be heard to roar. To prevent this, a small amount of the mother cow's dung should be applied to a calf's mouth before it sucks.[11]

One day, as Kirk was walking on a Dun-Shi (Fairy Hill), he fell and was presumed dead. After his funeral, he appeared to a relative and ordered him to go to a mutual cousin and say that he was not dead, but rather that he had been "taken" by the Fairies, and that there was only one way to free him. When a child who was born after his seeming demise was baptized, he would appear and the cousin should throw a dirk over his head when he appeared, so that he could return to the land of mortals.

Kirk did appear at a baptism, but the cousin was so startled to see him that he forgot to throw the dirk, and Kirk remains trapped with the Fairies to this day, within an old Scots Pine tree near the churchyard of Kirkton, Aberfoyle.[12]

10. McNeill, F. Marian, *The Silver Bough Vol. I*, P. 105
11. McNeill, P. 106
12. Ibid., P. 112

The Brahan Seer

The Brahan Seer, Coinneach Odhar Fiosaiche (Somber Kenneth of the Prophesies) was born on the Isle of Lewis in the early seventeenth century. One account of how he got his gift of Sight is this: his mother was in the hills guarding cattle near an ancient burial ground, when at midnight the graves suddenly opened and the dead emerged. One hour later, the dead went back to their graves but one Spirit remained behind.

Coinneach's mother placed her distaff, made of rowan wood, over the grave to prevent the Spirit from returning to its place of rest. A woman appeared demanding that the mother remove the rowan wood. The mother refused saying that she wanted an explanation as to why this one Spirit had lagged behind. The Spirit explained that she was a Norse princess who had traveled to Norway seeking her old home.

Appreciating the mother's courage, the Spirit told the mother about a special stone that would give her son the powers of prophecy, and when Coinneach was given the stone, he immediately gained prophetic powers (Dá – Shealladh, Second Sight). In differing accounts, the stone is blue, white, or holed.[13]

In another account, Coinneach received his gift from the Fairies, when as a boy he fell asleep upon a Fairy Mound. On waking, he discovered that a small, round, white stone with a hole in it had been placed on his chest. When he looked through the stone, he could see the past and the future and also divine people's true motives and intentions.[14]

Every prophecy that The Brahan Seer made subsequently came true. One hundred and fifty years before the Caledonian Canal was built, he prophesied that ships would sail around the Hill of the Yew Trees (Tomnahurich Hill) at Inverness. He foresaw the clearances of the Highlands and the end of the clan system, and said that one day there would be a house on every hill. He reported that Tomnahurich Hill, which was a Fairy Hill, would one day be under lock and key, and the Fairies chained within. The hill became a cemetery after his death.[15]

The Brahan Seer reportedly gave the magical ability to predict life or death to the Dripping Well at Avoch, Ross – a well with the reputed ability to cure deafness. Coinneach declared that by placing two lengths of straw or wood into the well, one would henceforth be able to tell if a person would live or die. If the straws or wood whirled around, the person would live, but if they remained static, the result would be death.[16]

When Kenneth MacKenzie, Earl of Seaforth, went to Paris and left his wife the Countess behind at Brahan castle, the wife became impatient with the Earl's absence, and consulted Coinneach regarding her husband. Coinneach refused to divulge what he "Saw" until the Countess threatened him. Then Coinneach admitted that he had "Seen" the count making love to another lady.

---

13. Ross, Anne, *Folklore of the Scottish Highlands*, PP. 45, 56
14. McNeill, F. Marian, *The Silver Bough Vol. I*, PP. 94-95
15. Ross, Anne, *Folklore of the Scottish Highlands*, PP. 45, 56
16. McNeill, F. Marian, *The Silver Bough Vol. I*, PP. 70-71

The Countess flew into a rage, accused Coinneach of witchcraft, and ordered his death by being drowned head first in a barrel of burning tar. But before the Brahan Seer died, he predicted doom for the House of Seaforth, which came to pass exactly as he foretold.[17]

Thomas the Rhymer and Tam Lin

Thomas the Rhymer or True Thomas (Thomas of Ercildoune) was given the gift of "Sight" after he met the Fairy Queen, kissed her, and served her for seven years. He was abducted by Fairies in the Eildon Hills in the thirteenth century.[18]

Tam Lin was the son of Thomas Randolph, the Earl of Moray, who according to a famous ballad was abducted by Fairies as a child. When he eventually married a human woman and conceived a child with her, his wife was forced to confront the Queen of the Fairies in a series of difficult trials.[19]

---

17. *McNeill, P. 95*
18. *Ibid, P. 111*
19. *Miller, Joyce, Magic and Witchcraft in Scotland, P. 21*

A
Highland
Herbal

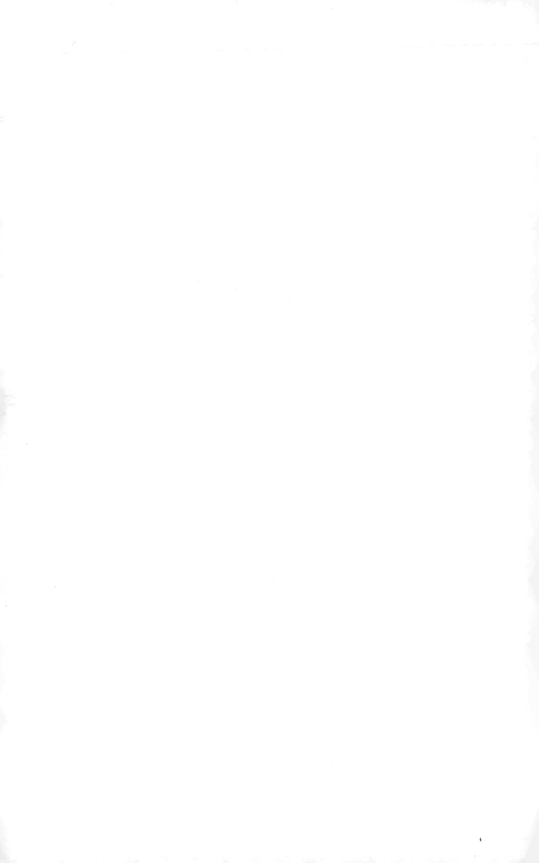

Medicinal Plants and Trees

Here is a selection of plants that were once used for healing and magic in the Highlands. I have included at least a brief mention of every plant covered in this text. Scotland has always been a cosmopolitan country and Highlanders were using herbs from many cultures from ancient times.

Using traditional herbs is a wonderful way to bond with the ancestors. You will be tapping into an ancient stream of wisdom handed down for millennia. But, before you begin to explore the green path of healing, there are a few things to be aware of:

If you have a medical condition, please consult a health practitioner before ingesting any of these plants. Modern drugs do not always interact well with plant medicines and certain conditions such as diabetes, high or low blood pressure, and pregnancy may be adversely impacted by the use of certain herbal medications. Just a few decades ago, it was nearly impossible to find information on herb and drug interactions and contra-indications, but now the internet has websites where you can easily cross reference an herb and a drug to see if there are any adverse effects.

To be most effective, magical and healing plants should be picked while speaking a prayer or invocation, or at the very least saying "thank you" to each plant you take. By tradition, it is best not to harvest using an iron implement because the Fairies despise iron. Whenever possible, use a knife or cutting tool made with flint, bone, crystal, or stone. (Please consult the Moon section above for the best times to plant and harvest herbal medicines).

Deciduous tree leaves must be harvested before Summer Solstice, as after that they will contain too many alkaloids (natural plant poisons that repel insects), and can be irritating to human tissues. Always gather bark from twigs and branches, never from the trunk of a tree, or you might kill the tree. Never "girdle" a tree, as this will surely kill it. The medicinal properties of trees are found in the thin living layer of tissue, just under the bark, called the cambium. The bark of the root also has medicinal properties, as may the leaves and flowers.

The part of the plant that you harvest will depend upon the season. Roots are gathered in the very early spring or in the fall, after the plant begins to die back. Gather flowers just as they begin to open. Gather leaves when they are fresh and new. Red or orange berries such as hawthorn, rowan berries and rose hips are best gathered after the first frost, as they will then be highly pigmented and contain the most Vitamin C. But after a second frost they will likely be ruined. Nature gives us a small window of opportunity and we have to be alert and watchful!

All doses indicated below assume a 150 pound adult is taking the herbal brew. A 75 pound child would get ½ the dose and so on. Adjust amounts according to body weight. Infants can get the benefit of herbs via their mother's breast milk (the mother should take the usual adult dose).

When giving herbs to infants, please check contra-indications carefully. Never feed honey to an infant as the bacteria could prove fatal.

Please use only organic herbs, as commercially harvested herbs contain too much pesticide, and always prepare the teas in a non aluminum pot with a tight lid. Never boil the herbs, always simmer gently, because volatile oils are lost via the steam.

As a general rule, roots, barks and berries are simmered (decocted), and leaves and flowers are steeped (infused) for about 20 minutes.

Herbal teas can be kept for up to a week in a glass jar with a tight lid, in the refrigerator. Avoid "wildcrafted" herbs as many medicinals are now becoming endangered species due to over-harvesting.

Please dry all plant material in the shade, never in the sun. When harvesting large amounts of plants, one drying method is to hang the plants upside down inside paper bags from a clothes line. That way the herbs will be protected from the sun and yet exposed to the air.

Herbal brews are generally most effective when taken in small doses throughout the day and not with meals. The usual dose (with some exceptions) is ¼ cup, four times a day, not with meals.

To Make a Poultice

Poultices are made by putting plants into a blender with a little water, pouring the liquid slush into a bowl, and adding powdered slippery elm bark or buckwheat flour (don't use wheat as many are allergic to it) to make a "pie dough" consistency. Roll the poultice out on a clean cloth with a rolling pin and apply the "pancake" to a burn, sprain, wound or skin irritation, for one hour. Remove and discard (do not re-use).

To Make an Herbal Salve

Salves are made by gently simmering herbs in butter or virgin cold-pressed olive oil (traditional Scottish healers used butter or lard) and adding hot, melted bees wax. Add just enough oil to barely cover the herbs and keep careful track of how many cups of oil you put in the pot. Simmer the herbs gently for 20 minutes, with a tight lid on the pot.

After the herbs have finished simmering, add the bee's wax. Use 3 or 4 tablespoons of hot melted bees wax for every cup of oil used. The oil and bees wax must BOTH be simmering hot when combined, or the salve won't harden.

Strain and put into very clean glass jars. A small amount of Tincture of Benzoin can be added as a preservative, but I have found that by using the green outer hull of walnuts in salves, no other preservatives are necessary (walnuts are anti-fungal). Store in a cool, dark place.

Making Tinctures

Alcohol tinctures are valuable because they last for many years (five or more). Place shredded plant material into a glass jar and barely cover with alcohol that is 80 proof or higher (whisky, vodka, gin, etc.) adding 10% spring water and about 1 tsp. of vegetable glycerin per quart of tincture. Some constituents extract in water, some in glycerin, and others in alcohol. In my experience tinctures that contain at least a small amount of glycerin and water seem to work best.

Seal with a tight lid and leave the plant material in the liquid only until the plant matter begins to wilt. Then strain and store in a dark brown or blue glass container with a tight lid or in a dark cupboard.

Harvesting Tips

When harvesting plant medicines the following rule applies: "Walk by the first seven, leave the eighth for the animals, you may take the ninth". (This is an old Native American saying). Do not gather a plant if there are less than nine plants left, even if the species is a "weed", because you want the "weeds" to be there next year for your use and enjoyment!

Be sure to research which species are endangered in your area and try to help the species you harvest by re-planting seeds, only taking a section of root and re-planting the rest, etc. Think in terms of the next seven generations each time you gather medicinal and food plants. When in doubt, don't pick! When planting flowers, herbs, shrubs and trees in your garden, do some research to find ones that are native to your area and help those species survive.

Please pay attention to the cautions listed in this section. Overuse or improper use of a plant may result in serious illness or worse. Before using any plant that is new to you internally or externally, try a small amount as a test to see if it agrees with your system.

If no Gaelic name is given that means the plant was introduced to Scottish gardens in very modern times.

IN THE EVENT OF A MEDICAL CONDITION, PLEASE CONSULT A MEDICAL PROFESSIONAL BEFORE INJESTING HERBAL REMEDIES.

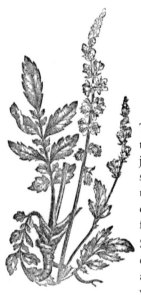

Agrimony

Parts used: the whole herb

Gaelic: *mur-druidheann, muir-droighinn, múr-dhroigheann*

Latin: *Agrimonia eupatoria*

The leaf tea is used to cleanse and heal the liver. Simmer the root and steep the leaves and take with honey for jaundice. The tea is taken internally for skin problems such as pimples and scrofula and applied externally to ulcers and sores (as a wash or compress). Use the tea as a drink for fevers and ague, and internally and externally for gout. The herb can be added to healing salves.

Steep 2-4 tsp. of the leaf or simmer 2 tsp. of the root per cup of water, for 20 minutes. Take 1/3 cup, three times a day. For external use: simmer 2-4 ounces in 1 quart of water for 20 minutes.

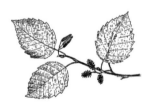

Alder

Parts used: bark and leaves

Gaelic: *Craobh-fhearn*

Latin: *Alnus glutinosa*

The leaves are made into a poultice for sore feet. A hot leaf poultice is applied to rheumatic parts. The bark decoction is used externally to wash inflammations and swellings and also makes a gargle for throat inflammation. Simmer the bark in vinegar to treat scabies, lice and scabs.

Simmer 1 tsp. bark or steep 1 tsp leaf per 1 cup of water. Take 1-2 cups a day in ¼ cup doses.

Lore: Alder is one of the 'Nine Sacred Woods' suitable to build the ritual fire at Bealltan and Samhuinn.

Alexanders, Black Lovage

Parts used: the herb

Gaelic: *lus nan grán dubh*
(plant of the black seeds)

Latin: *Smyrnium olusatrum*

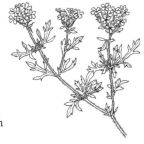

As a pot herb, Black Lovage is added to lamb broth for chest complaints and tuberculosis.

Caution: this plant is an emmenagogue (brings on the menses) and should be avoided in pregnancy. It has been used to expel the placenta after childbirth.

All-Heal, Self Heal

Parts used: the herb

Gaelic: *Dubhan ceann-cósach, Dubhan Pcean–dubh*

Latin: *Prunella vulgaris*

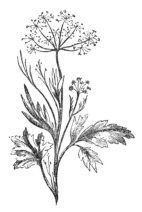

The herb is used in wound washes and salves, often with the addition of goldenrod (Solidago spp.) The tea is taken internally to heal injuries and obstructions in the liver, spleen, and kidneys and also benefits diarrhea. Use the tea as a gargle for sore throats and thrush. Steep 2 tsp. per cup of water for 20 minutes and take ¼ cup 4 times a day, or soak 1 tsp in 1 pint brandy for 3 days and take 2 tbsp. a day as needed.

Anise Seed

Parts used: the seeds

Gaelic: *ainis*

Latin: *Pimpinella anisum*

The seeds help digestion, promote appetite, and alleviate nausea, stomach cramps and gas. The tea increases breast milk in nursing mothers and relieves colic in infants. Strain the tea through an organic coffee filter to make an eyewash for sore eyes. Simmer 1 tsp. crushed seeds per 1 cup of water for 10 minutes and take ¼ cup 4 times a day.

For colic: simmer 1 tbsp in ½ pint milk for 10 minutes, strain and take while hot.

Caution: this herb should be avoided by pregnant women as it is an emmenagogue (brings on the menses).

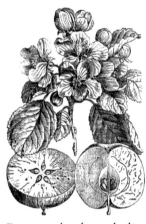

Apple

Parts used: the fruits and bark

Gaelic: *Ubhall*

Latin: *Malus sylvestris (crab apple), Malus domestica, Pyrus malus*

A syrup of apples, honey and rowan berries is used to cure coughs and chest complaints. Eat a roasted apple before bed and before a large meal to improve digestion and sleep. Peel and grate an apple for diarrhea (sour apples are most effective). For a laxative effect eat apples with the skin on them. Eating apples cleans the liver and wards off gout. Eating raw apples benefits the gums. Apply baked apple to sore throats, erysipelas, inflamed eyes. Blend raw apple cider with horse radish and drink to treat edema.

For rheumatic conditions dry the peels of organic apples and simmer to make tea (1-2 tsp. peel to 1 cup water, drink up to 3 cups a day). The twig bark can be simmered for fevers Caution: do not gather the bark after the first frost as it will contain cyanide. The seeds also contain cyanide which in large amounts can harm a small child.

Lore: Apples are associated with Avalon (Apple Land) and the Celtic Otherworld. An apple branch can take you to the Land of Fairy. To encounter Fairies, sleep under an apple tree at noon on Midsummer's Day. Apple divination: cut an apple in half and examine the seeds. If they are whole it means good luck. If one seed is damaged it means trouble. If more than one is cut it means severe misfortune.

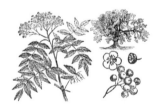

Ash

Parts used: seeds, leaves and bark

Gaelic: *craobh uinnsinn, nion*

Latin: *Fraxinus excelsior*

Gather the leaves in early June, dry, powder and store them for use throughout the year. Ash leaves are used to poultice snake bites. The leaf tea is laxative, and when the leaves are simmered in white wine they benefit jaundice. The bark tea is helpful for intermittent fever and ague, and it also cleans the spleen and liver and aids in rheumatism. The ripe seeds (called "keys") can be salted and pickled in vinegar as a substitute for capers.

Infuse 1 tsp. leaf per ½ cup of freshly boiled water. Steep for 3 minutes and take up to 1 ½ cups a day in ¼ cup doses. Simmer 1 tsp. bark per ½ cup water for 20 minutes. Take 1 cup a day in ¼ cup doses. Add mint or marjoram to improve the flavor.

Lore: When a child was born in the Highlands, the midwife would place a green ash stick in the fire. She collected the sap as it came out at the ends, preferably in a silver spoon, and fed a cooled spoonful to the newborn as its first food. Ash is one of the nine sacred woods of the Druids who used it to make healing wands.

Barley

Parts used: the grains

Gaelic: *eórna*

Latin: *Hordeum distichon, Hordeum vulgare*

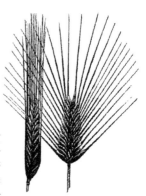

Boiled barley juice benefits the kidneys, stomach and throat. Barley meal and egg white are applied as a poultice to broken or fractured bones (followed by splinting). When the splints are removed, apply a salve made with Germander Speedwell (Betonica pauli), Saint John's Wort (Hypericum perforatum) and Goldenrod (Solidago spp.). Chop the fresh herbs and mix them into sheep's fat or butter, spread on a cloth and apply several times a day for a few days. Cooked barley can be applied externally to tumors and sores. Barley water helps to lower a fever.

Barley water: Wash the barley in cold water. Simmer 1 part barley for every 9 parts water for 20 minutes. Strain and drink in ¼ cup doses.

Betony

Parts used: the flowering herb

Gaelic: *lus beathaig*

Latin: *Stachys officinalis, Betonica officinalis*

This plant is useful for headache, including hangover. The leaves can be eaten in salads or made into tea. The tea benefits asthma, bronchitis, heartburn, and bladder and kidney problems. A very strong decoction will help to expel worms. The juice of the fresh herb is applied to wounds and ulcers; a poultice of the leaves is applied to sprains. Children who are weak or sickly can take ½ to 1 cup a day to build their strength.

Tea: steep 2 tsp. of the flowering herb per cup of freshly boiled water for 20 minutes. Take up to 1 cup a day, a swallow at a time.

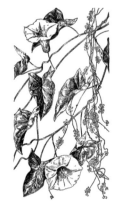

Bindweed, Hedge Bindweed

Parts used: the roots

Gaelic: *Dúil Mhail*

Latin: *Calistegia (= convolvulus) sepium*

This herb is a purgative that can be drastic in action. It should be used only with medical advice. It has been used as a purgative for constipation and lassitude of the bowels and must be combined with other laxatives and carminatives such as ginger and clove.

Lore: primrose (Primula officinalis) and hedge bindweed are picked on Bealltan morn, and woven into a wreath to avert evil.

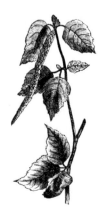

Birch

Parts used: the bark and fresh young leaves

Gaelic: *beith*

Latin: *Betula alba*

The bark of White Birch is simmered in spring water, then steeped with elderflowers to make a spring tonic. The bark tea makes a wash for chronic skin problems and can also be added to the bath. Wash the head with it to stop falling hair or apply the juice of the leaves to help with thinning hair. The tea is mildly sedative and helps with insomnia.

Leaf tea: steep 1 tbsp. per ½ cup water and take ¼ cup, 4 times a day.

Bark tea: simmer 1 tbsp. bark per ½ cup water; take ¼ cup, 4 times a day.

Lore: Plant a birch tree in the graveyard to guard the dead. Place a rod of birch in the child's cradle or in the coffin as a protective charm.

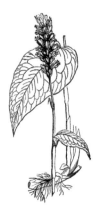

Bistort

Parts used: the roots

Gaelic: *glúineach an uisge, glúineag dhearg*

Latin: *Polygonum amphibium, Polygonum bistorta*

The roots have been used for bladder problems, diarrhea and dysentery and also make a mouthwash for gum and mouth inflammations. Use the tea as a wound wash or mash the fresh roots to make a poultice.

The powdered root is styptic when applied to a wound (stops bleeding). Simmer 2 tsp. root per each cup of water for about 20 minutes. Take 1 cup a day in ¼ cup doses.

Blackthorn, Sloe

Parts used: flowers, fruit, bark of the root

Gaelic: *áirneag, preas nan airneag, draighionn*

Latin: *Prunus spinosa*

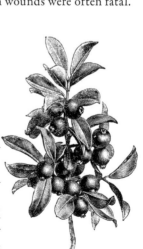

The flower tea is laxative and stimulates the appetite. It benefits the bladder and aids stomach cramps and skin problems. Infuse the flowers to make a tea for scabies (use externally). The flower tea is mildly purgative, strengthens the stomach and increases appetite, helps bladder and skin conditions, stomach cramps, edema and stones. The juice of the fresh berries (called sloes) is applied to mouth and throat inflammations (gather the berries after the first two or three frosts). The jam made from the berries is laxative and suitable for children (pick the fruits after several nights of frost). The root bark tea is helpful for fever.

Flower tea: steep 2 tsp. flowers per ½ cup water and take ½ cup, twice a day on rising and retiring.

Root bark tea: simmer 2 tsp. root bark per 1 cup of water for 20 minutes and take ¼ cup, 4 times a day.

Lore: staffs made of Blackthorn are magically protective when carried. In ancient times, they were made with thorns projecting out of them, to inflict a puncture wound on any would-be attacker. Such wounds were often fatal.

Blueberry, Bilberry, Blaeberry

Parts used: berries, leaves, bark of the root

Gaelic: *braoileag*

Latin: *Vaccinium myrtillus*

The berries are taken for diarrhea and dysentery and to dissolve kidney stones.

Caution: if you have kidney stones please see a medical practitioner.

In the Highlands they are eaten with milk, baked in tarts, and made into jelly (sometimes the jelly is mixed with whisky). A tea of the leaves or of the leaves and root bark is applied externally to ulcers and used as a gargle and mouth wash for ulcers in the mouth and throat. The leaf tea is helpful for diabetes- if taken for a long time it can improve vision and reduce the need for insulin.

To make the leaf tea: 2-3 tbsp. leaf per cup of water. Steep for 20 minutes and take ¼ cup four times a day. **Berries:** simmer 1 tsp. per cup of water for 20 minutes. Take 1-2 cups a day, cold. **Root bark:** simmer 1 tsp. per cup of water for 20 minutes and take 1 cup a day in ¼ cup doses.

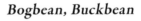

Bogbean, Buckbean

Parts used: the herb

Gaelic: *lus nan laugh, tríbhileach, pónair chapaill, mílsean monaidh*

Latin: *Menyanthes trifoliata*

The entire plant is simmered to make a spring tonic which can be bottled or frozen for winter use. For coughs take 1 tsp. three times a day. The leaf poultice is used for wound healing and the tea is taken simultaneously. The root helps the stomach and digestion. To improve appetite, take ½ cup of the root tea before meals. The root tea benefits stomach ulcers. The juice of the root is used for chest complaints, including tuberculosis. For jaundice and liver pain, take a tea of raspberry (Rubus ideaus), mint (Mentha spp), and bogbean (Menyanthes trifoliata) combined. Bogbean is useful to relieve constipation in both humans and animals and benefits asthma and heart conditions. The leaf tea is helpful for headache, fever, ague, intermittent chills and malaria. The dried leaf is smoked as an herbal tobacco substitute. Bogbean has been used in place of hops (Humulus lupulus) in beer brewing.

Leaf tea: use 1 tbsp. leaf per cup of water. Steep for 20 minutes and take ¼ cup, 4 times a day.

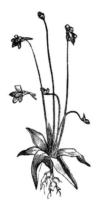

Bog Violet, Butterwort, Marsh Violet

Parts used: the leaves

Gaelic: *móthan*

Latin: *Pinguicula vulgaris*

The leaves are used to poultice sores and chapped hands. They are anti-spasmodic and anti-tussive and have been used to make a cough remedy for whooping cough. Gather the leaves in early summer just as the plant comes into flower and dry for later use throughout the year.

Lore: This most magical of Highland plants is worn in a golden amulet or as a charm to ward off evil and misfortune including: unrequited love, starvation, drowning, and the loss of a court case.

To make a love spell, a woman kneels on her left knee and gathers nine roots, knotting them together to make a "cuach" or ring. The woman puts the ring into the mouth of a girl who is seeking a lover, in the name of the Sun, Moon, and Stars and of the Three Worlds. When the girl meets the man she desires, she places the ring into her mouth and should the man kiss her while the ring is in her mouth, he will be bound to her forever. This kind of love spell does not guarantee happiness however, and just because a person is bound does not mean that they will love you or even like you!

Móthan is put under a woman in labor to ensure safe delivery and is carried by travelers as protection and can be secretly sewn into your clothing (women sew it into their bodice, men put it under their left arm). Feed the herb to an animal such as a goat or cow, and then drink its milk to gain magical protection. Place it under the churn or milk pail to prevent Fairies and sorcerers from stealing the milk. Weave a hoop of milkwort (Polygala vulgaris), butterwort, dandelion (Taraxacum spp.) and marigold (Calendula officinalis) and bind it with three threads made from fairy flax (Linum catharticum) and place it under the milk bucket, to stop ill intentioned Witches and sorcerers from "stealing" or spoiling the milk.

Bog Myrtle, Bayberry

Parts used: the leaves, branches, and cones

Gaelic: *rideag*

Latin: *Myrica gale*
(Myrica cerifera has similar properties)

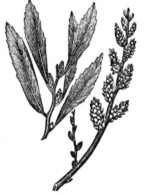

The tea is a worming agent for children. The wax, bark and leaves make an astringent brew that is a gargle for a sore throat, a douche for diarrhea and hemorrhage, and a poultice material for wounds, sores, and bruising.

Caution: the leaves are emmenagogue (bring on menstruation) and abortifacient (may cause a miscarriage) in large doses.

Bayberry was once used as a substitute for hops in beer making. A strewing herb for floors, it repels insects, including fleas and can also be used in the linen closet. The cones are simmered and a fragrant wax is skimmed off to be used in candle making. Simmer 1 tsp. of the bark per cup of water for about 5 minutes. Take ¼ to ½ cup, up to 2 cups a day.

Lore: The totem herb of the Campbells, it is said to repel evil Fairies.

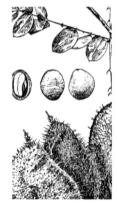

Bonduc Bean

Parts used: the seed

Gaelic: cnó Mhoire, crosphuing

Latin: *Guilandina bonduc*

The seeds wash up on the shores of the Western Hebrides after being carried north by the Gulf Stream, and are used to make a tea for children with diarrhea.

Lore: A charm for the woman in labor who holds the seed. The midwife may clutch the seed and make the sign of the (equal armed) Solar Cross over the laboring woman while reciting an incantation.

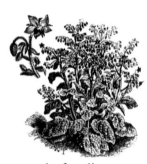

Borage

Parts used: the herb and flowers

Gaelic: *borrach*

Latin: *Borago officinalis*

"I borage bring courage" (traditional saying). A drink of borage is given to fighters to make them brave. The tea brings down a fever and helps restore strength after illness or poisoning. Calming to the nerves, the leaf and seed promote the production of breast milk. The tea helps with stress, depression and exhaustion. A poultice of the fresh herb is applied to inflammations.

Caution: this plant is diuretic and can cause contact dermatitis in some individuals. Not an herb for prolonged use.

Steep 1 tsp. dried flowers or 2-3 tsp. dried leaves per ½ cup water for about 5 minutes. Take ½ cup, twice a day.

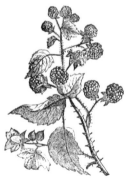

Bramble, Blackberry

Parts used: The fruit, root, and leaves

Gaelic: *dreas*

Latin: *Rubus fructicosus*

The bark of the root is decocted briefly and then steeped with pennyroyal (Hedeoma pulegioides) for bronchitis and asthma. The tea of the bark of the root helps edema, diarrhea, dysentery, and whooping cough. Erysipelas (strep infection of the skin) is treated with a leaf poultice and the leaf poultice can also be applied to burns, scalds, and piles.

Root Tea: simmer 1 ounce of root in 1½ pints of water for about 20 minutes. Take ½ cup every 1-2 hours as needed.

Leaf tea: steep 2 tsp. dried leaves per ½ cup water for about 20 minutes. Take up to 1 cup a day in ¼ cup doses.

Broom

Parts used: the flowering tops, seeds

Gaelic: *bealaidh*

Latin: *Sarothamnus scoparius, Cytisus scoparius*

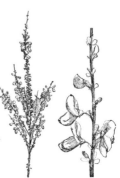

The flowering tops are gathered in early spring and used fresh or dried for later use. An infusion of the dried tops is mildly diuretic and helps cardiac edema. The seeds are emetic. For bladder and kidney ailments use 1 ounce of broom and ½ ounce dandelion root (Taraxacum officinale). Simmer the dandelion roots and broom in 1 pint of water until the liquid is halved, adding at the end ½ ounce dried juniper berries (Juniperus communis). When the mixture cools, add a pinch of cayenne pepper (Capsicum frutescens). Take ¼ cup four times a day.

Broom tea: Simmer 1 tsp. flowering tops or seeds per 1 cup of water. Take 1-2 cups a day.

Caution: large doses may lower blood pressure and even be fatal. Use only with expert supervision.

Lore: Broom, ragweed, and thorn are used by Witches to ride upon. When smoked, the flowering tops are supposedly mildly hallucinogenic.

Butterbur

Parts used: the root

Gaelic: *gallan mór*

Latin: *Petasites albus, Petasites vulgaris*

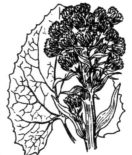

The root is helpful in fever and cardiac edema. The root is a heart tonic and diuretic and helpful for asthma, hay fever, colds, and calculi in the bladder. Simmer 1 ounce of root in 1 ½ cups water until 1 pint of liquid remains, and take ¼ cup, 4 times a day. The powdered root is added to wine and taken for fever. The dried, powdered root is also applied to ulcers.

Caution: prolonged use may harm the liver.

Lore: Butter was once wrapped in its leaves, which is how it got its name.

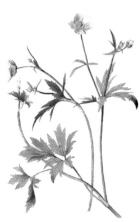

Buttercup, Crowfoot

Parts used: flower and leaf

Gaelic: *Follasgain, Lus an rócais*

Latin: *Ranunculus auricomus*

A poultice of the leaf and flower is used to draw blisters and remove warts and has been applied to gouty and rheumatic parts.

Caution: this plant is poisonous.

This herb should only be used with expert supervision.

Lore: Buttercups are worn in a bag around the neck to cure madness.

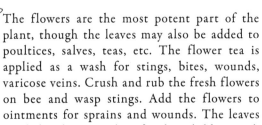

Calendula

Parts used: flower and leaf

Gaelic: *lus Máiri*

Latin: *Calendula arvensis*
(very similar to Calendula officinalis)

The flowers are the most potent part of the plant, though the leaves may also be added to poultices, salves, teas, etc. The flower tea is applied as a wash for stings, bites, wounds, varicose veins. Crush and rub the fresh flowers on bee and wasp stings. Add the flowers to ointments for sprains and wounds. The leaves and flowers can be eaten as salad and are very beneficial to children with scrofula (tuberculosis of the cervical lymph nodes). Calendula is cleansing to the lymph glands and beneficial in cancers. The flower tea tones the circulatory system and benefits jaundice, fevers, measles and internal infections. The tea also helps skin eruptions and measles, stomach cramps, colitis, diarrhea, boils and abscesses. It is used externally as a wash for ulcers, wounds, sores, sore eyes. Use the flowers in salves for sprains, wounds, burns, bruises, sores, boils, and pulled muscles. Freeze the fresh flowers, or make them into ice cubes, and use them throughout the year for sore throats (make a tea and gargle).

Flower tea: 1-2 tsp. of the flowers per ½ cup of water, steep 10 minutes, for internal or external use. Take ¼ cup, 4 times a day. Fresh juice: 1 tsp., 4 times a day.

Chamomile

Parts used: the flowers

Gaelic: *camobhil, camobhaidh*

Latin: *Anthemis nobilis*

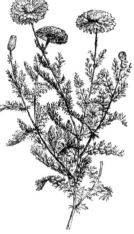

The tea is taken for poor digestion, flatulence, liver complaints and fever. The fresh flowers are chopped, added to butter (or hot oil and hot bees wax), and simmered gently to make a salve for cramps and painful joints.

A classic teething remedy: give the flower tea to a fretful, feverish bairn or bathe the child in a bath of the flower tea. Chamomile and mint (Mentha spp.) simmered with a bit of fresh organic lemon rind, makes a nice tea for insomnia. Apply the tea of the fresh plant to wounds and infections.

Flower tea: steep 1 tbsp. flowers per 1 cup water for about 20 minutes. For children the dose is 1 tsp. every ½ hour, for adults, ¼ cup 4 times a day.

To make a bath: steep 1 lb of flowers in 5 quarts of water for 10 minutes, strain and add to the bath.

Oil: steep fresh or dried flowers in oil for 24 hours, strain and rub on painful joints and swellings.

Carrot

Parts used: the root and seeds (wild)

Gaelic: *curran*

Latin: *Daucus carota*

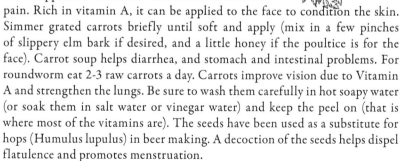

A carrot root poultice (domestic or wild carrot) can be applied to cancerous tumors and to muscle pain. Rich in vitamin A, it can be applied to the face to condition the skin. Simmer grated carrots briefly until soft and apply (mix in a few pinches of slippery elm bark if desired, and a little honey if the poultice is for the face). Carrot soup helps diarrhea, and stomach and intestinal problems. For roundworm eat 2-3 raw carrots a day. Carrots improve vision due to Vitamin A and strengthen the lungs. Be sure to wash them carefully in hot soapy water (or soak them in salt water or vinegar water) and keep the peel on (that is where most of the vitamins are). The seeds have been used as a substitute for hops (Humulus lupulus) in beer making. A decoction of the seeds helps dispel flatulence and promotes menstruation.

Caution: pregnant women and those desiring to conceive should avoid the seeds; they can prevent implantation of the egg in the uterus.

Seed tea: 1 tbsp. wild carrot seed per cup of water, simmered for about 20 minutes. Take ¼ cup, 4 times a day.

Carrot soup: simmer 1 lb. carrots in ¾ cup water until soft, mash and add 1 qt. broth. Carrot juice: 1-2 cups a day of the fresh root.

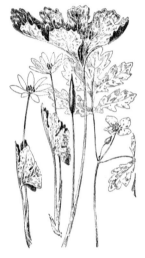

Celandine

Parts used: the flowering herb
(gathered in spring)

Gaelic: *searraiche, lus an torranain*

Latin: *Ranunculus ficaria*

The fresh juice is applied to growths on the ear, neck, piles, and breast lumps. For breast swellings, the roots are placed under the arms.

Caution: this can cause skin irritation. A very powerful liver cleanser, just a few drops of the fresh juice can be taken with water for this purpose, two or three times a day.

For piles: infuse 1 ounce of the herb in a pint of freshly boiled water and take ¼ cup, 4 times a day or add the herb to salves made with lard or with bees wax and olive oil, or apply as a poultice twice a day.

For abscesses: make a salve with celandine (Ranunculus ficaria) plus elder buds (Sambucus nigra), house-leek (Sempervivum tectorum), and plantain leaf (Plantago spp.)

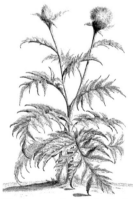

Centaury

Parts used: the herb

Gaelic: *ceud-bhileach*

Latin: *Centaurium erythraea*

The herb is a digestive aid and a general tonic for the digestive tract, blood, liver, and kidneys. Taken before meals, the tea improves appetite and helps rheumatism. The fresh juice or poultice of the fresh herb can be applied to wounds and ulcers. The tea helps lower a fever and can be mixed with Barberry (Berberis vulgaris) bark for jaundice. Centaury is also a worming agent. In Uist, pink centaury was once tinctured in whisky as a tonic.

Tea: steep 1 ounce of the dried herb in 1 pint of water and take ¼ cup four times a day, before meals.

Chickweed

Parts used: the herb

Gaelic: *fliodh*

Latin: *Stellaria media*

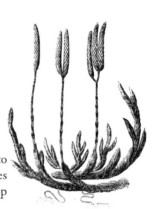

The fresh plant is mashed with a stone mortar and applied to sore breasts. It can be chopped, simmered, and taken as a weight loss tea, or added to healing salves. To help a person with a fever to get to sleep, wash their legs with a strong chickweed tea and then apply a warm poultice of the herb, or apply a warm fomentation to the neck and shoulders. Chickweed tea can be taken for insomnia. The herb is cooked and eaten like spinach.

Tea: 1 tbsp. fresh or dried herb per ½ cup water, take up to 1 cup a day in ¼ cup doses. For constipation: simmer 3 tbsp. in 1 qt water until ½ of the liquid remains. Take 1 cup every 3 hours until relief is obtained. Or take 1 tbsp. fresh juice 3 times a day, not with meals.

Club Moss

Parts used: the spores

Gaelic: *garbhag an t-sléibhe*
(little rough one of the moors)

Latin: *Lycopodium selago,
Lycopodium clavatum*

The plant was simmered by Highland women to make a skin tonic for the face and hands. The spores are styptic and can be applied to wounds to stop bleeding.

Caution: the plant is poisonous but the spores are not. The herb has been used in small amounts as an emmenagogue (to promote menstruation) but its action can be very violent. For this reason, the herb should only be used with expert advice. pregnant women should avoid the herb but not the spores.

Lore: according to Pliny, when the Druids gathered this plant they never used iron to cut it. It was taken by stealth, by a Druid dressed in a white garment. The Druid's feet were washed and bare, and the plant was plucked by the right hand, which had to extend through the left armhole. An offering of bread and wine was left for the earth as thanks. Carried as an amulet, the herb protects against accidents.

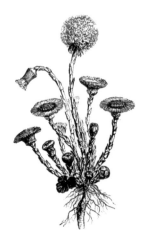

Coltsfoot

Parts used: the leaves and flowers

Gaelic: *cluas liath*

Lation: *Tussilago farfara*

The dry leaf can be smoked to benefit asthma, chronic bronchitis, and dry cough. The fresh leaves are juiced or made into syrup for coughs, colds, hoarseness, bronchitis, asthma and pleurisy. The tea is a helpful diarrhea remedy. Apply a poultice externally to insect bites, swellings, burns, ulcers and phlebitis.

Caution: overuse of this plant can be dangerous due to the high content of carcinogenic pyrrolizidine alkaloids.

Gather the flowers when they first open, and the leaves when mature.

Tea: steep 1-3 tsp. leaves or flowers per 1 cup of water for 30 minutes. Drink ¼ cup 4 times a day, warm. Juice: 1-2 tbsp., 3 times a day.

Comfrey

Parts used: the root and leaf

Gaelic: *meacan dubh*

Latin: *Symphytum tuberosum*

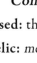

A paste of ground comfrey root and leaf can be spread on broken or fractured bones. The powdered root and leaf is used externally to stop bleeding and to poultice insect bites and stings. Cook the roots and leaves and apply when soft as a poultice for pulled and inflamed tendons, and to the chest for bronchitis and pleurisy. Alternatively chop the roots and stir with hot water to make a paste, spread on a cloth and apply for an hour and then discard. Repeat every 2-4 hours. Another method is to blend the leaves with water until liquid and add powdered slippery elm bark (Ulmus fulva) a bit at a time until a pie dough consistency is achieved. (Dried leaves can be reconstituted by pouring on a little freshly boiled water and then adding slippery elm bark). Roll out with a rolling pin onto a clean cloth and apply cold to burns, wounds, sores, ulcers, bruises, swellings, cuts, surgical incisions, fractures. Leave on for 1 hour and then discard the poultice. Comfrey leaves are a powerful addition to healing salves of all kinds.

Comfrey salve: simmer the chopped leaves in enough cold pressed olive oil to barely cover them for 20 minutes. Melt bees wax in a separate pot. When both are simmering add 3-4 tbsp. hot bees wax for every cup of oil used. (Never add cold bees wax to hot oil or cold oil to hot wax. If you do the salve will not gel). Stir and strain, into very clean glass jars. Apply to burns, chafing, dry skin, diaper rash, sun burn, and dry flaky eczema.

Caution: the roots and young leaves should not be taken internally due to a high content of carcinogenic pyrrolizidine alkaloids.

Corn
(cereal, grain)
Gaelic: *grán*

Barley is the true ancient staple of Scotland. Oats were introduced by the Romans.

Cowslip

Parts used: the flowers, root and herb

Gaelic: *múisean*

Latin: *Primula vera, Primula officinalis*

To make a cosmetic for the skin steep the flowers in white wine and use the liquid as a face wash. Use in salves for sunburn, freckles and wrinkles. The flowers are sedative and anti-spasmotic. The flower tea is useful for insomnia, migraine, nervous excitement, palsy, as a memory aid, and for muscular rheumatism.

Cowslip wine sleep aid: pour boiling hot sugar water over the blossoms, let stand until warm, add yeast and lemon. Allow to steep for two days, strain, store in a cask leaving a small hole open for the working. When it stops working, close it up for 6 weeks then bottle. A decoction of the root is an expectorant for mucus congestion, cough, and bronchitis. The leaves and flowers can be added to healing salves.

Caution: some people are allergic to this herb.

Flower tea: steep 2 tsp. flowers (add roots and leaves if desired) per ½ cup water. Take up to 1 cup a day, made fresh each time, in ¼ cup doses, 4 times a day.

Root tea: simmer 2 tsp. root per 1 cup water and take ¼ cup 4 times a day.

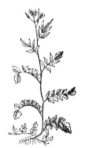

Cuckoo Flower

Parts used: the herb

Gaelic: *biolair ghriagain*

Latin: *Cardamine pretense*
(pratensis)

This herb is very high in Vitamin C and has been used for scurvy. It is also useful to bring down a fever and to soothe epileptic fits. It makes an expectorant tea for coughs. Very similar to watercress, it can be eaten in salads, cooked with nettles, or steeped as tea.

Lore: the name of the plant comes from the fact that its blooming accurately predicts when the cuckoo will first call in spring.

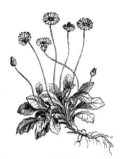

Daisy

Parts used: leaf and flower

Gaelic: *neóinean, an neónan mór*

Latin: *Bellis perennis,*
Chrysanthemum leucanthemum

Bellis perennis, the common daisy, is used in healing salves for bruises, swellings and wounds. The tea of this plant is helpful for colds, chest congestion, colic, and problems in the stomach and intestines where fermentation is the issue. It also benefits kidneys, liver and bladder and can be applied externally as a compress while being taken internally as a beverage. Gowan, or ox-eye daisy (Chrysanthemum leucanthemum) makes a tea for asthma. Its juice is simmered with honey to make a cough remedy which can also be used as a wound salve. The infusion promotes sweating and benefits bladder problems and edema.

Tea: steep 1 tbsp flowers per 1 cups of water. Take 1 cup a day in ¼ cup doses.
Juice: 1 tsp, 3 times a day. Apply externally to wounds and infection.

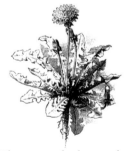

Dandelion

Parts used: the whole herb before flowering,
flowers, leaves and roots
(in fall)

Gaelic: *am beárnan Bríghde*
(notched plant of Bríghde)

Latin: *Taraxacum leontodon*

The root, which is gathered in fall when the plant begins to die back, is a liver and stomach tonic. The root is especially effective at removing excess moisture from the body such as edema of liver origin and benefits jaundice and other liver complaints.

Caution: the root stimulates bile production and should be avoided in gall bladder conditions.

The whole herb helps promote appetite. The leaves, gathered in spring, are a tasty pot-herb and an excellent addition to salads and can be eaten with bread and butter to relieve stomach ulcers. A type of coffee is made from the dried and ground roots. The milky sap can be applied to warts, daily until they disappear. The flowers contain calcium and the petals (not the sepals as they are too bitter) are added to salads and used to make wine. Warm dandelion tea helps indigestion, constipation, fever, and insomnia. The ancient Celts added chopped dandelion leaves and chopped hazel nuts (Coryllus avellana) to oatmeal as a food for invalids.

Leaf tea: steep 2 tsp. leaves per 1 cup of boiled water. Take 1 cup a day in ¼ cup doses, cold or at room temperature.

Root tea: simmer 4 ounces in 2 pints of water until half of the liquid is gone. Take 3 tbsp, 6 times a day.

Juice: in spring, add 1 tsp juice to milk, 3 times a day as a tonic. For rheumatism, gout and stiff joints: steep 2 tbsp fresh leaf and chopped root per ½ cup of water. Take ½ cup in the morning and again in the evening, plus 3 tbsp juice in an 8 ounce glass of water, once or twice a day. Also eat the fresh leaves in salad with olive oil, sea salt, and lemon juice.

Lore: the dandelion is sacred to Bríghde because the white sap resembles milk. Bríghde is a Goddess of motherhood whose festival, Oimelc, celebrates the lactation of the ewes.

Docken, Dock

Parts used: the root and leaf

Gaelic: *copag*

Latin: *Rumex obtusifolius*

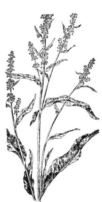

The root decoction is taken for scurvy and the fresh, peeled, and mashed roots are applied to bee stings, keeping the root poultice on for 4 hours and repeating until the swelling disappears. Simmer the roots in vinegar to make a wash for scabs and skin eruptions. The leaves are used to poultice burns, blisters, and nettle rash.

To make a salve for burns, scrapes, diaper rash, etc., the roots are simmered until soft with fresh butter or oil and mixed with hot beeswax (use 3 or 4 tbsp. simmering hot bees wax for every cup of butter or oil). Heat the beeswax in a pot until it simmers. In a separate pot bring yellow dock roots (Rumex crispus) and butter or olive oil to a simmer and cook (do not boil!) until the roots are soft. Combine the wax, oil and softened roots into one pot, bring to a simmer again, then strain and jar. Other herbs such as comfrey (Symphytum tuberosum), lavender (Lavandula vera), calendula

(Calendula officinalis) and chickweed (Stellaria media) may be added to the docken roots as they cook. Be sure you have a non aluminum pot with a tight lid so that the volatile oils are not lost.

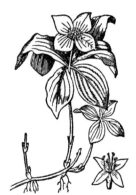

Dog's Mercury

Part used: the flowering herb

Gaelic: *lus Ghlinne Bhrácadail*

Latin: *Mercurialis perennis*

The tea makes a wound wash and the herb makes a poultice for swellings and old sores. The fresh juice mixed with vinegar is applied to warts, inflammations and sores. The plant is both emetic and purgative.

Caution: this plant must be used internally only with expert supervision. The fresh plant is poisonous and the poison is cumulative. (Drying and simmering removes the poison).

Dwarf Cornel

Parts used: the berries

Gaelic: *lus a' chraois*
(herb of gluttony)

Latin: *Cornus suecica*

The tea of the berries promotes appetite. The berries can be eaten as an appetizer and are a traditional winter food of the Eskimos.

Dwarf Elder, Ground Elder, Goutweed

Parts used: the herb and root

Gaelic: *lus an easbaig*

Latin: *Aegopodium podagraria*

A poultice plant for sciatica; it can also be applied as a fomentation by simmering the leaves and roots and soaking a cloth in the brew, then applying hot to the painful area. A diuretic and sedative, it is used internally as a tea to aid aching joints, gout, and sciatica. The mashed roots are applied to gout. To make the tea, simmer 2 tsp. roots or steep 2 tsp. leaves per cup of water. Take ¼ cup, 4 times a day.

Elder, Bourtree

Parts used: the roots, bark, young shoots, leaves, flowers, fruits

Gaelic: *ruis*

Latin: *Sambucus nigra*

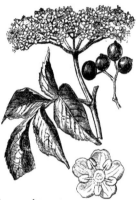

Elder flower water is used to wash the face as a skin tonic: simmer the flowers lightly for a few minutes then steep (a little Witch Hazel and alcohol can be added as a preservative). Elder flowers and pollen, almond oil and lard are used to make a healing salve for dry, flaky skin conditions (follow the salve making instructions at the start of this chapter). Taken internally the flower tea opens skin pores and promotes sweating, making it helpful for fevers and rheumatism. The young leaves (which must be gathered before Summer Solstice because after that they will contain too many natural pesticides) are used in salves for wounds and burns. The tea of the young leaves and shoots increases urine and helps edema. The bark and root are emetic and diuretic and must be used fresh.

Caution: large doses of the bark and root can lead to inflammation of the bowels and violent purging. Only use the leaves when they are very young and fresh.

The berry tea and wine are rich in iron, building to the blood, and a remedy for bronchitis, asthma, flu, and chest colds. The berries should be cooked before eating or juicing and can be made into a mildly laxative jam that will soothe intestinal irritations.

Bark or root bark tea: 1 tsp. fresh bark or root bark steeped in ½ cup boiled water. Take ¼ cup four times a day and no more *(see caution above)*.

Flower tea: steep 2 tsp flowers per 1 cup of water and take hot up to 3 cups a day. The flower tea is safe for children and babies to relieve fever. Elder berries can be baked into pies, scones and breads.

Lore: Elder has a protective female spirit that will protect you against sorcery as long as profound respect is shown to the plant. It is very bad luck to cut down an elder tree or to burn her wood. Use only twigs, leaves and berries or a small section of her root and be sure to thank the Elder Mother when you take any part of her dwelling. Whip handles for hearse drivers were once made of elder to guard against ghosts. Dried elderberries picked on Midsummer's Day are placed on the windowsill to prevent evil from entering. As with rowan, an elder cross is protective of the house and barn. Make one by binding two equal length twigs with red thread. Hang it over the door, place it by a window, or wear it on your person. The juice of the inner bark is applied to the eyelids to give someone "the Sight". Stand or sleep under an elder on Samhuinn or Bealltan Eve and you will see Fairies. Wear a sprig somewhere on your person to ward off evil Spirits.

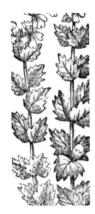

Eyebright

Parts used: the herb

Gaelic: *lus nan leac, glan ruis*

Latin: *Euphrasia officinalis*

Combine eyebright, black tea, and milk to make a soothing and cooling eye wash *(strain through an organic coffee filter before applying to the eyes)*. A tea of the fresh herb is used as eyewash for inflammation and eye strain. The tea also helps colds, sore throat, and hay fever.

Fresh herb tea: steep 1 tsp. fresh herb per 1 cup of water. Take 1-2 cups a day in ¼ cup doses. Simmer 1 tsp. dried herb in 1 cup of water for 5 minutes. Make a fresh batch daily.

In the case of eye infections such as conjunctivitis, "pink eye" and the like, add goldenseal (Hydrastis Canadensis) root to the eyewash. Use 1 tsp. root per pint of water, simmer for 20 minutes and strain through an organic coffee filter and add to the eyebright eye wash.

(Please note: Goldenseal is not a Scottish herb; it is an indigenous American plant).

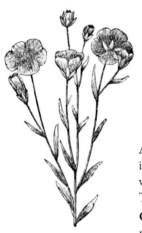

Fairy Flax

Parts used: the whole herb

Gaelic: *lion na mná* (or ban) *síthe*
(plant of the Fairy women),
lus míosach (menstrual plant), *lus caolach*

Latin: *Linum catharticum*

A strongly acting purge used for menstrual issues and as a laxative. It must be combined with a carminative such as mint (Mentha spp.). The tea helps jaundice and liver ailments.

Caution: pregnant women should avoid this plant. Large amounts can be fatal. Use only with expert supervision. The dried herb is infused using 1 ounce per 1 pint of freshly boiled water and taken in ¼ cup doses.

Fennel

Parts used: root and seeds

Gaelic: *lus an t-saoidh*

Latin: *Foeniculum vulgare*

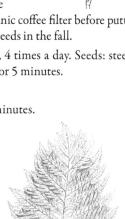

The root and seeds increase appetite and relive stomach cramps, gas, and colic. Boil the seeds in barley water (see Barley above) to increase breast milk in nursing mothers. Simmer the seeds to make an eyewash for eye strain and irritation (filter the liquid through an organic coffee filter before putting into the eyes). The root is gathered in the spring, the seeds in the fall.

Root tea: 2 tbsp. root per cup of water, take ¼ cup, 4 times a day. Seeds: steep 1 tbsp. seeds (crush slightly) in 1 cup of boiled water for 5 minutes.

Eye wash: simmer ½ tsp. seeds in 1 cup of water.

For colic: simmer 1 tsp. seed in ½ cup milk for 10 minutes.

Ferns
Common Fern, Polypody Fern, Female Fern, Brakeroot

Parts used: the root

Gaelic: *clach raineach*

Latin: *Polypodium vulgare*

The root benefits phlegm, wet lung conditions, catarrh, coughs, bronchitis, weak digestion, fever, and jaundice.

The root tea is helpful to expel tenia worms. Simmer 3 tsp. fresh or dried root per 1 cup of water until a syrupy consistency results. Take 2-8 tbsp. 4 times a day.

Hart's Tongue Fern

Parts used: the herb

Gaelic: *creamh na muice fiadhaich*
(wild pig's garlic)

Latin: *Asplenium scolopendrium*

The leaves are used in burn salves and as a tea that is tonic to the liver and removes sediment from the bladder. The tea is also helpful in bronchial afflictions.

Tea: simmer 2 ounces in 1 pint of water for about 20 minutes. Take ¼ cup, 4 times a day.

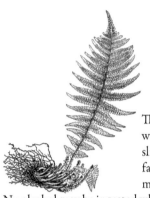

Male Fern

Parts used: the root

Gaelic: *Marc-raineach*

Latin: *Dryopteris felix-mas*

This fern is used for worming, specifically for tape worm. ½ ounce of the fresh root is mixed with slippery elm powder (Ulmus fulva) and taken while fasting. 1-2 hours after ingestion a strong purgative must be used to purge both the worms and the herbs. No alcohol may be ingested while taking this herb.

Caution: improper use of this plant can cause blindness, abortion, sterility and even death. It should only be used internally with expert supervision. It can be safely used externally as a foot bath for varicose veins. Collect the roots in autumn and simmer 1 lb. of the roots in water and add to a foot bath.

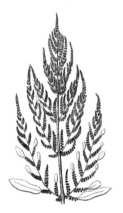

Royal Fern

Parts used: the root and young fronds

Gaelic: *raineach ríoghail*

Latin: *Osmunda regalis*

For knee injuries: chop and simmer the roots in water until soft. When cool, apply to the knee to relieve pain and swelling. Apply the roots to bruises, fractures, and trauma. The root tea benefits jaundice. Add the roots and young fronds to healing salves and ointments.

Tea: simmer 1 tsp. root per 1 cup of water for about 20 minutes or steep in freshly boiled water for 30 minutes. Take 1 tbsp. per hour.

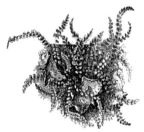

Spleenwort, Maidenhair Fern, Black Spleenwort

Parts used: the leaves

Gaelic: *dubhchasach*

Latin: *Asplenium spp.*

The infusion is used for coughs, tuberculosis, and insomnia.

Tea: steep 1 ounce of the leaf in 1 pint freshly boiled water. Add honey for coughs. The dose is 3 tablespoons.

Lore: Ferns are the sacred plant of Shetland, the homeland of the Trows (Fairies). On Samhuinn night the ferry-kairds (ferns) are seen to part as the Peerie-folk emerge on their travels. Ferns are also known as "Faeries' cairds" or "Trowie-cairds". "Cairds" are tools for carding wool. The Fairies hide the entrance to their Hills with luxuriant growths of fern.

Figwort

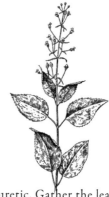

Parts used: the herb

Gaelic: *torranan, lus nan cnapan*

Latin: *Scrophularia nodosa*

The leaves are used to poultice wounds and bruises, piles, sprains, abscesses, swellings, gangrene, eczema, scabies, tumors, eruptions, and rashes. The root poultice is applied to tumors and sores. A tea of the leaf helps scrofula (tuberculosis of the cervical lymph nodes) and is diuretic. Gather the leaves in early summer and use the fresh leaves in salves and fomentations for bruises and minor wounds.

Tea: steep 1 tsp. plant per 1 cup of water. Take up to 2 cups a day, in ¼ cup doses.

Lore: gather at the incoming tide and use as a charm against the Evil Eye.

Flag
(Yellow)

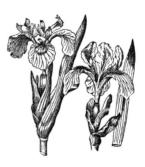

Parts used: the flowers and dried rhizomes

Gaelic: *seilistear*

Latin: *Iris pseudoacorus*

The dried roots are chewed to relieve sore throats, coughs, and hoarseness. The powdered root is taken as snuff for colds. Simmer the roots until soft and add a few drops of rosewater and apply to bruises. On delicate areas such as the face put a layer of silk between the poultice and the skin. The tea of the dried root is astringent and benefits diarrhea, liver, spleen, menstrual pain and colic. The flowers can be added to salves for ulcers and swellings.

Caution: pregnant women should avoid this herb as it has emmenagogic (brings on menstruation) properties. The plant is toxic in large doses and may raise blisters on the skin. Use only with expert supervision.

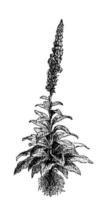

Foxglove

Parts used: the leaf

Gaelic: *lus nam bansíth*
(herb of the Fairy woman)

Latin: *Digitalis purpurea*

A remedy for cardiac edema and an important cardiac tonic (the modern drug Digitalin is derived from this plant) but due to its cumulative toxicity, modern herbalists prefer to use hawthorn (Crataegus oxyacantha) internally as a heart tonic.

Caution: drink the tea only with expert supervision. The plant is generally safe for external use; however, some people are highly sensitive to it and may experience headache, nausea, or rash from merely touching it. Before applying it liberally to the skin, test a small portion to see how your body reacts. A poultice of the moistened leaves is applied to erysipelas, erythema, eczema, wounds and boils. A hot poultice of foxglove leaf, butter, and garlic or onion can be applied to sore knees and for diphtheria. Apply to the knees and neck as needed.

Lore: The name is said to derive from the belief that the Fairies gave the flowers to the foxes so they could hunt silently at night by wearing the flowers as gloves.

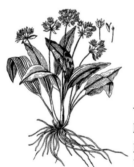

Garlic (Wild), Bear's Garlic, Ramsons

Parts used: the whole herb

Gaelic: *creamh*

Latin: *Allium ursinum*

Widely used in poultices for wounds and infections, the herb is anti-viral and anti-bacterial. Garlic helps remove plaque from the arteries, purifies the liver, and strengthens the immune system. It aids in the removal of pin worms and benefits diarrhea, constipation, colic, emphysema, bronchitis, and fever. It lowers blood pressure when used over time. It is most effective when taken fresh (the root can be dried for later use) and can be eaten in salads, as a cooked vegetable, or in soups.

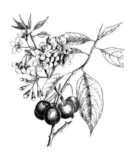

Gean, Wild Cherry

Parts used: the fruit stalks

Gaelic: *geanais*

Latin: *Prunus avium*

Simmer the fruit stalks as a drink for bronchitis, anemia, and diarrhea. Use ½ ounce per 1 pint of water.

Gentian, Field Gentian

Parts used: the root

Gaelic: *lus a' chrúbain*

Latin: *Gentiana campestris*

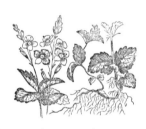

A bitter tonic used to improve the digestion when taken 30 minutes before a meal (it is even more effective if a bit of organic orange peel is added). The root tea helps stomach pain, heartburn, gas, indigestion, diarrhea and vomiting. It is used externally as a wound wash. The root has been used in lieu of hops (Humulus lupulus) to brew beer.

Root tea: simmer 1 tsp. root per 1 cup of water. Take 1 tbsp. every 2 hours or ½ hour before meals.

Germander Speedwell, Mountain Speedwell

Parts used: the herb

Gaelic: *nuallach*

Latin: *Veronica chamaedrys*

This herb is used with goldenrod (Solidago spp.) and Saint John's Wort (Hypericum perforatum) in wound salves (both herbs are magically protective as well). The tea is a blood cleanser and an expectorant for coughs; add honey to make a syrup for asthma and catarrh. Use the freshly expressed juice to benefit gout. Apply the herb as a poultice for itching and chronic skin conditions.

Tea: steep 2 tsp flowering herb per ½ cup water, take in ¼ cup doses, up to 1 ½ cups a day. Juice: 2 tsp. fresh juice in water or milk, 3 times a day.

Lore: the seeds of germander are worn as a protective charm. They were once worn around the neck of warriors who were going into battle.

Goldenrod

Parts used: the flowering tops and leaves

Gaelic: *fuinnseag*

Latin: *Solidago virgaurea*

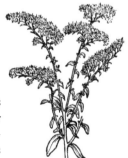

This herb is used in wound salves with Saint John's Wort (Hypericum perforatum) and germander (Veronica chamaedrys) or mixed with fresh all-heal (Prunella vulgaris) and butter. The tea is helpful for kidney inflammation, kidney and bladder stones, arthritis, eczema, whooping cough, excessive menstruation, diarrhea, and internal hemorrhage.

Caution: if you have stones in the kidney or bladder please seek expert advice before using this plant.

Apply the leaves as a poultice for insect bites and stings, wounds and sores. Pound to a paste with valerian root (Valeriana officinalis), add to fresh butter and apply to bruises.

Tea: steep 1 ounce of the flowering top in 1 pint of water for 20 minutes, or simmer 1 tbsp. flowering tops in ½ cup water for 2 minutes and then steep. Take ¼ cup, 4 times a day. Make a fresh batch daily.

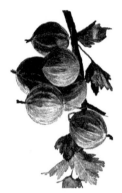

Gooseberry

Parts used: the fruits and leaves

Gaelic: *grósaid*

Latin: *Ribes grossularia*

The tea helps with sediment in the urine and is also beneficial for teen-aged girls, when taken just before the periods. The juice of the berries is rich in calcium, sulphur, and Vitamins A, C, B1.

Leaf tea: use 1 ounce of dried leaf per pint of water, steep for 20 minutes and take 1/3 pint, 3 times a day.

Lore: use the thorns to puncture warts and sties (lay a golden ring around the wart as you do this). Pick 10 thorns, use one to puncture the wart or sty, then point the others towards the blemish and throw them over your shoulder, one at a time.

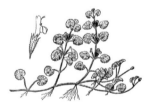

Ground Ivy

Parts used: the flowering herb and leaf

Gaelic: *iadhshlat thalmhainn*

Latin: *Nepeta glechoma*

Take as tea with honey for coughs, bronchitis, and headaches. The tea benefits liver, kidneys, and digestion and is helpful for diarrhea. Use the tea as a wash for sore eyes (filter through an organic coffee filter before applying to the eyes). Use the herb as a poultice, or combine with mashed yarrow (Achillea millefolium) and chamomile (Anthemis nobilis, Matricaria chamomilla) flowers to poultice abscesses and tumors. Use the tea as a wound wash for sores and ulcers. Dry the leaves to make a snuff for asthma and headaches. A few drops of the fresh juice can be given to a child with an upset stomach (add to water, milk, or juice).

Tea: steep 1 tsp. herb per ½ cup freshly boiled water, add honey to taste. Take ¼ cup, 4 times a day.

Caution: this herb can be poisonous in large doses.

Groundsel

Part used: the whole plant

Gaelic: *am bualan*

Latin: *Senecio vulgaris*

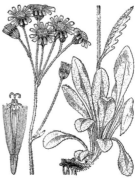

Wash the plant carefully and lay in a bowl. Pour boiling water over it, cover and allow steeping then soak a cloth in the hot liquid. Apply the hot cloth to a boil, covering with a second cloth to help hold in the heat. For swellings, bruises, inflamed breasts, apply cold. The cold infusion also helps soothe chapped hands. Taken internally, a weak infusion is purgative; a strong infusion is emetic and emmenagogue (brings on menstruation). The tea can be used to bring down a fever. For gout, mash the herb, mix with lard, and apply to the feet.

Caution: pregnant women should avoid this plant, it can be abortive. The plant can be poisonous to livestock, keep away from horses and sheep. This herb can be harmful to the liver and must be used with expert supervision.

Lore: groundsel root is a magical aid in dairying. Put it under the milk pail to prevent the milk being "stolen" by sorcery.

Hawthorn, May Tree, Whitethorn

Parts used: flowers, leaves, and fruits

Gaelic: *sgiach, sgitheach*

Latin: *Crataegus monogyna, Crataegus oxyacantha*

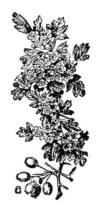

Steep the flower buds and fresh young leaves in spring, to make a tea for sore throats. Tincture the flowers and leaves in early spring or the red berries in the fall (the berries are most potent when gathered just after the first frost but by the second frost they may be ruined) to make a heart tonic that will help to balance blood pressure. The berries can also be simmered to make a sore throat tea.

Caution: this herb lowers blood pressure over time.

Flower tea: steep 2 tsp. buds per 1 cup of water, take up to 1 ½ cups a day in ¼ cup doses.

Berry tea: simmer 1 tsp. crushed berries per ½ cup water for about 20 minutes. Take up to 1 ½ cups a day in ¼ cup doses.

Lore: the totem plant of the Ogilvies. Where oak, ash and thorn grow together, your are likely to see Fairies. A lone hawthorn tree standing on a hill or near a source of water is likely an entrance to the Fairy realm and should never be harmed or disturbed. A hawthorn growing by a holy well should never be cut or dishonored and nothing should be removed from it, including fallen wood. Hawthorn flowers should never be brought into the house except on Bealltan Eve when they can be placed in front of the door before sunrise. Medicines can be made from the flowers if appropriate respect and thanks are given to the Tree Spirit. Those who seek contact with the Fairy Realm will sleep beneath a solitary hawthorn growing on a hill, on Bealltan or on Midsummer's Eve.

Hazel

Parts used: the nuts

Gaelic: *calltainn*

Latin: *Corylus avellana*

An important food in ancient times and thus given many mystical associations, hazel nuts are a rich source of carbohydrates, protein, phosphorus, magnesium, potassium, copper, and fatty acids. The powdered nuts can be mixed with mead or honey water to help ease chronic coughs. Add pepper (Piper nigrum) to the drink to help draw mucus from the sinus passages. The dried and powdered husks and shells are simmered in red wine to help stop diarrhea. Hazel nut milk is given to sick children and to those who can't tolerate cow's milk. Soak the fresh nuts in water overnight, blend and stain out the "milk".

Lore: hazel rods are cut on Midsummer's Day to be used for dowsing and water witching, and to find veins of gold, coal, lead, and lost or hidden objects. If two nuts are found in one shell it is very unlucky to eat them. Hazel nuts are sacred to Goddesses because of the milk in the green nut and because hazel nut milk is given to sick children. Hazel is also associated with the Gods of thunder, fire and lightning because its wood is used to make fires by friction. There is a magical well at the bottom of the ocean where the Salmon of Wisdom eat the nuts that fall from nine magical hazels known as the Well of Segais or Connla's Well. It is the source of all inspiration and knowledge. For every nut they eat, the salmon get a spot (possibly a reference to an ancient system of initiation). Any person who eats of the Salmon of Wisdom becomes at once a seer or a poet. Some speculate that the red flesh of the salmon may actually be a veiled reference to the ingestion of Amanita muscaria, a red-capped mushroom with white spots.

Heather

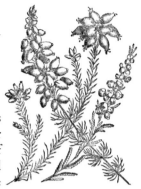

Parts used: the flowering herb, fresh or dried

Gaelic: *fraoch*

Latin: *Calluna vulgaris,
Erica cinerea, Erica tetralix*

Heather tea is soothing to the nerves and promotes sleep. Apply the flowering tops as a poultice or compress to the head for headache or insomnia, stuff pillows and mattresses with them to obtain restful sleep. In ancient times the very best mattresses were stuffed with heather. A decoction of the flowering tops helps chest conditions and coughs and also benefits indigestion, cystitis, diarrhea, and hay-fever, nervous conditions, depression, gouty and rheumatic pains, and heart complaints. It is, and was, a veritable pharmacy for those living in cold, damp and boggy areas. The tea helps nursing mothers increase breast milk. Heather liniments are applied to arthritis and rheumatism and a hot poultice of the flowers is applied to chilblains. Heather is slightly diuretic and anti-microbial. It can strengthen the heart but slightly raises blood pressure. Steep 1 tsp. shoots per ½ cup freshly boiled water or simmer 4 tsp. shoots per ½ cup water for 5 minutes. Take ¼ cup twice a day.

Lore: the Picts are said to have made ale from heather, without the use of hops (Humulus lupulus). Here is a recipe from Wilma Paterson of the Isle of Skye: 1 gallon heather tops, 2 lb. malt extract, 1 1/2 lb sugar (or 1 lb honey), 3 gallons water, 1 ounce yeast. Cut the heather when it first comes into bloom; simmer in 1 gallon of water for about 1 hour. Strain through a jelly bag onto the sweetener and the malt extract, stir until dissolved. Add the remaining water and when lukewarm, the yeast. White heather is especially sacred and magical and brings good luck. It grows only on the grave of a Fairy or on ground where no blood has ever been shed. Heather tops should be gathered at dawn for greatest magical potency.

Helleborine, White Helleborine

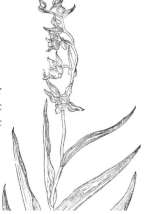

Parts used: the root

Gaelic: *eileabor geal, eileabor leathann*

Latin: *Epipactis latifolia, Epipactis helleborine*

The dried, powdered root is used as a snuff for colds. Modern studies reveal that this plant may have anti-viral, anti-fungal, and antibiotic properties.

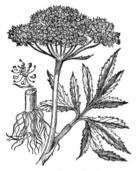

Hemlock, European Water Hemlock, Cowbane

Parts used: the herb

Gaelic: *fealladh-bog*

Latin: *Cicuta virosa*

This is the plant that was used to execute convicted criminals (Socrates for one) in ancient Greece.

Caution: this plant is poisonous and fatal to humans and cattle. Do not attempt to use this plant without expert supervision.

Herb Robert

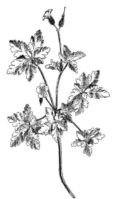

Parts used: the herb (remove any fruits)

Gaelic: *lus an ellain* (plant for hives)*, lus an róis*

Latin: *Geranium Robertianum*

The herb is chopped and simmered to make a hot poultice for hives, erysipelas (strep infection of the skin), and skin cancer. Apply a hot poultice of the leaf to bladder pain, fistulas, and bruises. Apply a cool poultice of the fresh herb to inflammations. The tea makes an astringent wash for mouth inflammation and when diluted can be used as an eye wash (strain carefully through an organic coffee filter before using it in the eyes). The tea is beneficial to diarrhea, gastritis, enteritis, and gout. Steep 1 tbsp. dried herb per 1 cup of water for 10 minutes. Take ¼ cup, 4 times a day.

Holly, English Holly, Mountain Holly, European Holly

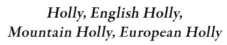

Parts used: leaf

Gaelic: *Cuileann*

Latin: *Ilex aquifolium*

The dried leaf is brewed as tea for coughs, fever, bronchitis, arthritis, rheumatism, gout, urinary stones and complaints. Steep 1-2 tbsp. dried leaf per cup of freshly boiled water. Take ¼ cup, 4 times a day.

Caution: the berries are poisonous.

Honeysuckle

Parts used: flowers, leaves, seeds

Gaelic: *féithlean*

Latin: *Lonicera periclymenum*

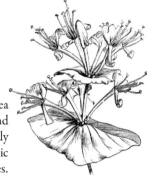

Crush and then steep the flowers to make a tea for bronchitis, headaches, shortness of breath, and asthma of nervous origin. Use the flower tea externally as a wash for sunburn. The flower tea is anti-spasmodic and soothes hiccoughs. Add the flowers to burn salves.
The tea of the leaf is laxative and can be used as a gargle for sore throats. Simmer the flowers and leaves briefly in honey to make a syrup that will help coughs and asthma.

Horehound, White Horehound

Parts used: the herb

Gaelic: *grábhan bán*

Latin: *Marrubium vulgare*

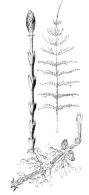

The whole herb is infused to make an expectorant tea for asthma, bronchitis, and coughs. Horehound is helpful for fevers, calms the heart, and balances secretions of the internal organs and glands. Taken warm it is a diuretic and helps with a fever, taken cold it is a stomach tonic. Use the tea externally as a wash for skin afflictions. Steep 1 tsp. herb per ½ cup water, taking up to 1 ½ cups a day in ¼ cup doses.
Juice: take 1 tsp. fresh juice, twice a day.

Horsetail, Shave Grass, Scouring Rush

Parts used: the plant

Gaelic: *clois*

Latin: *Equisetum arvense*

This silica rich plant can be used to scour pots and pans. Simmer the plant in water to make a wash for wounds and skin irritations, and for mouth and gum sores and inflammations. The tea is useful for lung conditions, including tuberculosis. The tea is also taken for leg and stomach ulcers, bladder issues, edema, profuse menstruation, leucorrhea and can be used as a douche for female complaints. The juice of the herb helps anemia resulting from stomach ulcers because it is a clotting agent for the blood.

Caution: overdosing with this herb can lead to poisoning.

Steep 2 tsp. dried herb per ½ cup water; take up to 1 cup a day in ¼ cup doses or simmer 1 tsp. fresh or dry herb per ½ cup water for 5 minutes and strain.

For internal hemorrhage: take 2 cups in tablespoon doses throughout the day. Juice: take 1 tsp. in water.

For external use: as a wash make a stronger tea.

Lore: The magical name for this plant is Faeries' Spindles.

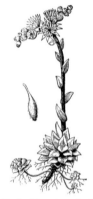

Houseleek

Parts used: the fresh leaf and juice

Gaelic: *lus nan cluas (ear plant)*

Latin: *Sempervivum tectorum*

The juice and leaves are used to poultice skin diseases, burns, shingles, gout, inflammations and traumas. The leaf is simmered into salves for inflammations and burns. Mix the juice with honey and apply to thrush and mouth ulcers. To remove corns and warts, apply the juice daily, and at night apply a houseleek poultice. Or slice a leaf in half, and apply the inner surface to the wart. The leaves are steeped to make a tea for fever. The juice is dropped into the ears to ease pain. Apply the leaf poultice to the forehead and temples for insomnia and headache. Apply the poultice to the crown of the head to stop nosebleed. Rub the fresh leaf onto bee stings and nettle rash.

Caution: large doses of the juice are emetic and purgative: only use the juice externally. The leaves must be used fresh, never dried.

Leaf tea: steep 1 tsp. fresh leaf per 1 cup water; take ¼ cup, 4 times a day.

Lore: growing on the roof, the plant protects the house from storms, lightning, fires, and sorcery.

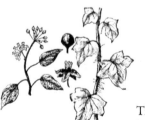

Ivy, English Ivy

Parts used: the leaf and twigs

Gaelic: *eidheann*

Latin: *Hedera helix*

Tincture the leaves in vinegar to treat corns, add the leaves to burn salves. Simmer the leaves in water to make a wash for ulcers, wounds, burns, boils, dandruff, and skin irritations, using about 1 tsp. herb per cup of water. The twigs are simmered in butter to make a sunburn salve.

Caution: this plant causes contact dermatitis in some individuals and so only use it externally.

Lore: On the eve of a Fire Festival (Samhuinn, Oimelc, Beallran, Lúnasdal) pin three leaves of ivy onto your night gown to dream of your future lover. Bind ivy, woodbine (Asperula odorata) or bramble (Rubus fructicosus), and rowan (Sorbus aucuparia) into a wreath and hang it over the house or barn to bring protection from witchcraft, the Evil Eye, and cattle diseases. Make a wreath of milkwort (Polygala vulgaris), butterwort (Pinguicula vulgaris), dandelion (Taraxacum spp.), and marigold (Calendula officinalis), and bind it with a triple cord of ivy, placing it under the milk pail to prevent the milk from being charmed away. Ivy is one of the last plants to bloom in the fall and provides food for bees late into the season, and for this reason it symbolizes abundance. It was once used in marriage bouquets and crowns to symbolize the female spirit, while holly was used to symbolize the male essence.

Juniper, Mountain Yew

Parts used: the dried, ripe berries

Gaelic: *samhan, aiteann, Aiteal*

Latin: *Juniperus communis*

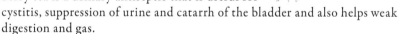

The berries are used to flavor drinks (the distinctive flavor of Gin is from juniper berries), as a poultice for snake bite, in massage oils for rheumatism and arthritis. A tea of the berries benefits chest congestion and relieves edema resulting from heart, kidney, or liver disease. The berry tea is a urinary antiseptic that is useful for cystitis, suppression of urine and catarrh of the bladder and also helps weak digestion and gas.

Caution: the berries are emmenagogue (bring on menstruation) and should be avoided by pregnant women. Do not take the tea for more than two weeks as it can cause kidney irritation. Avoid the tea if you have weak kidneys or a kidney disease.

Tea: use 1 tsp. crushed berries per ½ cup water, steep for 10 minutes. Take ¼ cup two or four times per day.

Lore: Burn juniper branches before the entrance to the house and barn on New Year's morning, as an act of ritual purification. The tips of the branches can be burned throughout the year to bring peace and harmony to the home. To work magically, the plant must be pulled out by the roots, the branches tied into four bundles and taken between five fingers, while chanting a prayer.

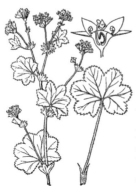

Lady's Mantle

Parts used: the dried herb and root

Gaelic: *copan an driúchd, trusgan* (dew cup)

Latin: *Alchemilla vulgaris, A. alpina*

Used in the Highlands to poultice wounds, this plant is styptic (stops bleeding) due to a high amount of tannins. It is helpful for excessive menstruation, bleeding between periods, children's diarrhea, and colitis with bleeding. Use it as a douche for candida. The roots are used externally only, to stop bleeding.

Caution: pregnant women should avoid this plant. Gather when the leaves are dry from June to August. For external use, double the amount of plant matter.

A. vulgaris: steep 1 tbsp per cup for 15 minutes; take ¼ cup, 4 times a day.

A. alpina: simmer 1 tbsp per 1 cup water for 5 minutes. Take ¼ cup, 4 times a day. Silvery Lady's Mantle (A. alpina) is particularly good for relieving gas.

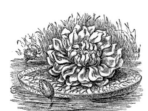

Pond Lilly, White Pond Lilly

Parts used: the roots and leaves.

Gaelic: *duilleag bháite bhán, bioras*

Latin: *Nymphaea alba, Nymphaea, odorata*

To remove corns, simmer the roots in vinegar until soft, and apply to the corn for 3 or 4 days. The root is astringent, benefits diarrhea and reduces sexual desire. Combine the roots with powdered slippery elm bark to poultice boils, ulcers, and skin inflammations. Simmer the roots as a wash for skin irritations, a gargle for sore throat, a douche for chronic vaginal discharge, cervical ulceration, and fibroids. The roots and leaves are used to poultice wounds cuts and bruises.

Caution: if the plant is gathered fresh be sure to soak it in water with a few tablespoons of vinegar for at least 20 minutes, to get rid of parasites.

Root tea: 1 tsp. per cup of water, simmer for 2 minutes and take ¼ cup, 4 times a day.

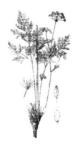

Lovage, Sea Lovage

Parts used: root, leaf, seeds

Gaelic: *siunas, sunais*

Latin: *Ligusticum Scoticum*

The plant is used to flavor broths and is eaten in salads. It is added to lamb's broth to help cure serious chest complaints and tuberculosis. The leaves can be eaten raw or cooked as a pot herb. The stems are candied. The stems are blanched and eaten like celery, and the young shoots and leaves can be eaten cooked or raw.

Lore: The plant is reputedly an aphrodisiac, and Spanish nuns were once forbidden to grow it in convent gardens.

Marigold, Pot Marigold
(see Calendula)

Marjoram
Parts used: the herb

Gaelic: *oragan, lus Mharsaili*

Latin: *Origanum vulgare*

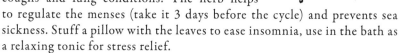

This herb is applied as a fomentation to pains in horses. The tea of the fresh herb helps indigestion, colic, headache and nerves. It is expectorant and mildly anti-viral, which helps coughs and lung conditions. The herb helps to regulate the menses (take it 3 days before the cycle) and prevents sea sickness. Stuff a pillow with the leaves to ease insomnia, use in the bath as a relaxing tonic for stress relief.

Caution: pregnant women should avoid this herb.

Tea: steep 2-3 tsp. herb per 1 cup of water. Take up to 2 cups a day, in ½ cup doses.

Mint
Parts used: the herb as it comes into bloom

Gaelic: *meant*

Latin: *Mentha spp.*

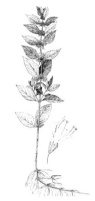

Mint is a popular beverage tea which improves digestion and dispels gas. For pains in the side after jaundice combine mint, bogbean (Menyanthes trifoliata), and raspberry (Rubus spp.). Add a strong mint and lemon balm (Melissa officinalis) tea to the bathwater to heal nerves and sinews. Mint can be used to poultice bee and wasp stings. The tea makes a gargle for mouth sores and sore gums. A strong tea of spearmint (Mentha spicata) is used to bathe chapped hands and for fevers. To soothe flu and to ward off a cold, combine peppermint (Mentha piperita) with elder flowers (Sambucus nigra) and yarrow (Achillea millefolium) or boneset (Eupatorium perfoliatum). For abdominal cramps, diarrhea and nausea take the hot tea in milk or water. Peppermint eases heart palpitations. For nervous problems combine peppermint with wood betony (Stachys officinalis) as a tea. For teething children combine ½ ounce mint, ½ ounce skullcap (Scutellaria lateriflora) and ½ ounce pennyroyal (Mentha pulegium) and steep for 30 minutes in a pint of freshly boiled water. Sweeten and give to the child in teaspoon doses.

Caution: do not give honey to an infant as the bacteria could prove fatal.

Mint tea: 2-3 tsp. leaf per 1 cup of water, take 1-2 cups a day for no more than 8 days. Then stop for a week.

Lore: senna (Cassia spp.), mint (Mentha spp.) and rue (Ruta graveolens) are plaited and worn as a bracelet, necklace or crown to repel evil. Scatter mint leaves around food to deter mice, they loathe the smell. Oil of peppermint is repulsive to rats. In my personal experience, mint is a wonderful motivator that attracts success with finances and other projects. Add the oil to shampoos, soaps and the bath water while visualizing your intent.

Mistletoe, European Mistletoe

Parts used: leaves and twigs

Gaelic: *uil'- íoc, druidh-lus, súgh dharaich*
(All-heal, The Druid's Herb, Juice of the Oak)

Latin: *Viscum album*

Caution: be sure you are using only Viscum album. Other species are very harsh and abortive and can be poisonous to humans.

The stems and leaves are used for fevers and heart conditions, mixed with ivy (Hedera helix). Mistletoe is a tonic for epilepsy and convulsive nervous conditions including urinary and heart conditions of a nervous origin, and it helps stop internal bleeding. It is used for very high fevers such as typhoid. It reduces blood pressure and slows the pulse after an initial rise. It enhances the immune system and fights tumors: a preparation is made from it called Iscador, which is used to shrink cancerous tumors. Combine mistletoe with skullcap (Scutellaria lateriflora) and valerian (Valeriana officinalis) for nervous conditions; with motherwort (Leonurus cardiaca) and hawthorn (Crataegus oxyacantha) for myocarditis; with blue cohosh (Caulophyllum thalictroides) for irregular menstruation; with hawthorn (Crataegus oxyacantha) and lime flowers (Tillia spp.) for hypertension.

Caution: the berries are poisonous. Large amounts of this herb can damage the heart. I have successfully used this plant to help a person with the neurological effects of Lyme disease, but they still had to use standard antibiotics to purge the organism from their system.

Steep 1 tsp. twigs and leaves per 1 cup of freshly boiled water, for about 20 minutes. Take ¼ cup, 4 times a day.

Lore: mistletoe is sacred to the God of Love Balder, which is why it is common to kiss under it at the Winter Solstice. It is placed in the marriage bed to promote fertility. It is one of the most sacred plants of the Druids, when found growing on an oak. Of interest, modern studies have shown that the most potent anti-tumor activity is seen in the plants that are found growing on old oak trees (the plant can also be found growing on old apple trees and other tree species). A sprig of mistletoe is cut on Samhuinn Eve with a new dirk after circumambulating the tree three times deiseil. Thus collected, it makes a charm against Witchcraft and brings good luck in battle. It can be placed in the bairn's cradle to prevent abduction by Fairies (be sure to put it in a place where the bairn won't eat it, for example under the mattress).

Monkshood, Aconite, Wolf's Bane

Parts used: the leaf and root

Gaelic: *fuath a' mhadaidh* (wolf's bane)

Latin: *Aconitum napellus*

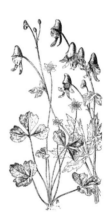

This herb is poisonous. Its common name, wolf's bane, tells the tale. It is anti-bacterial, antifungal, anti-viral, and historically was used for fevers.

Caution: do not attempt internal use without expert supervision. Even a small amount can be fatal. Add the leaves and root to liniments for arthritis pain and gout.

Motherwort

Parts used: the flowering tops and the leaves

Gaelic: *lus-leíghis* (healing herb)

Latin: *Leonurus cardiaca*

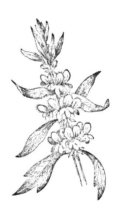

This plant is calming to nervous heart problems and heart palpitations. It relieves stomach pains and gas, while it dispels depression, and aids in nervous irritability during menopause. It is also helpful in fevers that produce delirium and a nervous state, chest congestion, shortness of breath, neuritis and neuralgia. Use the tea externally as a wash for fresh wounds.

Caution: it can cause contact dermatitis in some people. Steep 1 tsp. of the flowering tops and leaves per ½ cup of water and take ¼ cup a day.

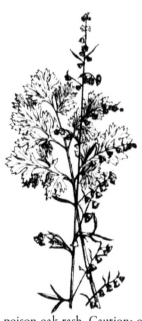

Mugwort

Parts used: flowering herb and the root
(in the fall)

Gaelic: *liathus*

Latin: *Artemisia vulgaris*

A pot herb when eaten young, dried mugwort can be smoked as herbal tobacco for those trying to wean themselves from cigarettes. Mix it with spearmint (Mentha spicata), sumac (Rhus glabra) leaves (harvested when red in the fall), coltsfoot (Tussilago farfara) and mullein (Verbascum thapsus) leaf to make an herbal smoking blend. For anorexia, gather mugwort and nettles (Urtica dioica) in spring, and take them as broth or as cooked greens. Mugwort tea is helpful for heart palpitations, PMS and to regulate the menses. It makes a bath for gout, rheumatism and tired legs. Apply a fresh poultice or the juice to poison oak rash. Caution: overdose can cause poisoning. A mild infusion helps the digestion and the appetite and is helpful at the onset of a cold or fever. Take it as tea, or add it to the bathwater.

Caution: this plant is an emmenagogue (brings on the menses) and should be avoided by pregnant women.

Juice: 1 tsp. of the fresh juice can be taken in water for fever.

Tea: steep 1 tbsp. of the dried herb per ½ cup water for 20 minutes. Take 1/8 cup, 4 times a day.

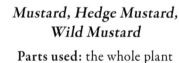

Mustard, Hedge Mustard, Wild Mustard

Parts used: the whole plant

Gaelic: *sgeallag, praiseach gharbh*

Latin: *Sisymbrium officinale*

Wild mustard is eaten as a cooked green when young. Mustard, the kind you can buy at the supermarket, is also a powerful healing agent. Powdered mustard is added to the bath to relieve cold symptoms (steep 7-9 ounces for a full bath), or steep your feet for five minutes in a mustard foot bath (steep 3-4 ounces for a foot bath). Then, drink a hot toddy and get into bed immediately.

Classic Hot Toddy:
1 in malt whisky
2 in boiling hot water, poured over a silver spoon
1 generous tsp of heather honey
1 slice of lemon

(Cinnamon stick, clove and/or freshly grated ginger can also be added to a hot toddy)

For pneumonia and pleurisy, apply a mustard poultice to the lung area. To make the poultice: mix powdered mustard with water to make a paste and spread on a linen cloth. Place gauze over the plaster then lay the plaster on the skin.

Caution: mustard plasters can cause skin irritation. Watch carefully to make sure the skin does not burn. Leave the plaster on until the burning sensation becomes too painful, wipe away any remaining plaster with an herbal salve, and cover the area with a dry cotton cloth. Any residual irritation will disappear in a few days. Never apply a mustard plaster to sensitive areas. For those with delicate skin, cut the mixture with rye, rice or buckwheat flour to lessen burning.

Tea: a strong infusion of the herb helps with loss of voice and sore throats. Mustard is an antiseptic and a sterilizing agent. It can even be used to remove nasty scents from old jars, bottles, etc. by soaking them in a mustard and water mix.

Nettles

Parts used: the herb,
(collected just before flowering)

Gaelic: *deanntag, feanntag*

Latin: *Urtica urens*

The young greens are added to soups, made into clear broth, or cooked as a pot herb. Nettle broth (cál deanntaig) is helpful for coughs, upset stomach, and rheumatic complaints. Nettles are warming to the system and very rich in iron, support the kidneys and bladder, and nourish the blood. The root tea is beneficial for chest complaints such as tuberculosis and other persistent coughs, and for kidney centered edema. The leaf poultice is applied to wounds to stop bleeding.

Caution: nettles have an acid that burns the skin. Collect the herb using garden gloves, or rubber gloves, and rinse with clear cold water. The acid that causes the burning will wash off very quickly and easily.

To make a nourishing food for invalids, or for a spring tonic, mix the spring gathered greens with oatmeal. Nettle juice is helpful to stop internal bleeding and can be applied to a cloth to stop nosebleeds. The juice of the root or leaf mixed with honey helps asthma and bronchitis. The fresh leaves are steeped to make a wash for burns and skin irritations. Burn and inhale the dried leaves for asthma and bronchitis. Decoct the seeds and then add them to the leaf tea for tuberculosis and intermittent fever. Simmer nettles with violet leaves (Viola odorata) and whey to benefit fevers and nerve conditions. Cook nettles with egg whites to promote restful sleep. Add dried nettles to the fodder of sickly horses, feed cooked nettles to pigs, and add nettles to chicken feed to increase egg production. The stems are pounded and woven into cloth; cut and dry the stems, then steep them, and allow rotting until the outer part of the stem is weakened; separate the outer fibers from the bast fibers, and then hackle until soft enough to spin by drawing the fibers repeatedly through long, sharp spikes set into a board. The more hackling, the softer will be the resulting fiber*. Spin with the fibers to make "nettle–cloth" or use the cord to make ropes and twine for fishnets. Nettles are also used to make paper and nettle beer.

Nettle tea: steep 2-3 tbsp leaf per 1 cup of water. Juice: take 1-2 tbsp. with water. (*Leona Stonebridge Arthen, master dyer and weaver, personal conversation)

Lore: The Romans practiced "urtication" or flailing themselves with nettles, to keep warm.

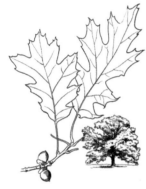

Oak, White Oak

Parts used: the bark, acorns, leaves and galls

Gaelic: *darach*

Latin: *Quercus alba*

A tea is made from the decocted inner bark or leaves. The leaves must be gathered before Summer Solstice, because after that they will contain too much natural plant poison. White Oak is the most palatable of the oaks when used internally, though other oaks can be used for wound washes and other external applications. White oak tea is helpful for sore throats and chest congestion, intermittent fever, internal bleeding, and as a wound wash. The tea is also helpful for diarrhea, dysentery, and makes a gargle for bleeding gums and sore throat, a douche for leucorrhea, and a wash or compress for piles. For fever, mix the spring gathered leaves or inner bark with chamomile flowers (Anthemis nobilis). Oak galls (the round excrescences produced by insects) are even more astringent and can be made into a tea for dysentery, diarrhea and cholera, to stop bleeding and to bathe hemorrhoids. Dry and powder the acorns to dust old ulcers and infected wounds.

To make an oak bath: simmer 8 ounces of the bark in 7 pints of water for 20 minutes and add to the bath water.

To make a wound wash, wash for piles, etc.: simmer 1-2 pounds of inner bark in 2 quarts of water until the liquid is halved.

Oak tea: simmer 1 tsp. inner bark per ½ cup water, for 20 minutes. Take ¼ cup, 4 times a day.

Lore: oak is the king of the trees and very sacred to Druids. It is revered as a tree that spans the three worlds, with its roots that go down as far as the tree is high.

It attracts lightning, marking it as a tree of the Gods. The parasitic mistletoe that grows on oak partakes of its life-sap, making it equally sacred. Women can hug an oak to ensure easy childbirth. When swearing an oath it is traditional to say: "By oak and ash and thorn". It is said that where oak and ash and thorn (hawthorn) grow together, you are likely to see Fairies.

Oats

Parts used: the grains and straw

Gaelic: *corc*

Latin: *Avena sativa*

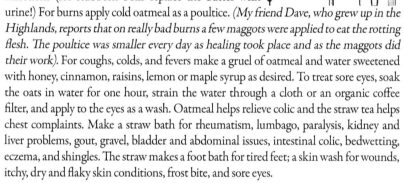

Oats have been a household staple since Roman times. Apply hot oats and butter as a poultice to boils and infections (for stubborn boils replace the butter with urine!) For burns apply cold oatmeal as a poultice. *(My friend Dave, who grew up in the Highlands, reports that on really bad burns a few maggots were applied to eat the rotting flesh. The poultice was smaller every day as healing took place and as the maggots did their work).* For coughs, colds, and fevers make a gruel of oatmeal and water sweetened with honey, cinnamon, raisins, lemon or maple syrup as desired. To treat sore eyes, soak the oats in water for one hour, strain the water through a cloth or an organic coffee filter, and apply to the eyes as a wash. Oatmeal helps relieve colic and the straw tea helps chest complaints. Make a straw bath for rheumatism, lumbago, paralysis, kidney and liver problems, gout, gravel, bladder and abdominal issues, intestinal colic, bedwetting, eczema, and shingles. The straw makes a foot bath for tired feet; a skin wash for wounds, itchy, dry and flaky skin conditions, frost bite, and sore eyes.

Oat straw tea: simmer the straw in water for one hour, add honey to taste.

Oat bath: simmer 2 pounds of straw in 3 quarts of water for 30 minutes, strain and add to the bath. Or tie 1 pound of oatmeal into gauze and soak it in very hot water. Pour the water into the bath and use the gauze pack as a sponge.

Lore: to cure warts take nine times nine (eighty one) oat stems and bundle them into nine bunches of nine stems each, and hide them under a stone. As they wither, so will the wart.

Onion

Parts used: the bulb

Gaelic: *uinnean*

Latin: *Allium cepa*

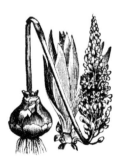

For pneumonia, boil two onions and place one under each armpit. For bad knees, chop onions and garlic, mix with a small amount of chopped foxglove leaf

(Digitalis purpurea) and butter, and use the mixture to poultice the knee. For diphtheria, apply the same poultice to the neck. Eat fresh onions daily to ward off heart attack and stroke, and to lower blood pressure. Onions (and garlic) are very cleansing to the arteries. Drop 2 or 3 drops of the juice into the ears for ear ache. Apply raw onion as a poultice to burns. Apply roasted onions as a poultice to hard tumors and to gout. Onions (also leeks, garlic and chives) reduce the risk of stomach cancer. Onions help restore sexual desire after a long illness and after severe stress. Eaten with bread they can help relieve an upset stomach and gas. Mix the juice of fresh onions with honey for coughs, and apply the juice or a poultice of the mashed bulb to infected wounds (I have seen raw onion slush stop gangrene from spreading. The person soaked their gangrenous foot in a bucket of chopped and blended onion several times a day for an hour each time, took the herb echinacea internally, and applied calendula ointment to the wound).

Lore: cut an onion in half and hang one half outside of the window. Leave the other half above the door of the sick room to absorb disease.

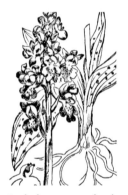

Orchids

Parts used: the root

Gaelic: *dá-dhuilleach, úrach bhallach*

Latin: *Listera ovata, Orchis maculata*

The Twyblade or Twayblade (from two leaves or blades) orchid (Listera ovata) is used in formulas to heal the stomach and bowels. The spotted orchid (Orchis maculata, Dactylorhiza maculata) is used to poultice the flesh when splinters, glass, or dirt are embedded in it. Orchids are reputed to have aphrodisiac qualities; their roots soothe and nourish the whole body and can be added to tonic formulas. A poultice of the root cures scrofula (tuberculosis of the cervical lymph nodes) and is applied to tumors.

Lore: Witches use the fresh roots in love spells. A withered root is used to curtail desire or affection. The purple orchis Lus an Tálaidh (the enticing plant) has two roots, the larger root is male and the smaller root is female. Pull the plant by the roots before sunrise while facing south. Assign a name to a root, either for a man or for a woman. Place whichever root is to be used in spring water before sunrise. If it sinks, the person named will be your future spouse. The root can also be dried and powdered and put in your pillow to dream of your future spouse. If you take the root of the appropriate sex and have a person of the opposite sex consume it, they will be made to fall in love with you.

Caution: before you inject any part of an orchid make sure it is from an organic source. Restaurants may offer orchid flowers as a garnish, for example, but they are probably heavily contaminated with pesticides. The other root will cause antipathy. For this reason, in the Highlands the plant is called grádh is fuadh (love and hate). **A note of caution:** any love that is manipulated or coerced by magic will fade away after marriage.

Parsley

Parts used: the dried root,
seeds and leaves, juice

Gaelic: *pearsal*

Latin: *Carum petroselinum*

Parsley is a diuretic herb that is warming to the system
and an activator of the thyroid. It is helpful for edema,
bladder issues, amenorrhea, colic, inflamed prostate and menopausal hot flashes.

Caution: pregnant women and those with kidney disease should avoid this plant,
and it should not be taken during a fever.

Apply a poultice to the breasts of nursing mothers to dry up breast milk (also have
them drink sage tea (Salvia officinalis) at the same time). Parsley strengthens hair,
nails, skin, the liver and gall bladder. It benefits jaundice, asthma, coughs and
gallstones. Added to green juices such as wheat grass, it is very supportive of the
lungs. Apply the herb as a poultice for wounds. The seeds contain Apiol, a carotene
precursor, Vitamins C, E, Folic Acid (B9), bioflavonoids, iron and other minerals.

Tea: simmer 1 tsp. per 1 cup of water for 5 minutes and take ¼ cup, 4 times a day.

Seed tea: simmer 2 sp. per 1 cup of water and take ¼ cup, 4 times a day. Juice: 1-2 tsp.
in water or mixed with carrot juice or other green juices, such as wheat grass.

Pellitory of Spain

Parts used: the herb and dried root

Gaelic: *lus na Spainnte*

Latin: *Anthemis pyrethrum*

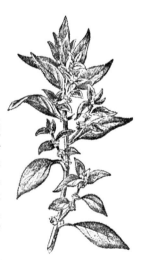

The tea is useful for fevers, or you can take 1
ounce of the juice, one hour before an expected
bout of intermittent fever. It will gradually
dispel the fever by the third dose. The root is
used in salves for gout, sciatica and bruising.
For paralysis of the tongue and lips, neuralgic
or rheumatic afflictions of the face and head,
gargle the tea daily or chew the root daily for
several months.

Leaf tea: steep 2 tsp. dried herb per 1 cup water
for 20 minutes.

Root tea: simmer 2 tsp. dried root per 1 cup of water for 20 minutes. Take
¼ cup, 4 times a day.

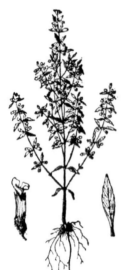

Pennyroyal

Parts used: the herb

Gaelic: *peighinn ríoghail*

Latin: *Mentha pulegium*

Simmer raspberry root (Rubus spp.) and then steep with pennyroyal leaf for asthma and bronchitis. Pennyroyal helps gas, colic, stomach upset and nausea, fever, measles and whooping cough. It promotes menstruation and eases cramps and pain.

Caution: pregnant women should avoid this herb as it can be abortive.

The tea is used as an external wash for rash, itch, and skin eruptions.

Tea: steep (do not simmer or the volatile oils will be lost) 1 tsp. herb per cup of water for about 20 minutes. Take ¼ cup, 4 times a day.

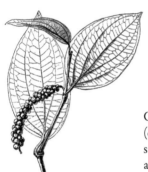

Pepper, Black Pepper

Parts used: the dried, unripe fruits

Gaelic: *peabar*

Latin: *piper nigrum*

Ground pepper is applied as styptic to stop bleeding (cayenne pepper or Capsicum frutescens, does the same – keep both on hand in the kitchen in case of accidents). Black pepper has antiseptic properties, is anti-bacterial and insecticidal (a reason why it was liberally used to preserve foods in ancient times). It helps constipation, aids digestion, nausea and gas, and is useful for diarrhea. Add it to febrifuge teas. The decoction of the seeds is used as a wash for tinea capitis, a fungal infection of the hair and scalp.

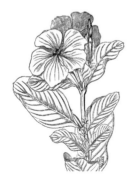

Periwinkle, Lesser Periwinkle

Parts used: the leaves and flowers

Gaelic: *faochag*

Latin: *Vinca minor*

The leaves are astringent and used in salves and washes for bruising and skin irritations, skin cancer and bleeding piles. The leaves may be chewed and placed in the nose, or packed into the mouth, after a tooth is pulled, to stop bleeding. The tea also helps excessive menstrual flow and it is soothing to the nerves (it is slightly sedative). It improves memory after head injury, stroke and other neurological issues; aids diarrhea, lung congestion, and hemorrhages. It can be beneficial for colitis and diarrhea. Gargle the tea for sore throat and tonsillitis, and take it internally for piles. The flowers are gently laxative when used fresh and may be made into a syrup with honey (simmer gently) and given to children or adults.

Caution: do not take more than the recommended amounts. Overdose could result in toxicity varying from mild abdominal cramping to skin flushing and serious cardiac complications. Stop taking it if you develop a headache.

Leaf tea: steep 1 tsp. of leaves per cup of water for about 20 minutes. Take ¼ cup, 4 times a day (not with meals).

Pine

Parts used: resin, needles, buds, shoots

Gaelic: *pin-chrann, giuthas*

Latin: *Pinus spp.*

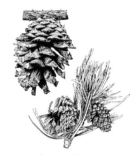

A salve is made with pine resin which is gathered as it drips down the outer bark of the tree. It can be used fresh or dry. To make the salve melt the resin in lard (or olive oil) and bees wax. Heat gently until everything is melted and spread onto a linen cloth and use it to plaster boils and sores. The warm plaster is kept on for 12 hours, and then discarded. Bathe the affected part and apply a second plaster. Scotch pine or Norway pine (Pinus sylvestris) needles and shoots are simmered to make an antiseptic wound wash or an anti-viral and expectorant tea for coughs and fevers. The resin can also be burned when dry and powdered in a mortar and pestle. It makes a nice incense when ignited on a charcoal briquette.

Plantain

Parts used: the whole herb

Gaelic: *cuach Phádraig, slánlus*

Latin: *Plantago major, P. lanceolata*

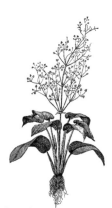

Fresh plantain leaves are chewed or ground to poultice bites, wounds, skin problems and hemorrhoids; and are steeped to make a douche for leucorrhea. The ground or chewed leaves are styptic for wounds.

Caution: in general it is best to soak fresh wild plants in water to which a few tablespoons of vinegar or sea salt have been added for 20 minutes to remove parasites before chewing or ingesting.

Chew the fresh leaves and pack them around infected teeth and gums to pull out pus and suppuration. Plantain can be added to healing salves and poultices. For tonsillitis, apply a plantain poultice to the neck. Plantain is soothing to insect stings. The lower side of the leaf is said to draw infection when laid on a sore. For diarrhea, vomiting, profuse menstruation or any other acute discharges, simmer the leaves in water into which a piece of red-hot quartz has been dropped. In a burn salve, use a mixture of plantain leaf, black currant leaf (Ribes nigrum), elder buds (Sambucus nigra), angelica (Angelica archangelica) root, and parsley (Carum petroselinum). For a skin healing salve, combine plantain, celandine (Chelidonium majus), elder buds and young leaves (Sambucus nigra), and houseleek (Sempervivum tectorum). The tea benefits diarrhea, piles, coughs, mucus congestion, gastro-intestinal problems, worms, bladder problems and stomach ulcers. Chew the roots to temporarily relieve toothache.

Tea: steep 1 tsp. leaf per ½ cup water for 20 minutes and take ¼ cup, 4 times a day.

Seeds: for thrush, simmer 1 ounce of the seeds per 1½ pints water until 1 pint remains. Add honey and feed in tablespoon doses, 4 times a day.

Juice: 5 tsp. a day of the fresh juice is taken in milk or soup for lung conditions, bowel and digestive problems, worms, bladder complaints, stomach ulcers.

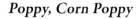

Poppy, Corn Poppy

Parts used: flowers and seeds

Gaelic: *meilbheag*

Latin: *Papaver rhoeas*

Put the seeds into a clean handkerchief, tie it, and allow the bairn to suck on it, to help with teething and to bring restful sleep (see Chamomile). Simmer the heads in honey or wine to make a syrup for coughs and for insomnia. Infuse the petals for asthma, bronchitis, catarrh, whooping cough, and angina. This is a wild variety of poppy that is only slightly narcotic, unlike the opium poppy of Asia Minor.

Tea: steep ½ ounce of the dried petals per 2 pints of water. Take ¼ cup, 4 times a day.

Lore: the smoke from yellow poppy is used to repel evil Spirits.

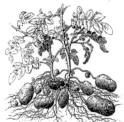

Potato

Parts used: the roots and plant

Gaelic: *buntáta*

Latin: *Solanum tuberosum*

Introduced into the Highlands and Western Isles in 1725, by 1840 about ¾ of all food consumed in those areas was the potato. As a result, the potato famine of 1840 hit hard. Put a slice of raw potato on a black eye. For nose bleed, put raw potato slices on the back of the neck. For fever and chest complaints, make a poultice of cooked, mashed potato and fresh, grated ginger. Apply the warm poultice to the lung area to break up congestion and draw out fever. Raw potato juice can be applied to gout, rheumatism, lumbago, sprains, bruises, and synovitis (joint inflammation).

To bathe rheumatic parts: simmer 1 pound of unpeeled potatoes, cut in quarters, in 2 pints of water until only 1 pint of liquid remains. Apply the hot liquid to swollen rheumatic parts. Or steep the cut up roots with the fresh stalks and berries for several hours in cold water and apply as a cold compress. Mash raw potato in a mortar and apply to burns and scalds.

For frost-bite: mash baked potato with oil and apply.

Lore: Carry a slice of raw potato in your pocket to cure rheumatism.

Primrose

Parts used: the root and herb

Gaelic: *sóbhrag*

Latin: *Primula vulgaris*

Apply a primrose leaf poultice to burns, cuts and boils. Add the leaves to healing salves. The root tea can be taken in tablespoon doses for headache. The whole plant is sedative and helpful for nervous conditions.

Flower tea: steep 1 ounce of the petals per 1 pint of water and take ¼ cup, 4 times a day.

Root tea: simmer 1 tablespoon root per cup of water for about 20 minutes. Take in tablespoon doses for nervous headaches.

Puffball
(Mushroom)

Parts used: the young mushroom and the powdery inner spores of the mature mushroom

Gaelic: *caochag*

Latin: *Bovista nigrescens*

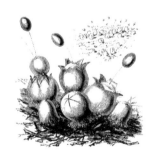

A very ancient food and medicine, we have evidence that this was a healing agent used by the Picts from sites such as Skara Brae in Orkney. The young mushrooms are eaten as food. The powdery inner tissues of the mature mushroom are applied to wounds to stop bleeding. The sliced, fresh young mushrooms can be placed on a burn. Smoke from burning puffballs is used to stupefy bees in order to safely collect honey.

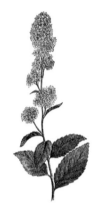

Queen of the Meadow, Meadowsweet

Parts used: the herb

Gaelic: *Crios Chu-chulainn*

(CuChulainn's belt)

Latin: *Filipendula ulmaria*

According to tradition, the hero and warrior CuChulainn was cured of a fever by soaking in a meadowsweet bath. Use the herb for headaches and fevers. It contains salicylic acid (the active ingredient in both willow bark and aspirin) which makes it anti-inflammatory. Taken as tea, it helps flu, lung conditions, gout, rheumatism, arthritis, edema, bladder and kidney problems, and diarrhea. Use it as an external wash for wounds and eye irritations (be sure to filter it through an organic coffee filter before putting it into the eyes). Steep 2 tbsp. of the herb per cup of water for about 20 minutes and take ¼ cup, 4 times a day, or simmer 2 tbsp of the dried root per 1 cup of water for about 20 minutes and take ¼ cup, 4 times a day.

Juice: 1 tbsp. a day, taken in water.

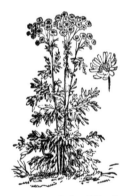

Ragwort, European Ragwort

Parts used: the herb

Gaelic: *buaghallan*

Latin: *Senecio jacobea*

To ripen a boil or a tumor, chop the herb and mix it with butter. Apply the warmed poultice to swollen and hard breasts, and to tumors and boils, to ripen them.

Caution: this plant can harm the liver and should not be taken internally.

Lore: it is said that Witches and Fairies travel by riding the stalks.

Raspberry

Parts used: the leaves and fruits

Gaelic: *preas súbh chraobh*

Latin: *Rubus idaeus*

Simmer mint (Mentha spp.), bogbean (Menyanthes trifoliata) and raspberry leaves to make a tea that relieves the after effects of liver ailments. Raspberry leaf tea should be taken throughout pregnancy to ease morning sickness and to relax and strengthen the uterus in preparation for childbirth. The leaf tea also benefits diarrhea, is used as a gargle and a mouthwash, and as a wash for wounds, sores, and rashes. The juice of the berries is cooling to fevers. Mix the berry juice with red wine and red wine vinegar, simmer with a few sprigs of parsley, to make a tonic for the heart (take a few tablespoons daily).

Leaf tea: steep 2 tbsp. leaf per ½ cup water and take ¼ cup, 4 times a day.

Rhubarb

Parts used: the roots and stalks
(the leaves are poisonous)

Gaelic: *luibh na purgaid*

Latin: *Rheum rhaponticum, Rheum palmatum*

Eat multiple servings of cooked rhubarb stalks to relieve "itching in the flesh" (eczema, acne, urticaria, etc.). The root is laxative, but not for prolonged use. A cold extract of the root increases appetite (soak the root in cold water for 10 hours). For a laxative effect take ¼ cup, twice a day.

Root tea: simmer 1 tsp. chopped root in ½ cup water.

For diarrhea: simmer ¼ tsp. root in ½ cup water and take ¼ cup, twice a day.

Caution: pregnant and nursing mothers should avoid this plant.

Rose

Parts used: red flowers, hips, leaves, stalks

Gaelic: *rós*

Latin: *Rosa spp.*

For erysipelas (strep infection of the skin), make a decoction of the rose wood and leaves and apply it. Rose leaves can be chopped and simmered gently with butter and that can also be applied by spreading it on a clean cloth. At the same time, a tea of stonecrop (Sedum album) or Herb Robert (Geranium Rrobertianum) is taken internally. The dried petals of red roses (please be sure you are using an old fashioned variety with a strong fragrance, not a modern scentless genetically altered variety!) are infused for headaches and to make a heart and nerve tonic that is purifying to the blood. Simmer the petals to make a wash for mouth sores. Simmer (never boil) red roses in red wine to make a remedy for uterine cramps and for exhaustion. Apply the rose and wine decoction to the forehead as a compress for headaches. Warm it and pour it into a sore ear. Rose honey can be used for sore throats – simmer the petals or fresh hips gently in the honey (be sure to use only the peel of the hips, remove the seeds and hairs). Rose vinegar makes a compress for headaches. Gather the petals before the flower opens fully.

Rose tea: simmer 2 tsp hips per cup of water for about 20 minutes or steep 2 tsp. blossoms per cup of freshly boiled water for 20 minutes.

Rose honey: pound the petals and/or fresh hips with a little boiling hot water. Strain and then simmer the liquid with honey.

Rose vinegar: steep the petals of red roses in vinegar, but do not heat.

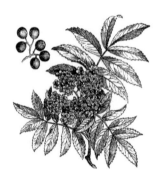

Rowan, European Mountain Ash

Parts used: the berries

Gaelic: *caorann, fid na ndruad*
(The Wizard's Tree)

Latin: *Sorbus aucuparia*
(note: while S. aucuparia has red berries, Sorbus Americana, American Mountain Ash, has identical properties and orange berries. They can be used interchangeably)

The juice of the ripe red berries is laxative and makes a gargle for sore throats. Simmer the berries and strain the liquid to make a Vitamin C rich gargle for tonsillitis. The fresh berry juice is slightly laxative, but once cooked the berries become astringent and anti-diarrheal. In the Highlands, a syrup is made with rowan berries, honey and apples, to treat colds. The berries are made into a jam that benefits diarrhea and is safe for young children.

Rowan Berry Jam
1 part ripe berries (gather after the first frost)
½ part sugar or ¼ part honey
1 part apples

Take 1 tbsp. of the jam, 3-5 times a day for diarrhea in adults and children.

Juice: 1 tsp. fresh berry juice can be taken in water.

Dried berries: soak 1 tsp. dried berries per 1 cup of water for 10 hours and take ¼ cup, 4 times a day.

Lore: possibly the most ubiquitous magical plant of the Highlands, every house once strove to have a rowan tree nearby. Twigs, wreaths and crosses of rowan were placed in the home and barn as protective charms and furniture, cradles, boats, tools, carts, and houses were made of rowan wood to bring luck and protection from evil sorcery.

"The Hags came back, finding their charms,
Most powerfully withstood,
For Warlocks, Witches cannot work,
Where there is rowan tree wood."
(Laidley Worm, Traditional)

Rowan twigs bound with red thread were tied to an animal's tail to protect it from the Evil Eye.

"Rowan tree and red thread gar the Witches tyne their speed". (make, lose) (Traditional)

Put a sprig of rowan on your hat for luck, or sew a tiny equal-armed Solar Cross of rowan, bound with red thread, into your clothing. Carry rowan to ward off rheumatism.

Rowan berries are said to be the food of the Tuatha Dé Danann (the Fairies) which is why they are often seen near stone cairns and circles in Scotland. Rowan wood was once used to make the cross-beam in the chimney called the "rantree" (rowan tree). The churn staffs, the distaff of the loom, the pin of the plough, and parts of the watermill, were all made from rowan to bring magical aid and protection. Rowan was planted near the house door and trained to grow in an arch over the barn door or the farm gate, to keep evil from entering. At the Fire Festivals, a rowan wand was placed on all the door lintels and a piece in every pocket. Rowan wood was used to build the ritual fires upon which bannocks were baked on holy days. Coffins were made of rowan wood to prevent the dead from returning to haunt the living. Make a wooden knife or athame of rowan wood to use in your rites and ceremonies. It will protect your circle from all harm. Why use a metal athame or knife when the Fairies despise iron?

Rue, Meadow Rue

Parts used: the herb

Gaelic: *rú beag*

Latin: *Thalictrum minus,
Thalictrum alpinus*

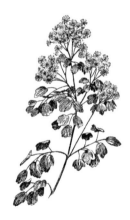

The infusion was used for worms.

Caution: this plant belongs to a poisonous family and should only be used with expert supervision.

Sage

Parts used: the leaf
(collected just before flowering)

Gaelic: *sáiste*

Latin: *Salvia officinalis*

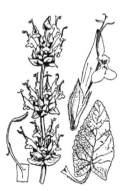

A poultice of the leaves can be applied to cuts and bruises, insect bites, and stings. The tea of the leaf dries up breast milk and helps dieters stop their cravings for sweets, such as chocolate. The tea is very drying and useful for wet lung conditions, and makes a gargle for a sore throat or tonsillitis. Use the tea for night sweats, nervous conditions, depression, vertigo, to regulate menstruation, diarrhea, and bowel inflammations. Chop the herb and mix it with oats to worm a horse. Chew the leaves, and then insert them into the ear of a sheep or cow to restore eyesight.

Sage tea: steep 1 tsp. per ½ cup of freshly boiled water for 30 minutes. Take ¼ cup, 4 times a day.

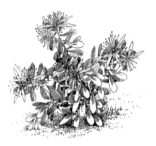

Saint John's Wort

Parts used: the herb

Gaelic: *lus na fala (blood wort),*
achlasan chalium chille
(armpit package of Saint Columba)

Latin: *Hypericum perforatum,*
Hypericum pulchrum

Place a poultice of the herb in the armpits to relieve nervous conditions and terrors. Use the herb in salves and butter ointments with germander (Betonica pauli) and goldenrod (Solidago spp.) to treat wounds, burns, bruising and skin problems. A tea of the herb can be used as a wash to staunch bleeding. Taken internally, Saint John's Wort tea calms bladder hysteria, bed wetting and insomnia, cramps and other menstrual disorders. The flower tea is useful for mild depression, nervous afflictions, anemia, headache, jaundice and chest congestion.

Caution: use only in the dark half of the year when you are least likely to have sun exposure on large patches of skin. In the Northern hemisphere that would be roughly October to April. Prolonged use of the plant causes photo-sensitivity in both humans and livestock, and it may also be poisonous to livestock. [For those who have found the herb helpful in Seasonal Affective Disorder or mild depression, I recommend switching to Kava-Kava (Piper methysticum) and Damiana (Turnera aphrodisiaca) in the light half of the year].

Herb tea: steep 1 tsp. dried herb per ½ cup freshly boiled water for 5 minutes. Take ½ cup (warmed) on waking and ½ cup before bed.

Lore:

> "Trefoil, vervain,
> St John's Wort, dill,
> hinders Witches in their will".
> *(Traditional)*

If found unsought, wild Saint John's Wort can prevent fevers and abduction by Fairies, especially if it is found on Saint John's Eve. It is named for the fact that, in Britain it blooms around Saint John's Eve (near the summer solstice). The ancient Celts smoked it over the Midsummer fire to make a protective charm.

Scabious, Devil's Bit

Parts used: the dried herb

Gaelic: *ura bhallach*

Latin: *Scabiosa succisa, Scabiosa pratensis*

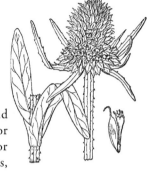

Apply the root poultice to itching body parts and to toothaches. The root is simmered in wine for fever, and for internal bruising as from a fall or a blow. The herb tea benefits coughs and fevers, purifies the blood, and makes a gargle for a sore throat or tonsillitis. Use the tea externally as a wash for skin eruptions, pimples, sores, and dandruff. Apply the fresh juice to wounds and old sores. Add the plant to salves for the same.

Herb tea: use 1 ounce of the dried herb per 1 pint of boiled water, steep for 20 minutes.

Root tea: simmer 1 ounce of the chopped roots in 1 pint of wine. Take ¼ cup every 2 hours until perspiration starts.

Scurvy-Grass, Spoonwort

Parts used: the fresh leaves and juice

Gaelic: *am maraiche* (the sailor), *carran, pláigh na carra*

Latin: *Cochlearia officinalis*

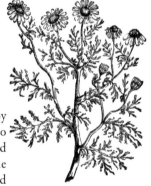

Rich in Vitamin C, this plant was used by fishermen and Vikings on long voyages to prevent scurvy. It was eaten at breakfast to ward off disease and to strengthen the stomach. The herb makes a poultice for cramps and boils, and taken internally the tea benefits edema, rheumatism and venereal diseases. A few teaspoons of the fresh juice can be added to orange juice or other fresh juices to make a spring tonic. This herb must be used fresh to be effective.

Tea: infuse 2 ounces per 1 pint of freshly boiled water for about 20 minutes and take ¼ cup, 4 times a day.

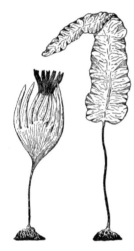

Seaweeds

Parts used: the whole plant,
still clinging to a rock, and
gathered in a non polluted, pristine ocean

Gaelic: *feamainn*

Latin: *alga*

Seaweeds are some of the only sources of exotic trace minerals still available for the human diet. As agriculture has adulterated the soil with chemical fertilizers and pesticides, and as precious top soil has run off into streams, rivers, and the sea, it is nearly impossible to get all necessary nutrients from land vegetables alone. Everyone needs to supplement their diet with seaweed of many colors: green, yellow, red, and brown. Seaweed should be alive when collected, that is, attached to a rock or the sea floor.

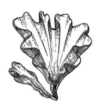

Linarich *(Sea Lettuce)*

Gaelic: *lúireach (cloak)*

Latin: *Ulva lactuca, Monostroma grevillei*

Bake in an iron pan and then put over a goiter, holding it in place with a bandage.

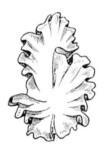

Slake, Laver

Gaelic: *slócan*

Latin: *Porphyra umbilialis*

Cook and eat with butter.

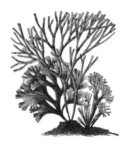

Carrageen

Gaelic: *cairgein*

Latin: *Chondrus crispus*

Gather at low tide, lay out in the sun and rain, so that it is washed and bleached. Use it in stews, puddings, and jelly, to thicken and set.

Channelled Fucus
Gaelic: *feamainn chírean*
Latin: *Fucus canaliculatus*

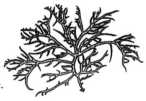

Simmer in ocean water and apply to a rheumatic knee.

Dulse
Gaelic: *duileasg*
Latin: *Palmaria palmata*

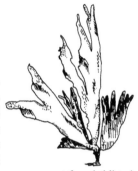

Dulse can be eaten raw, or boiled and topped with butter. Dulse soup is particularly helpful for stomach problems. Dulse improves vision and relieves colic and constipation when simmered. Drink the liquid while also eating the plant. A dulse poultice can be applied to the temples to relieve headache and migraine. Dry and powder it and take it in capsules while fasting to drive out worms. After childbirth, a poultice of the fresh plant is placed on the abdomen to expel the placenta.

Sea-Tangle
Gaelic: *stamh*
Latin: *Laminaria digitata*

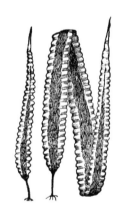

To promote appetite, simmer the plant and drink the infusion with butter added. Apply the seaweed to goiter and swellings. Seaweeds, especially brown ones like Laminaria digitata, protect the body from radiation poisoning by ensuring that the thyroid gland does not take up radioactive iodides. L. digitata is a brown kelp that grows in abundance around the shores of Scotland.

Senna
Parts used: *the leaves and fruits*
Latin: *Cassia acutifolia,*
Cassia angustifolia, Cassia fistula

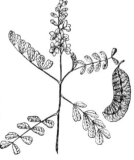

Senna is a strong laxative that must be mixed with cinnamon (Cinnamomum zeylandicum), coriander (Coriandrum sativum) or ginger (Zingiber officinale) to prevent gripping. Cassia angustifolia is the mildest in action. One teaspoon of cream of tartar may be added to senna tea.

Leaves: infuse 3½ ounces of the leaf with ½ tsp. coriander, cinnamon, or ginger in 1 quart of boiled water for 15 minutes, strain and take when cold, 1-4 tbsp. per dose.

Pods: steep 6-12 pods of Cassia fistula in about 5 tablespoons of cold water. For an elderly person or a young child use 3-6 pods.

Caution: do not use this herb if bowel inflammation, prolapsus ani, or hemorrhoids exist. Nursing mothers should avoid this herb as it will pass on to the infant via breast milk.

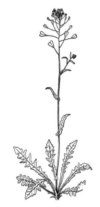

Shepherd's Purse

Parts used: the herb and juice

Gaelic: *sporran na fala, lus na fala*

Latin: *Capsella bursa-pastoris*

Apply the tea or powdered herb to wounds, and after surgery to stop bleeding. This plant regulates blood pressure and heart action. It also regulates menstruation and can be used to promote contractions in labor, and to strengthen bowel movements.

Tea: steep 1 tsp. fresh or 2 tsp. dried herb per ½ cup freshly boiled water. Take ¼ cup, 4 times a day. Juice: 1 tsp. twice a day

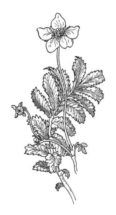

Silverweed, Cinquefoil

Parts used: the herb

Gaelic: *brisgean, barr brisgein*

Latin: *Potentilla anserina*

The roots can be eaten roasted or raw. When eating raw roots, please be sure to soak the roots in water into which a few teaspoons of salt or vinegar have been added for about 20 minutes to remove parasites. Grind the raw or roasted roots into flour to make a famine food that was once popular during the clearances (especially so because sheep won't touch it). The tea made with water or milk helps diarrhea and dysentery. To relieve cramps, mix the herb with equal parts of lemon balm (Melissa officinalis) and chamomile (Anthemis nobilis, Matricaria camomilla) in a tea. Silverweed makes an external wash for skin irritations and a gargle for mouth sores and sore throat.

Tea: simmer 2 tsp. herb per 1 cup of water or milk, steep for 20 minutes and take ¼ cup, 4 times a day.

Sneezewort

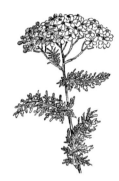

Part used: the leaf, gathered before flowering

Gaelic: *luibh bhán*

Latin: *Achillea armica*

The leaf decoction helps stomach ailments and a leaf poultice can be applied to wounds to stop bleeding. This plant is closely related to yarrow and has similar properties (see Yarrow below).

Sorrel

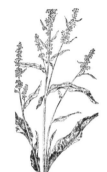

Part used: the fresh herb

Gaelic: *samh, sealbhad, puinneag, puinneagan*

Latin: *Rumex acetosa, Rumex spp.*

The fresh leaf is used in soups, and eaten raw on a journey to relieve thirst. It is a cooling herb for fevers and tuberculosis. Chew or mash the fresh leaves and apply to wounds and bruises. Dog Sorrel, sealbhag nan con, is eaten in salads. Mountain sorrel, Deer sorrel, sealbhag nam fiadh (Latin: Oxyma digyna) is also esculent. Meadow sorrel (Latin: Rumex acetosa) root tea is taken to stop bleeding in the stomach or excessive menstruation. The tea of the leaves and stems is diuretic and helpful for gravel or stones, mouth and throat irritations, ulcers, gingivitis, and bad breath. Use the leaf tea as a wash for skin ailments.

Caution: this plant is a kidney irritant if consumed in large quantities or taken for a long time. Persons with kidney diseases should avoid it.

Root tea: simmer 1 tsp. root per 1 cup of water for 20 minutes. Take ¼ cup, 4 times a day.

Leaf tea: steep the leaves and stalks for 20 minutes using 1 tsp. per cup of water and take ¼ cup, 4 times a day.

Spearwort, Spinewort

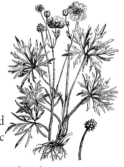

Part used: roots, stems

Gaelic: *glas-leum, lasair-theine*

Latin: *Flammula jovis, Ranunculus flammula*

The bruised plant is applied to raise blisters and inflammations. The poultice is applied to syphilitic sores, cancers, and prurient ulcers.

Caution: this is a poisonous plant that should only be used with expert supervision.

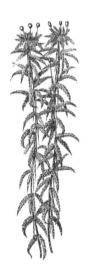

Sphagnum Moss, Bog Moss

Part used: the spongy green mat

Gaelic: *cóinneach dhearg*

Latin: *Sphagnum cymbifolium*

When dried, the moss is absorbent and antiseptic. In ancient times, it was used to diaper babies, line cribs, and dress wounds. It absorbs twice as much moisture as cotton and was used to make women's menstrual pads (in very ancient times the moss was stuffed into soft buckskin pads). For wounds, soak the moss in garlic juice and water, and apply. For sore feet, simmer alder leaves (Alnus glutinosa) and sphagnum moss, and then use the resulting tea to soak and rub the feet.

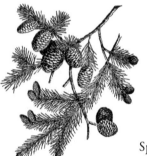

Spruce, Norway Spruce, Lakelander Spruce, Scandinavian Spruce

Part used: the young shoots

Gaelic: *giuthas lochlannach*

Latin: *Picea excelsa*

Spruce beer sweetened with molasses provides a mineral rich tonic for fevers and colds. A tonic tea is made by simmering the branch tips in water and adding molasses as a sweetener. The warm tea (with the molasses) is iron rich and antiseptic, and can be taken for coughs and flu. The branch tip tea promotes sweating and helps in fevers, and is also used to make a vapor bath for bronchitis. Simmer the new growth or needles to make a bath that is calming to the nerves.

Steep: 2 tsp. new growth per ½ cup water for 10 minutes.

Simmer: 4 ounces of the shoots per 1 quart of water for 20 minutes. Take ¼ cup twice a day.

Bath: make a strong tea using 1-5 pounds of needles or new growth.

Spurge

Part used: the resinous sap and leaf

Gaelic: *lus-léighis* (healing herb)

Latin: *Euphorbia peplus*

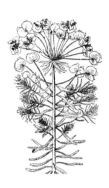

The milky sap is caustic and is applied to warts. Caution: this plant is poisonous and a violent purgative. The herb may have been used in ancient times for skin cancer. The leaf tea has been used for cholera, diarrhea, dysentery, and as an astringent douche for leucorrhea.

Caution: extreme care must be taken with this plant. It can be irritating to both skin and respiratory passages. It should only be used with expert supervision.

Stonecrop, Wall Pepper, Houseleek

Part used: the herb

Gaelic: *grábhan nan clach*

Latin: *Sedum acre*

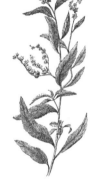

The tea is taken for erysipelas inwardly, and is used externally as a wash for ulcers, edema and intermittent fever. In very small doses, it is helpful to lower blood pressure.

Caution: large doses are emetic and purgative. The plant can cause skin irritation and blisters in sensitive people. Use only with expert supervision. This plant can be abortive, avoid during pregnancy.

Tansy

Part used: the herb

Gaelic: *lus na Frainge*

Latin: *Tanacetum vulgare*

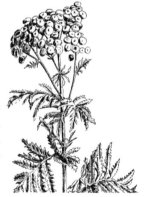

Tansy has been taken as tea or tinctured in whisky to make a vermifuge, and the leaves and flowers have been used as a wash for skin eruptions and bruises. However, it is probably too dangerous for home use. To keep flies away, tansy is mixed with elder leaves (Sambucus spp.) and used as a strewing herb.

Caution: this plant can be poisonous even when used externally. Overdose can be fatal or cause convulsions. Use only with expert supervision.

Tea, Black Tea

Part used: the dried leaf

Gaelic: *tí*

Latin: *Camellia thea, Camellia sinensis*

In the Highlands, Black Tea was taken with cloves (Caryophyllus aromaticus), nutmeg (Myristica fragrans), or caraway seed, (Carum carvi) using ½ tsp. tea plus ½ tsp. seeds or spice, for two people. "Tea" is calming to the nerves and a mild anti-depressant. Both black and green teas are anti-tumor and diuretic. Apply cooled tea bags to tired eyes, sunburn, and to the temples and forehead for headaches. Native herb teas included agrimony (Agrimonia spp.), raspberry leaf (Rubus spp.), lemon balm (Melissa officinalis), dandelion leaf (Taraxacum officinale) and wood betony (Stachys officinalis).

Caution: Black Tea should be avoided by those with peptic ulcers as the tea increases acidity in the stomach. Black Tea can reduce iron and protein absorption and overuse may lead to insomnia and B1 deficiency.

Thistle

Part used: the leaves, stem and root

Gaelic: *gíogan, cluaran, cluas an fleidh*

Latin: *Onopordon acanthium, Carduus heterophyllus, Sonchus oleraceus*

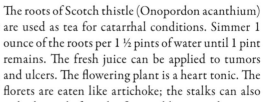

The roots of Scotch thistle (Onopordon acanthium) are used as tea for catarrhal conditions. Simmer 1 ounce of the roots per 1 ½ pints of water until 1 pint remains. The fresh juice can be applied to tumors and ulcers. The flowering plant is a heart tonic. The florets are eaten like artichoke; the stalks can also be peeled and eaten. Gather the leaves before the flowers bloom, and remove the prickles before cooking. The Melancholy thistle (cluas an fleidh) (Carduus heterophyllus) is decocted in wine to dispel depression. Sow thistle (Sonchus oleraceus) is the best tasting genus. The young spring gathered leaves are eaten raw or cooked. Add the leaves to salads and soups. Cook the stems like asparagus after removing the outer skin.

Lore: "the flower of Scotland", the thistle was adopted as the national symbol after the battle of Cargs. A Danish invader had attempted to make a surprise attack on a Scottish clan, but he stepped barefoot on a thistle, and his howls of pain foiled the attack. The thistle symbolizes strength and tenacity through adversity, thriving in the wild, damp landscape of Scotland.

Thyme, Wild Thyme, Mountain Thyme

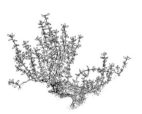

Part used: the herb

Gaelic: *lus an rígh*

Latin: *Thymus serpyllum*

A tonic for the nerves, thyme is taken as tea or made into a pillow for those with nightmares. The flowering tops are used to scent clothing and household linens. Thyme is drying and a tonic for the lungs: use it for throat and bronchial illnesses. The tea also benefits painful menstruation, diarrhea, and gastritis, lack of appetite, anemia, headache and hang over. For coughs the fresh plant works best. Mix the tea with honey and take it for heart trouble. Heat the fresh herb gently in honey and use it for whooping cough. The herb is antiseptic and can be used as a mouthwash, gargle or wound wash. The wash can also be applied to tumors, bruises, and rheumatic complaints. Drink the tea while fasting to purge hook worms and ascarids. Add the tea to the bath water, for swellings, sprains, bruises, rheumatism, paralysis and nervous exhaustion. Thyme is used in salves for shingles. Over time, the tea can cause revulsion for alcohol along with nausea, diarrhea and sweating. This "cure" will probably need to be repeated a few times.

Caution: overuse of this plant can lead to poisoning and hyper stimulation of the thyroid gland.

Tea: steep 2 tsp. fresh or 1 tsp. dry herb per 1 cup of water for 5 minutes.

Bath: make a strong decoction and add it to the bath water.

For alcoholism: ¼ cup herb steeped in 1 quart freshly boiled water for 30 minutes. Take one tbsp. every 15 minutes.

Tobacco

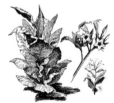

Part used: the leaf, dried and/or cured

Gaelic: *tombaca*

Latin: *Nicotiana tabacum*

The dried and shredded leaf can be applied to wounds to stop bleeding. A leaf can be rolled and inserted into the rectum as a laxative to evacuate the bowels. Apply a moist tobacco poultice to piles. The poisonous alkaloid in tobacco, nicotine, has antiseptic properties, but when smoked, it causes nausea, cardiac irregularities, arterial degeneration, impaired fetal development, emphysema, lung cancer and other cancers. The leaf should be applied sparingly to the skin and with caution. Too frequent use can lead to poisoning and even death. This plant was originally a sacred herb of Native America that was later introduced into Europe. It was meant to be a sacrament in prayer ceremonies, not for recreational or habitual use. An elder Witch and mentor of mine, Ted Mills, made me promise to warn all young people about the dangers of this highly addictive plant. Ted died of emphysema in his sixties, as a result of being a chain smoker.

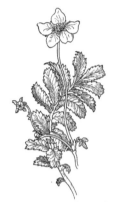

Tormentil

Part used: the fresh or recently gathered root, the herb

Gaelic: *leamhnach*

Latin: *Potentilla erecta, Potentilla tormentilla*

The roots are simmered in water or milk for diarrhea and chewed for sore lips. The tea makes a gargle for sore or ulcerated throats, a douche for leucorrhea, a tea for dysentery and jaundice, and for conditions where diarrhea and constipation alternate. Use the strong tea as a wash for piles, eye inflammations, ulcers, sores. For internal use, add a bit of cinnamon stick (Cinnamomum cassia, which is the bark usually marketed commercially as "cinnamon" because it is better tasting than Cinnamomum zeylanicum, or real "Cinnamon") at the end of decocting. Apply the fresh juice of the root to wounds and sores, add the juice and/or root to healing salves.

Root tea: use 1 tbsp. root per 1 cup of water, simmer for 20 minutes. Take 2 tbsp., 4 times a day.

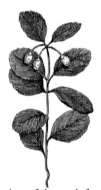

Trailing Pearlwort, Procumbent Pearlwort

(see Bog Violet, Butterwort, Marsh Violet above)

Gaelic: *Móthan*

Latin: *Sagina procumbens*

Lore: Some authorities believe that trailing pearlwort is the famous móthan, a potent charm against fire, sorcery and attacks from Fairy women. Pearlwort is a tiny, pale green flowered plant that is a member of the pink family and native to Britain. It stays green until late autumn and is evergreen in mild winters. It is placed over the door for luck and to prevent anyone in the house from being "taken" by Fairies. It is put on the right knee of a woman in labor so that the bairn will not be abducted at birth. It can be fed to a cow, and when the milk is imbibed, the same protections are passed through the milk. The cow's calf is sained by drinking the milk. The plant can be offered at a holy well in place of silver, by pressing the juice into the water. To make a love charm, go down on the left knee and gather nine roots of the herb and braid them into a ring. Place the ring into the mouth of anyone seeking a lover in the name of the "Sun, Moon and Stars". The juice of the plant can be held in the mouth for the same purpose. If the suitor can obtain a kiss from the object of their desire while keeping the plant in their mouth, a bond will form.

Vetch, Kidney Vetch

Part used: the flowering tops

Gaelic: *meóir Mhoire, cas-on-uain*

Latin: *Anthyllis vulneraria*

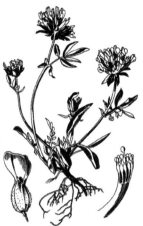

For wounds, cuts, and bruises make a wash, and then cover with a poultice, applying a fresh poultice every hour. The tea can be used internally as a purgative and will help stop vomiting in children.

Tea: steep 1 tsp. fresh or dry flower heads in ½ cup water. Take ¼ cup, 4 times a day.

Vetch, Tuberous Vetch

Part used: the roots and seeds

Gaelic: *carra-meille, carrachan*

Latin: *Lathyrus montanus, Orobus tuberosus*

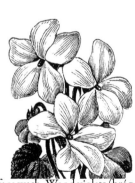

The dried roots are chewed like licorice and their flavor stays in the mouth, warding off hunger and thirst for long periods. This is, and was, a classic traveling food. The roots were once used to flavor alcoholic beverages such as heather ale. The frequent chewing of the roots prevents drunkenness. The tubers are boiled or roasted like chestnuts, and the seeds can be eaten cooked.

Caution: the seeds can be toxic to the nervous system if eaten in large amounts. The seeds are only safe when eaten sparingly, and should never exceed thirty percent of the diet.

Violets

Part used: the plant
(collect the roots in the fall)

Gaelic: *sail chuach, bróg na cuthaid*

Latin: *Viola odorata (Sweet violet, Garden violet),*
Viola canina
*(Dog violet, so called because
it has no scent or Wood violet)*

Simmer the whole herb in goat's milk to make a cosmetic face wash. Wood violets (bróg na cuthaid) are simmered in whey to ease a fever. The leaf poultice is applied to the skin of sore breasts, and violet leaves are taken as tea and used externally to poultice cancers of the colon, throat and tongue. The tea of the herb benefits headaches and phlegmy conditions when taken internally. For a fever, simmer violet leaves and nettles (Urtica spp.) in whey. This mixture will also benefit the nerves. Sweet violet or Garden violet (Viola odorata) leaf tea is helpful for respiratory conditions and headaches and makes a gargle for sore throat and mouth inflammations. Sweet violet tea of the roots and flowers (simmer the roots then steep the flowers in the hot liquid) helps coughs, insomnia and nervous conditions. The flowers and seeds are mildly laxative and in large doses the roots are emetic. The syrup of the flowers is laxative, can be used to flavor or color medicines, and was used traditionally to benefit fevers, epilepsy, insomnia, jaundice, sore throat and headaches. Violet flowers can also be made into jelly. Rich in iron, young violet leaves and flowers are added to salads in the spring. The leaves are cooked like spinach as a pot herb and the fresh leaves are used in salves and poultices for wounds.

Leaf tea: steep 1 tsp. plant matter per ½ cup water for 20 minutes, strain and take ¼ cup, 4 times a day.

Root tea: simmer 1 tbsp. root per ½ cup water.

Syrup: pour boiling hot water over an equal volume of flowers, steep for 10 hours and strain. Re-heat the liquid, adding an equal amount of fresh flowers, and let stand for 10 hours. Strain again, and repeat the process several times. Then, bring the final batch of liquid to a simmer, cool, and add honey until a syrup consistency results.

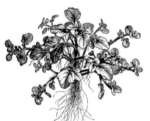

Watercress

Part used: the leaf, root, young shoots and juice

Gaelic: *biolair*

Latin: *Nasturtium officinale*

A liver cleanser, watercress is used to clean and nourish the blood and to lower fevers.

The plant helps gout, stomach upsets, phlegm in the chest and eczema. It has expectorant properties, is high in Vitamin C, and strengthens the immune system. It is rich in trace minerals. Apply fresh watercress to the scalp when hair is lost due to fungus infection.

Tea: steep 1 tsp. young shoots per ½ cup freshly boiled water, for 10 minutes. Take ½ cup, 3 times a day. To ensure potency of the vitamin content, make a fresh batch each time.

Juice: 1 tsp., 3 times a day.

Caution: when gathering this plant in the wild, be sure to soak it in water with a few tablespoons of vinegar or sea salt added to remove flukes and parasites, especially if there are sheep in the vicinity. Prolonged and excessive use can lead to kidney damage. Avoid this plant if you have weak kidneys. Do not take daily or use consistently for more than four weeks. Avoid during pregnancy. The juice must be diluted with water or milk for internal use.

Waterlilly, White Waterlilly

Part used: the root, flower and leaf

Gaelic: *duilleag-bháite bhán, lili bhan, ruamalach*
(beacon or warning)

Latin: *Nymphaea alba, Nymphaea odorata*

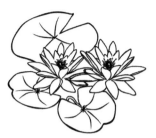

The roots are simmered in vinegar and applied to corns for three days. The root tea can be taken for internal bleeding such as heavy menstruation. The root is anaphrodisiac (removes desire), an astringent for diarrhea and helpful for irritable bowel and prostatitis. The roots are used in poultices for wounds, boils, ulcers, and skin inflammations (add powdered slippery elm bark (Ulmus fulva) to the root poultice). The root decoction makes a wash for skin irritations, a gargle for sore throats, an eye wash (be sure to filter carefully with an organic coffee filter before putting it into the eyes) and a douche for leucorrhea. The leaves are used as a tea and a compress for fevers, and a syrup of the flowers benefits insomnia.

Caution: be sure you have the fragrant white waterlilly, as other species are poisonous.

Leaf tea: steep the leaves using 1 tsp. per cup of water for 20 minutes. Root tea: simmer 2 tsp. per cup of water for 20 minutes.

Douche: 2 ounces of leaf and 2 ounces of root per 2 pints of water simmered for 2 minutes and used while warm.

Lore: In the Highlands, the roots were used to make a black, grey or chestnut colored dye depending on the mordant used. Water Lily was said to strengthen Fairy spells and could cause a person to be Fairy struck.

Willow, White Willow

Part used: the inner bark, taken from a twig or branch

Gaelic: *Saille*

Latin: *Salix spp., Salix alba*

Many species of willow are found in Britain and in the Americas. All willows have salicin which converts to salicylic acid in the body, the "active ingredient" of synthetic willow bark (otherwise known as "aspirin"). The inner bark is stripped from a twig and simmered in water to make a medicinal tea that will address all the ills usually dealt with by modern "aspirin": aches and pains, inflammation, fever, toothache, muscle strain, etc. Willow bark is slightly antiseptic and can benefit rheumatism, upset stomach, sore throat and swollen tonsils. It makes an external wash for burns and wounds, and the foot bath will deodorize sweaty, stinky feet. Willow bark can be taken in capsules to benefit heart conditions. It is slightly sedative and can help with insomnia.

Caution: those who are allergic to aspirin should avoid this herb, and over use can cause internal bleeding. There are mixed reports on the safety of this herb for young children. It is probably wise to avoid giving it to very young children in order to prevent Reyes syndrome which can result from aspirin type drugs.

Bark tea: simmer 1-3 tsp. inner bark per cup of water for 20 minutes. Take ¼ cup, 4 times a day. The White Willow, salix alba, is the most palatable species for internal use.

Lore: willows are widely used in basketry, screens, and caneing and to make a brown or tan dye for wool. Willow wood is a traditional wood used to make harps, and for this reason, willow is sacred to poets. Willow is one of the "nine sacred woods" used to kindle sacred fires at Bealltan and Samhuinn.

Woodbine
(see Honeysuckle)

Lore: woodbine is cut at the waxing moon and made into a hoop through which sick children are passed three times, to cure them.

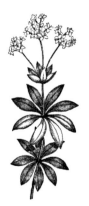

Woodruff, Sweet Woodruff

Part used: the herb

Gaelic: *lus na caithimh*

Latin: *Asperula odorata*

The herb is used to relieve coughs, chest conditions and fevers when taken as tea. The tea also helps jaundice and those with a tendency to develop gravel and stones in the bladder. It is soothing for migraine, neuralgia, nervous conditions and insomnia, and helps with stomach pain, regulates the heart, and is diuretic.

Caution: large amounts can cause dizziness and vomiting.

Tea: steep 2 tsp. of the dried herb per 1 cup of water. Take ¼ cup, 4 times a day.

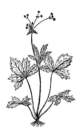

Wood Sanicle, European Sanicle

Part used: the leaves

Gaelic: *bodan coille*

Latin: *Sanicula europea*

The plant is used both internally and externally as an infusion for wounds, infections, scrofula (tuberculosis of the cervical lymph nodes), and ulcers. The tea helps catarrh in the lungs, stomach and bowels, makes a gargle for sore throat and mouth inflammations, and is used to stop bleeding, both internally and externally.

Tea: steep 2 tsp. per ½ cup water for 10 minutes. Take ½ cup a day in ¼ cup doses.

Wood Sorrel, Shamrock

Part used: the fresh herb
(gathered in the spring)

Gaelic: *seamrag, greim saighdeir*
(a soldier's mouthful)

Latin: *Oxalis acetosella*

Gathered in spring, the herb can be eaten in small amounts. It is added to soups and salads and taken as tea for fevers including typhus. Caution: do not eat large amounts of this plant as it contains oxalic acid that can harm the kidneys and cause internal bleeding and diarrhea. Persons with weak or diseased kidneys should avoid this plant. The cold tea helps indigestion and liver complaints. It is used externally as a wash for skin conditions.

Tea: steep 1 cup of the herb per quart of freshly boiled water for 3 minutes. Take ¼ cup, 4 times a day, for a few days.

Lore: where shamrocks are plentiful there is sure to be Fairy activity in the area. Sheep Sorrel (Rumex acetosella) is known as Fairy Money.

Wormwood

Part used: the leaves and flowering tops
(gathered in the fall before the first frost)

Gaelic: *burmaid*

Latin: *Artemesia absinthum*

Gather the herb in the fall and hang it upside down in a cloth or paper bag to dry. The flowering tops make a vermifuge tea that must be taken on an empty stomach to be effective. The tea helps indigestion and stomach pain, lack of appetite, gas and heartburn. It stimulates the liver and gall and improves blood circulation. The tea can be taken during labor for pain and is applied externally as a compress or fomentation for sprains, bruises and skin irritations.

Caution: excessive or over use of this plant can result in poisoning.

Vermifuge: steep 2 ounces of dried herb per pint of freshly boiled water for about 20 minutes. The dose is 1 tsp. for a child and 1 tbsp. for an adult, no more, taken on an empty stomach.

Tea: steep 2 tsp. leaves and/or flowering tops per 1 cup of water. Take ½ cup a day in tbsp. doses.

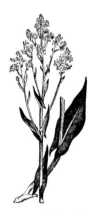

Woad
(from Anglo-Saxon "Wad")

Part used: the leaf

Latin: Isatis tinctoria

Woad was once used to poultice the spleen when there was pain in that area. Woad can be added to salves for weeping ulcers and to stop bleeding. Woad tests positive for antifungal activity against T. mentagrophytes (athlete's foot) and has some antiseptic properties.

Lore: Julius Caesar recorded that the British indigenous tribes used the herb to paint their bodies blue when they went naked to their rituals, however modern researchers who have experimented with the plant believe that it could not have been used to paint the body – they believe that the Picts were probably wearing tattoos which were done with copper (Lindow Man II, the preserved bog body in the British Museum has traces of copper pigment on his skin for example). The leaf produces a blue, green, yellow or a pink color in wool depending on how long the wool is steeped and which mordants are used.

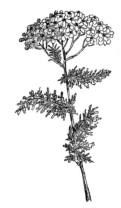

Yarrow

Part used: the herb and juice

Gaelic: *earr-thalmhainn,
lus chasgadh na fala*

Latin: *Achillea millefolium*

Yarrow is used in salves for wounds and in poultices as a styptic (stops bleeding). The tea helps cramps in the stomach, lack of appetite, gastritis, enteritis, and benefits the liver and the gall bladder (by stimulating bile production). It is helpful for internal hemorrhage and eases colds and fevers. It is a specific for stomach flu because it purifies the bowels. Add peppermint (Mentha piperita) and elder flowers (Sambucus nigra) to yarrow tea in equal amounts, to make a stomach flu remedy. The tea also makes a douche for leucorrhea, and a strong decoction is used externally as a wound wash, to bathe sore nipples and chapped hands. The fresh juice of the spring gathered leaves is a tonic for the whole system and builds the blood. The juice can also be used to stop bleeding, bloody cough, rectal and urinary bleeding, nosebleed, and excessive menstruation. Add the very young leaves (when the plant is no more than 3 inches tall) to salads.

Caution: extended use of this plant can cause photosensitivity. Yarrow contains thujone, a toxic compound.

Tea: steep 1 tbsp. dried herb per cup of water. Take ¼ cup, 4 times a day.

Wash: simmer 2 tbsp. per cup of water for 20 minutes.

Fresh juice: take 1 tsp. in water, up to 4 times a day.

Lore: a woman rises before dawn and gathers the plant to place it under her pillow and dream of a future lover. If she sees him with his back turned towards her they will not marry, but if she sees him facing her, then marriage is certain. Yarrow is a sacred plant that must be gathered while chanting:

> *I WILL pluck the yarrow fair,*
> *That more brave shall be my hand,*
> *That more warm shall be my lips,*
> *That more swift shall be my foot;*
> *May I an island be at sea,*
> *May I a rock be on land,*
> *That I can afflict any man,*
> *No man can afflict me.*
> (Traditional - Carmina Gadelica, Volume II, number 164)

Yew

Part used: the needles

Gaelic: *ioua*

(this is the old Pictish/Gaelic word for yew),

iubhar, ioghar

(iogh means "pain", thus, the one which causes pain)

Latin: *Taxus baccata*

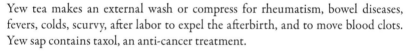

Yew tea makes an external wash or compress for rheumatism, bowel diseases, fevers, colds, scurvy, after labor to expel the afterbirth, and to move blood clots. Yew sap contains taxol, an anti-cancer treatment.

Caution: all parts of this tree are poisonous except for the red flesh of the berries. This plant can kill you and must be used only with expert supervision. Fifty needles could be fatal to an adult if injected.

Lore: the leaf and bark are highly toxic and fatal to both humans and cattle. The sap was used by the ancient Celts to poison arrows while the wood was used to make deadly long bows. The oldest tree in Europe is the Fortingall Yew, near Loch Tay in Scotland. Yew trees were held to be very sacred by the Druids, and according to tradition, the Druids bathed the dead in baths of yew to bring them back to life (possibly an ancient cancer treatment). Yew is the clan badge of the Frazers. The island of Iona was once named Ioua (Yew) and was a sacred island of the Druids before being taken over by Columba and his monks. Yew trees are associated with immortality because they are very long-lived and are frequently planted in graveyards in Britain (this is also done because yew is poisonous to sheep – it keeps farmers from pasturing their sheep near the graves).

Highland Herbal Sources:

Bartram, Thomas, Bartram's Encyclopedia of Herbal Medicine, Marlowe and Company, New York, 1998

Beith, Mary, Healing Threads, Polygon, Edinburgh, 1995

Foster, Steven and James A. Duke, Eastern/Central Medicinal Plants, Houghton Mifflin, New York and Boston, 1990

Grieve, M. A Modern Herbal, Vol. I, II, Dover Publications, New York, 1971

Gruenwald J et al, PDR for Herbal Medicines, Medical Economics Company, Inc., Montvale, NJ, 1998

Hoffmann, David: Medical Herbalism. Rochester, VT: Healing Arts Press, 2003

Hopman, Ellen Evert, A Druids Herbal – For the Sacred Earth Year, Destiny Books, Rochester, VT., 1995

Hopman, Ellen Evert, A Druids Herbal of Sacred Tree Medicine, Destiny Books, Rochester, VT., 2008

Hopman, Ellen Evert, Tree Medicine-Tree Magic, Phoenix Publishing Inc., Custer, WA, 1991

Livingstone, Sheila, Scottish Customs, Barnes and Noble Books, New York, 1997

Lust, John, The Herb Book, Bantam Books, New York, 1974

Marwick, Ernest, The Folklore of Orkney and Shetland, Birlinn Limited, Edinburgh, 2005

McNeill, F. Marian, The Silver Bough Vol. I, MacLellan, Glasgow, 1977

Miller, Joyce, Magic and Witchcraft in Scotland, Goblinshead, Musselburgh, Scotland, 2005

Potterton, David, ed., Culpepper's Color Herbal, Sterling Publishing Co. Inc., New York, 1983

Websites consulted:

Carmina Gadelica, Vol 2, Am Mothan, Sacred-texts.com, http://www.sacred-texts.com/neu/celt/cg2/cg2055.htm

Carmina Gadelica, Vol 2, Yarrow, Sacred-texts.com, http://www.sacredtexts.com/neu/celt/cg2/cg2047.htm

Scottish Plant Uses, Flora Celtica, Alphabetical Listing of Genera, http://rbg-web2.rbge.org.uk/celtica/dbase/genera/GENERA.HTM

O'God, Heather: Calluna vulgaris & the ericas, Druidry.org, http://druidry.org/obod/trees/Heather.htm

L., Pinguicula vulgaris-L., Plants For a Future, http://www.pfaf.org/database/plants.php?Pinguicula+vulgaris

L., Onopordum acanthium – L., Plants For a Future, http://pfaf.org/database/plants.php?Onopordum+acanthium

Scottish Plant Uses, Senecio vulgaris, Flora Celtica, http://193.62.154.38/ cgibin/nphreadbtree.pl/parent=/filename=usedata/firstval=11/ SID=440.1185305064?SPECIES_XREF=Senecio+vulgaris

Scottish Plant Uses, Taxus baccata, Flora Celtica, http://193.62.154.38/ cgi-bin/nph-readbtree.pl/usedata/maxvals=10/firstval=1?SPECIES_ XREF=Taxus+baccata

Scottish Plant Uses, Nymphaea alba, Flora Celtica, http://193.62.154.38/ cgi-bin/nph-readbtree.pl/usedata/maxvals=10/firstval=1?SPECIES_ XREF=Nymphaea+alba

Ní Dhoireann, Kym, The Problem of the Woad, http://www.cyberpict.net/ sgathan/essays/woad.htm

Dictionary of the Scots Language, http://www.dsl.ac.uk/dsl/

Fishing Magic, Boats, and The Lore of the Sea

The Lore of Boats

Many exacting traditions and prohibitions surround the dangerous act of setting out to sea in a boat. For example, sailors must be careful to never name the place to which they are headed by its real name, lest the Spirits know where they are going and cause mischief. Certain birds such as the stormy petrel are a bad omen when seen, as is a raven when perched on the mast. A raven in such a position implies that sorcery or Witchcraft is afoot. Wild geese setting out to sea imply good weather, while wild geese flying towards shore presage an approaching storm. Curlews are a very bad omen, while swallows are a sure sign of good weather.

A stranger must never walk over the ropes of fishing tackle, and should they do so by accident, must re-trace their steps to undo the harm. To protect against sorcery, Spirits, Fairy mischief, the Evil Eye and the like, a horseshoe should be nailed to the mast.[1]

Ideally the boat should be made from one of the nine sacred woods. A boat made entirely of oak will go faster than any other boat at night. Old wood must never be used in boat construction, and knots in the wood should be carefully examined before using any planks. Swirling shapes in the wood that look like water, called "windy knots", might attract storms, whereas fish shapes in the wood, called "fishy knots", are very lucky and might attract fish by sympathetic magic.[2]

A red thread is ritually tied around the first nail used in a boat's construction for luck, and a woman should apply the first mop of tar (after that, the mop must always be stored with its head up). A gold coin should be hidden beneath the mast

1. Ross, Anne, Folklore of the Scottish Highlands, P. 101
2. Marwick, Ernest, The Folklore of Orkney and Shetland, P. 72

and a horseshoe nailed on for luck (see above). The boat is always referred to as a "she", for which reason it was traditionally thought to be unlucky to have a woman on board during a voyage, because the woman or the boat might get jealous.[3]

When launching a new boat, or starting a new fishing season, barley should be sprinkled on deck for luck, and a bottle of spirits broken across the bow saying: "May the Gods bless this boat and all who sail in her". Everyone should cheer and chant the boat's name and follow the ritual with a feast of bread, cheese, beer and whisky.

The nets must be sprinkled with whisky before use and also held over a ritual fire to be purified by smoke. Everyone who takes part in the making or mending of the nets should be rewarded with a dram of whisky.

When pulling the boat down to the sea in preparation for launch, the boat must travel continuously without halting. After launch, if the boat is forced to return to shore it is very unlucky. Boats traveling together must not be counted, nor should fish, until everyone and everything is safely back on land.[4]

The crew should always board on the right side of the boat and the boat should leave the harbor deiseil, even if this is inconvenient. It is very unlucky to leave the harbor wrang-gaits or tuaithiuil (against the sun). A fishing boat should make three circles deiseil when setting out to sea, and while doing so, the water should be silvered with a coin to calm the waves.

No one should ask where the boat is headed or discuss the matter (see above). No one should call to the boat from shore. No food should be eaten on the boat until all the lines are out, and the first fish caught must be thrown back in honor of Shony, God of the Sea.[5]

Certain people and animals presage ill-luck for a voyage. If a red-haired woman, a priest, a chimney sweep, a flat-footed person, a person with a squint, a cat, rat, otter, or pig is encountered before shoving off, a fisherman must go back into the house and leave the back door backwards before setting sail. Another way to undo the damage of having your path crossed by any of the above persons or beasties is to draw a cross with a knife and then spit.[6] Farmers and fishermen once had metal crosses made of studs built into the soles of their boots so that they automatically made a cross when they walked.[7]

Offerings should be made to Shony on holy days such as the Fire Festivals, Solstices, and Equinoxes. At Samhuinn, offerings such as ale and oatmeal gruel are made to Shony and other Gods of the Sea. When offering a gift of ale and food, one person should walk into the sea and recite the following:

"Shony, I give you this cup of ale hoping you will be so kind as to send us plenty of sea-weed for enriching our ground in the coming year".
(Traditional) (other requests can be added as needed)

3. *Livingstone, Sheila, Scottish Customs, P. 106*
4. *Marwick, Ernest, The Folklore of Orkney and Shetland, P. 76*
5. *Livingstone, Sheila, Scottish Customs, PP. 106-107*
6. *Livingstone., P. 109*
7. *personal conversation*

Then everyone should celebrate with feasting, singing and dancing, long into the night.[8]

At Hogmanay, the boat should be sained by carrying a lit torch around it three times deiseil. If a boat returns with a good catch, money or fish should be given to the crippled, the poor, and the mentally disabled.[9]

Magical Protection of Boats and Ships

Certain objects are carried by sailors as magical aids on any voyage. A child's caul or golden earrings will bring protection from drowning. A lump of coal or a cowrie shell are very lucky on board as is a red flannel cloth (the cloth is also useful for sore throats).

Certain words must not be uttered on a ship: the words kirk (church), salt, minister, priest, pig, rabbit, hare, fox or rat must never be spoken aloud. The mere uttering of the word "pig" can raise a storm, and if salt is accidentally spilled it must be tossed over the left shoulder. If a taboo word is spoken, someone must immediately touch iron to undo the bad luck.

On shore and on ship, egg shells must be carefully crushed so that sorcerers can't use them to raise a storm. Also, a wife must never do laundry on the day her man sets out to sea, lest he be washed away through sympathetic magic. [10]

Once a ship is at sea, if it is necessary to calm the waves, "silver the water" with the offering of a silver coin, or wave a hand softly in the opposite direction of the wave swells. Wrapping a seal skin around the mast will also calm the waters. But if a person falls overboard they must be recovered or the sea will not calm.

Whistling on board a ship can raise a storm. If a ship is becalmed, whistling gently can bring a needed wind. To call up a wind, stick a steel bladed knife into the mast in the direction from which the wind is needed. [11]

Fishing Magic

Bait must be gathered with care and immediately covered with seaweed, and kept away from the cat (no part of the fishing gear must ever smell of cat). When gathering limpets for bait, they should be knocked off the rocks with a single stone, and when the bait bucket is full, the stone flung away. If it breaks into pieces, the catch will be good, but if it does not break, it is better to stay home.

To remove the limpets easily from their shells, place them in a bucket of very hot water.

It is bad luck for a fisherman to throw fish bones into a fire or to fish on a full stomach, because fishing while hungry encourages the fish to bite by sympathetic magic.

8. *Livingstone, Sheila, Scottish Customs, P. 108*
9. *Livingstone, P. 109*
10. *Ibid., PP. 108-109*
11. *Ibid., P. 110*

No one should see the fisherman leave the house, or call out to him, or wish him luck as he sets out, lest jealous Spirits or people take notice. [12]

The fisherman should place a bit of grain in the bottom of the fish basket to attract luck. On the way to the boat, he should pick up a stone on the beach and say "May I come safely back to where this came from", and if a stone is accidentally dredged from the sea it must always be carried back to land. A fisherman must always return to shore with some part of his clothes wet. [13]

Fishing lines must always be cast, and the fish brought in, on the starboard side. Once a fisherman has caught three fish his luck will improve. If the fish are cleaned on deck, the deck must not be swabbed or the good luck might be washed away - rain and seagulls must be left to do the cleaning. If a man returns with a poor catch, his wife should berate him and kick the bag in which the fish are stored, to drive out the bad luck. [14]

At the end of the season, free smoked fish are distributed to waterside pubs, and horse and boat races are held in celebration. Any fish caught at Yule are distributed as gifts to widows and orphans. [15]

12. *Marwick, Ernest, The Folklore of Orkney and Shetland, P. 75*

13. *Marwick, P. 76*

14. *Ibid., PP. 76-77*

15. *Livingstone, Sheila, Scottish Customs, P. 106*

Farming, Fertility, and Harvest Customs

The Plow, the Seed and the Grain

The farming year proper begins at Oimelc with the first plowing, when the farmer drinks a cup of ale or whisky and pours another on the plow saying: "Gods speed the plough" and "May Bríghde bless the plough". No work should follow the blessing - a feast and dance are held to celebrate the beginning of the agricultural cycle. A ring is hidden in the punch and whoever finds it will be next to wed.

The first plowing should be done in the Waning Moon, with reverence for the act of penetrating the Earth. Before starting, a small remnant of the last year's harvest is fed to the plow horse, and bread, cheese, and a drink are given to the plow man. The plow man returns the favor by toasting the family.

A bit of the last year's harvest is buried in the soil of the first furrow, and a bit of the earth from the first furrow is rubbed on to the horse's neck or the horse's ears are anointed with butter. The plow and horse are sained with a sprinkling of salt water before the first row is cut.[1]

In some areas the plow and harness were once anointed with stang (urine) to saine them. A stang tub stood by every cottage door because the stale urine was used to clean yarn and blankets, and to set color into cloth, and to dress leather.[2]

A dian stane (luck stone), a round red or brown stone with a hole bored into it, is hung on onto the plow. It is a Sun symbol that is positioned so that it always hangs on the side of the plow that faces the Sun. Each time the end of a furrow is reached the dian stane is moved to the opposite side.

If lightning strikes a furrow during the spring plowing, it is very good luck. When a farmer goes to a neighbor's farm to plow, the neighbor must jump over

---

1. *Livingstone, Sheila, Scottish Customs, PP. 99-100*
2. *Marwick, Ernest, The Folklore of Orkney and Shetland, P. 65*

the plow before work can begin, for luck.[3] These kinds of jumping rituals are sympathetic magic because as high as the farmer leaps, so high will the grain grow.

Once the furrows are ready for planting, the seeds are sewn (to ensure germination an egg and an iron nail made by a black smith should have been stored with the seeds all winter). The sower should always walk deiseil to sow the seed which is pulled from a basket or a cloth slung around the neck.

At Summer Solstice, the fields are sained by a torch which is lit from the ritual fire and carried deiseil around the edges of the fields to purify them. Celebrants jump the flames to be blessed and to encourage the grain to grow as high as their leaping, by sympathetic magic. Feasting and dancing follow.[4]

When reapers first arrive at a farm they drink a toast. Then, the farm owner lays their hat on the Earth and lifts their sickle while facing the Sun. A small portion of grain is cut and the farm owner whirls it three times deiseil over their head as a chant is begun to bless the harvest.[5]

The Consecration of the Seed

"...The Feast day of Michael, day beneficent,
I will put my sickle round about
The root of my corn as was wont;
I will lift the first cut quickly;
I will put it three turns round
My head, saying my rune the while,
My back to the air of the north;
My face to the fair sun of power..."

(Traditional, from Carmina Gadelica 88)[6]

While the reapers work, a "bandster" (usually a woman) makes the bands to tie the sheaves. If a band breaks she owes the reapers a kiss.[7]

When but one last sheaf remains, the reapers line up to throw their sickles at it. When the "hare" is finally cut, all race to the farmer to win a wee dram (of whisky). The winner of the race will be the next to marry.

If the last sheaf is taken early, it is called "the Maiden" (the Land Goddess in her youthful aspect). If late in the season, it is called "the Cailleach" (the Old Woman of winter, the veiled one, the ancient Land Goddess). It is dressed in clothing appropriate to a maiden or a crone, and given a place of honor at the harvest supper table where it is toasted and thanked.[8]

Some houses keep the Cailleach or the Maiden in the farm kitchen for luck, maintaining a small collection of such figures for years. A Corn Mother, Rye Mother, Pea Mother, Flax Mother, etc., may be made to honor the fertile Spirit of each of these different crops.[9]

3. Marwick, P. 65

4. Livingstone, Sheila, Scottish Customs, P. 100

5. Livingstone, P. 100

6. Carmichael, Alexander, Carmina Gadelica – Hymns and Incantations, P. 97

7. Livingstone, Sheila, Scottish Customs, P. 100

8. Livingstone, P. 101

9. Lamb, Gregor, Carnival of the Animals, P. 25

A portion of the last sheaf of the harvest is kept to be buried in the first furrow plowed the next spring.

Of course, every farm and homestead must have a section of land that is never plowed and where no human ever goes (The Gudeman's Croft). Wild weeds and grasses are allowed to grow there undisturbed, as a shelter for the Brownies and other Fairies.

Wheat Weavings and Corn Dollies

The tradition of making a "Corn Dolly", or female figure from the last sheaf of the harvest, has very ancient roots. The wheat weaving does not have to be a human figure, it can be a cornucopia, a horn of plenty to be hung over the door for luck, or it can be a plaited weaving that is given to a lover or neighbor as a gift, for luck and to celebrate the end of the harvest.

In some areas the Corn Dolly is shaped like a dog. In Orkney, where it is called the "bikko" (bitch) from the Old Norse "bikkja", a straw dog is placed at the door of the last farmer to bring in the harvest, usually accompanied by a satirical note. The Orkney, "staw" dog (pronounced "stray") is a life sized dog made of straw and twisted straw ropes wound over a wooden frame, or made entirely of straw.[10]

On the Isle of Skye in the West of Scotland, the last sheaf embodies a Spirit goat called the gobhar bacach (cripple goat) and the woman who carries it home must pretend to limp (in Shetland, the Fairies are said to dance with a limp and their dance is called the "haltadans").

The goat is passed from house to house and must be gotten rid of as quickly as possible or it will bring bad luck. It is carried in secret by the last farmer to thresh, to a neighbor who is still threshing, and if the farmer is caught bringing the goat it spells trouble, because no one wants to receive it. The constant passing of the taunting goat has the effect of speeding up the harvest.[11]

The goat has deep spiritual meaning in ancient Indo-European religion. In the Rig Veda of India (a collection of Vedic hymns from 1200-900 BCE), the goat is paired with the sacred horse, a solar animal that is offered as a sacrifice. At the horse sacrifice, a goat companion accompanies the horse to announce the offering to the Gods:

The Sacrifice of the Horse

"When, as the ritual law ordains,
The men circle three times,
Leading the horse that is to be the oblation
On the path to the gods,
The goat who is the share for Pusan
Goes first, announcing the sacrifice to the gods."

(Verse 4)[12]

The goat is a fitting symbol to announce the great sacrifice of the Earth in the harvest season.

10. *Lamb, P. 11*

11. *Ibid, P. 59*

12. *O'Flaherty, Wendy Doniger trans., The Rig Veda, P. 90*

Straw Men and Scare Crows

While the last sheaf of grain is usually associated with the Land Goddess or with a female animal such as a bitch or a mare, in some areas, it is made into the figure of a straw man, a bull, a cock, a hare, a boar, or a billy-goat.

In northern Orkney, a scarecrow of straw is occasionally made at the end of the reaping. The "straw man" is seen as a magical helper for the farm, his function is to protect the farm from the trials of winter. Such a figure must never be dressed.

> *"When Broonie got a cloak or hood (Brownie)*
> *He did his master nae mair good."* (no more good)
>
> (Traditional)[13]

Harvest Home

The feast to celebrate the end of the harvest is called the "kirn" or harvest supper. A feature of the meal is a punch into which small symbolic objects are dropped. If someone scoops a ring into their cup they will soon have a lover. If someone gets a button they will remain a spinster or a bachelor. To fish up a coin means good luck.

The altar is decorated with sheaves of wheat or other grains, and samples of the best fruits and vegetables of the farm. Harvest fruits and vegetables, and offerings of newly canned foods are brought to the local pantry for the poor.[14]

Dairy Magic

Magical woods are hung over the entrance to the cow barn for protection, and whoever does the milking is sure to leave a bowl for the Brownie who lives in the barn. Milk is also poured onto a hollow stone for the Fairies.

A coin is placed in the milk pail for luck and to keep the milk from curdling. Wreaths of marigolds (Calendula officinalis) and dandelions (Taraxacum spp.) are placed under the milk pail to keep the milk from thinning. Figwort (Scrofularia nodosa) cut during the incoming tide, or a small bag with an iron nail made by a black smith and a small piece of pearlwort (Sagina procumbens), is carried around the milk pail three times deiseil and then slipped under the pail.

To determine if you have "honest milk", lay a penny carefully on top of the cream. If it sinks, the milk is still in its natural state, but if it sits on top, that means the milk has a spell on it.[15]

Before churning butter, a cabbage leaf or a coin is placed under the churn to prevent Trolls from spoiling it. An incantation must be recited while

---

13. Lamb, Gregor, *Carnival of the Animals*, P.13
14. Livingstone, Sheila, *Scottish Customs*, PP. 101-102
15. Livingstone, PP. 102-103

churning.[16] If a visitor enters the dairy while butter is being churned, they must lend a hand or the butter may refuse to set.

If the dairy appears to be bewitched, boil pins in a pot, and the offending sorcerer will suffer pain and release the spell. (To keep your local Witch happy, especially if they have helped you throughout the year, it is always a good idea to leave a portion of peat, hen's eggs, or fresh thatch at their door).[17]

Here is a traditional riddle from Shetland:

> *A marble wall*
> *As white as milk,*
> *All lined with skin,*
> *As smooth as silk,*
> *Neither doors nor windows*
> *A person behold,*
> *Yet the thieves break through*
> *And steal the gold.*[18]

16. *Marwick, Ernest, The Folklore of Orkney and Shetland, P. 78*

17. *Livingstone, Sheila, Scottish Customs, P. 103*

18. *Marwick, Ernest, The Folklore of Orkney and Shetland, P. 123 (answer – an egg!)*

Domestic Life

Money

In Scottish communities after making a deal, a wee dram (of whisky) is often taken to seal the bargain. "Deal money" always involves giving something back, to ensure good will amongst neighbors. When money changes hands, the recipient of the cash should always give back a little for the children of the buyer. If land is sold, the buyer should gift the former land owner's spouse with a piece of jewelry or other small token. When an apprentice completes their first project, they must provide ale-money for their co-workers.[1]

Food and Whisky

The ancient tradition of hospitality is a hallmark of Scottish domestic life. Celtic hospitality is generous in all areas, but in the Highlands, it reaches legendary proportions. A portion of any meal may be set aside for the Fairies or for any unexpected guest or stranger who happens by. Strangers are welcomed into the home to sleep over when they need a bed, for you never know when a stranger may be a God or Goddess in disguise.

But there are still times when folk may not wish to be disturbed. When a group of men enter a house on business or to drink, the door is left open and a rod placed across the opening as a sign that no person without rank may disturb them.[2]

Ancient Scottish indigenous cuisine featured salmon, trout, shellfish, wild boar, venison, fruits, nuts, berries, roots and leafy greens, pure water, cattle,

---

1. Livingstone, Sheila, *Scottish Customs*, P. 112
2. Ross, Anne, *Folklore of the Scottish Highlands*, PP. 106-108

goats, and sheep. In 1988, the Royal museum of Scotland served a Mesolithic-Neolithic meal that featured indigenous delicacies such as salted hazelnuts, oatcakes with crowdie (gruth in Gaelic, crowdie is a type of creamy curd cheese), watercress and other herbs, brose meal pancakes (brose meal is peas meal) stuffed with mushrooms and juniper berries, smoked venison with yoghurt and rowan berries, laver bread, smoked salmon, and parsnip and carrot croquettes.

The ancient Scots and Picts ate seaweeds and barley, and dishes such as salmon baked with honey and herbs, and fish cooked with salt, cumin, and vinegar.[3]

Uisge-beatha (the waters of life) or whisky has long been the ubiquitous drink of Scotland, regarded as a noble liquid suitable to offer to the Gods. In ancient times, warriors were given alcohol as they set off to battle to give them courage. Being drunk was not a disgrace (but being overweight was, and it could result in a fine).

I had the good fortune to spend a week in a home in County Fife some years ago. Every evening after dinner, the whole family, from grandparents to grandchildren, sat in the parlour sipping whisky and sharing the day's news. I was told that it is a grave sin to dilute the drink with anything as polluting as water or ice, however, three drops of water (no more) could be added to a glass of whisky to release the flavor and aroma.

Whisky was once used to heal wounds, treat colds and grippe (the flu), sharpen memory, dispel melancholy, preserve youth, cure tooth ache, remove gum infections, burst swellings in the throat, help sciatica, reduce deafness, relieve hoarseness, cure headache by rubbing the head with it, and calm trembling limbs. A small amount was added to milk, gruel, jellies, jams, and teas. Whisky could be flavored with fennel (Foeniculum vulgare), thyme (Thymus serpyllum), mint (Mentha spp.), anise (Pimpinella anisum), juniper, (Juniperus communis) or cranberries (Vaccinium spp.).[4]

Oatmeal is the other ubiquitous healing agent and food, as the many recipes I have offered in this book attest. There is a drink that actually combines these two most basic ingredients of Scottish fare: whisky and oats, known as "Atholl Brose" which dates back to at least 1475 CE. In that year, the Earl of Atholl went after Iain Macdonald, Lord of the Isles, because he was fomenting rebellion against the king. Upon learning that MacDonald habitually drank from a certain well, the Earl had it filled with whisky, oatmeal, and honey. The MacDonald drank from the well, became inebriated, and was captured.[5]

Atholl Brose
4 bottles whisky
1 whisky bottle full of cream
1 pound medium/coarse oatmeal
1 pound heather honey
1 tablespoon brandy

3. Beith, Mary, Healing Threads, P. 18

4. Beith, P. 59

5. Traditional Scottish Recipes, Atholl Brose, Rampantscotland.com, www.rampantscotland.com/recipies/blrecipe_brose.htm

Put the oatmeal and whisky into a large container and cover with a clean linen cloth. Allow it to soak for 72 hours. After soaking, the whisky is strained off and put into a jug or glass container. Only the clear liquid should be siphoned off. Place the remaining oatmeal in a linen cloth and twist to squeeze out any remaining liquid, a small amount at a time. Mix the cream with the brandy (the brandy prevents the cream from curdling) and pour the cream very slowly into the whisky. Stir continuously with a wooden spoon as the liquids are combined. Slowly stir in the honey (warm the honey slightly beforehand to make pouring easier).[6] The left over oatmeal is cooked and eaten with milk, butter or cream.

House and Home

When building a house, an "earth-fast stane" must be included somewhere in the walls. This is a stone that is partly in the earth and partly above, and around which the wall is built. A handful of "haley stones" (holy stones) should also be incorporated into or under a wall, for example crystals, quartz, or a flint knife.

A piece of iron is inserted over the door to prevent "evil" from entering, such as iron nails or a small equal armed cross made of iron nails forged by a black smith, or a horse shoe are especially good for this purpose.[7] Of course, this raises a philosophical quandary. It is well known that the Fairies detest iron. Do you really want to keep them out?

A pint of ale or beer is given to each male or female worker as the foundation stone is laid, and a bit of ale or beer is also poured onto the earth as an offering for the Spirits (at one time a bit of bull's blood was mixed with the first mortar). When the last stone is set in place, a feast is given and a dram offered to every worker. Failure to do this freely will bring bad luck on the building.[8]

Once the house is finished, a cat should be brought in, because if evil Spirits are about, they will enter the cat, thus saving the family. And every house should have a "knockin-stane", a large stone bowl used to grind grain with a wooden pestle. These stanes (stones) go back to Pictish times and are preserved as family heirlooms, carried to each new home by successive generations of the family.

When leaving a house, the departing occupants must be sure to ritually sweep the place clean so that their good fortune goes with them.[9]

House Blessing Rite

"Beating the house" is an old Celtic custom. Upon moving into a new house and on Hogmanay, you should take a fresh loaf of bread and pound it against the front door for luck. Or, take a fresh branch of evergreen, and circumambulate the house three times deiseil, while saying:

---

6. *Atholl Brose, The Original One and Only Recipe, Cabarfeidh.com, www.cabarfeidh.com/atholl_ brose.htm*
7. *Marwick, Ernest, The Folklore of Orkney and Shetland, P. 79*
8. *Livingstone, Sheila, Scottish Customs, P. 111*
9. *Marwick, Ernest, The Folklore of Orkney and Shetland, P. 79*

Good luck to the house,
Gook luck to the family,
Good luck to every wall,
Good luck to every rafter,
Good luck to every door and window,
Good luck to the wife,
Good luck to the husband,
Good luck to the children,
Good luck to the sheep,
Good luck to the cows,
Good luck to the cat,
Good luck to the dog, etc.

The evergreen is then taken into the house and kept all year for luck.

Sacred Birds and Animals

ertain birds and animals appear with regularity in Celtic legends and
stories and on Pictish carved stones. Here is a small overview of some
animals and birds and their ancient symbolism. Every traditional clan
once had their own plant and/or an animal totem. The clan was under a geas
(magical prohibition or taboo) never to eat their animal totem, and the warriors
tucked a bit of their totem plant into their bonnet as magical protection and for
identification purposes.

Do a little research into your own genealogy and find out if your family is
under the guidance and protection of a certain plant, bird, or animal. If not,
pick a plant and an animal for your clan. Feed, honor, and protect your totem
and it will bring you spiritual guidance and protection in return.

Sacred Birds

Albatross — When seen at sea this bird is an omen of death.[1]

Cuckoo — It is unlucky to hear a cuckoo before breakfast. If one appears
near the house on a quarter day it is a sign of death.[2]

Crane — Eating a crane's flesh is taboo. In the Highlands, a bed ridden
person who was thought to have lived too long could be put to death by
saying into the keyhole of their bedroom: "Will you come or will you
go? Or will you eat the flesh of cranes?" It was a bad omen for a warrior
to see a crane while on the way to a battle. Cranes were featured on
Gaulish warrior's helmets and shields as a military symbol.

---

1. *Livingstone, Sheila, Scottish Customs, P. 133*

2. *Livingstone, P. 133*

When Finn MacCumhail's father was killed in a battle and Finn himself was tossed over a cliff, his grandmother came in crane form, and saved him. The ancient "Hag of the Temple", Cailleach an Teampuill, had four sons who appeared as cranes. They could be turned back into human form only if blood from the Connra bull, owned by the Cailleach Bhéara, was sprinkled on them. The Celtic Sea God Manannán had a magical "Crane Bag" made from the skin of a woman who was magically transformed into a crane. It held all of the God's most precious possessions.

Miadhach is a woman who was transformed into a crane by her father, Eachdhonn Mór. She still lives in crane form and is now one of the world's oldest animals. "Corrgainecht" is a type of magic where the magician takes the crane's stance: standing on one foot, with one hand extended and one eye closed (Cranes are semi-aquatic animals who live between the worlds of earth, air and water. The crane stance shows that the magician is operating both in this world and in the Otherworld). To hear a crane or heron at night is a bad omen.[3]

Crow — The Mórrígan often appears as a hooded crow (See raven below).

Eagle — In Gaul, the eagle was a symbol of Taranis, the Thunder God. Eagles are found on Pictish symbol stones. The divine Celtic Warrior God Lugh (Lugus, LLeu) transformed himself into an eagle. Eliwlod, son of Madog, Arthur's nephew, spoke to Arthur in eagle's form. By tradition, the grave of Arthur on Snowdon is guarded by a pair of eagles. Sixty oracular eagles are said to gather at Loch Lomond each year to prophesy the future. In Irish tradition, the eagle Druim Brecc is said to be one of the oldest animals on earth. In Welsh lore, it is the eagle of Gwernabwy that is one of the oldest animals.[4]

Falcon — The Fili, Irish sacred poets whose job was to prophesy the future for the king or queen, wore capes of bird feathers. The northern Goddess Freyja had a falcon's skin that Loki the Trickster God borrowed to do magic. Eagle-skins and swan-skins also had magical properties.[5]

Goose — The goose is a martial bird sacred to the ancient British. A flock of geese on a lake at night might be a coven of Witches, especially on the first Thursday of the lunar month. The Celtic Horse Goddess Epona sometimes rides upon a goose (the original Mother Goose). In Romano-Celtic areas, geese often accompany images of Mars, the Roman God of War. The goose is also associated with Taranis, the Gaulish Thunder God, who is also a Military God.[6] Geese are fierce protectors and can guard a house as well as any dog.

Lark — In Scotland the lark is called "Lady Hen". In Orkney, it is said that anyone who steals a lark's eggs will get three black spots on their tongue because the lark also has three such spots on their tongue.[7]

3. Ross, Anne, Pagan Celtic Britain, PP. 279, 283, 285
4. Ross, P. 275
5. Lamb, Gregor, Carnival of the Animals, P. 126
6. Ross, Anne, Pagan Celtic Britain, P. 270
7. Lamb, Gregor, Carnival of the Animals, P. 135

Magpie — To see one solitary magpie is unlucky, especially if it is seen before breakfast.[8] As the old rhyme relates (when counting magpies):

> *One for sorrow,*
> *Two for mirth,*
> *Three for a wedding,*
> *Four for a birth,*
> *Five for silver,*
> *Six for gold,*
> *Seven for a story,*
> *Never to be told (ie a secret)*
> *(Traditional)*

Owl — In Scottish Gaelic, the owl is called Cailleach Oidhche (the night hag) and is generally associated with Goddesses. In Welsh tradition Lleu had a magical wife created for him out of flowers by the magician Gwydion. When his wife, Blodeuwedd, plotted with her lover Gronw to kill him, Llew escaped by transforming himself into an eagle and flying into a magical oak. After regaining his human form, Llew turned his wife into an owl.[9]

Raven — The appearance of a raven is a sign of death.[10] Ravens are associated with Goddesses of War such as the Mórrígan (Great Queen, Phantom Queen), because they and the crows are often first on the field to pluck out the eyes and eat the flesh of dead warriors. The Mórrígan is a triple Goddess whose three aspects are Badb Catha (battle crow or vulture), Macha (raven woman) and Nemain (battle frenzy). She appears to warriors who are about to die as the "washer at the ford', a woman washing their blood stained clothing. She mated with the Daghda as they both straddled a river. She also parted a river so that an army could cross it.

The Gaulish Raven Goddess Nantosuelta (winding river) appears as a raven in Her warrior context, and as a dove in the context of motherhood, hearth, and home. The Gaulish Goddess Epona is sometimes shown accompanied by a raven. The northern God Odin is accompanied by ravens, symbolic of His Otherworldly wisdom.

The city of Lugudunum (Lyon) in ancient Gaul was sacred to Lugus (Lugh), and was built on a site where a flock of ravens had landed. This was considered a good omen because ravens are such wise birds and also associated with battle, as well as with prophecy - fitting attributes for Lugus, master of every art: of magic, craft, and war. In Gallo-Roman iconography, a deceased person is often shown holding a raven. The Welsh hero Bran (Raven) is a battle leader whose severed head continued to entertain people, even after his death. The Welsh hero Owein had a band of magical raven-warriors. Cú Chulainn, the warrior-hero son of Lugh, was accompanied by two ravens though he

8. *Livingstone, Sheila, Scottish Customs, P. 133*
9. *Ross, Anne, Pagan Celtic Britain, P. 274*
10. *Livingstone, Sheila, Scottish Customs, P. 133*

often had to do battle with flocks of Otherworldly ravens. The hero Caoilte and his followers had to kill three magical ravens that appeared to them at Samhuinn.

The Druids prophesied the future by observing the movements of ravens, their flight and their calls. Ravens appear in tales as bearers of evil tidings, and Witches are said to take the form of ravens. When a raven appears there is danger in the offing. It is especially bad if a raven lands on the roof. But ravens with white feathers are a very good omen.[11]

Swan — Swans symbolize purity and the Otherworld and must never be killed. To see seven swans flying is a wonderful omen of wealth and good fortune.[12] Swans are associated with the Sun, water, and healing. When a God or a Goddess appears as a swan in Celtic legend, they can always be identified by the golden or silver chain around their neck. Humans may also be magically transformed into swans and will be seen wearing a gold, silver or bronze chain. Swans pull the carriage that carries the Sun across the sky.[13]

Wren — The wren is called the "King of all Birds", even though it is amongst the smallest. According to tradition, the birds once had a contest to see who would be king. Each bird: the goose, the eagle and so on, boasted that it would fly longest and highest. The mighty eagle flew higher than any until, when it was exhausted and could fly no higher, a tiny wren popped out of its feathers, flew highest and won the day. This story illustrates that intelligence wins in the end, over brute strength. The wren is also called the "Spirit of the Hedge". The hedge separates fields and is a liminal space (between the worlds). The wren is also known as "The Druid Bird" because it lives between two worlds and wins by intelligence rather than brawn.

In ancient times, the wren was hunted during the twelve days of Yuletide. It was caught, tied to a pole, and carried around the village, especially to the homes of lovers and newlyweds. In some areas, the wren was carried on a tiny bier with an apple placed on each corner, symbolic of Abhalloch (Avalon, the Otherworld). At every home, the inhabitants would make an offering to the "dead king" and were given a feather for luck. Finally, the bird was interred in a wild area or by the sea.

Sometimes, instead of a dead bird, an apple or a clove studded orange was decorated with wheat and greenery and carried from house to house to bring luck and the Sun's blessings to all.

In Ireland, boys carry a holly or gorse bush decorated with ribbons and declare that there is a wren inside of it. Usually there is nothing in the bush, or a live bird is trapped in a glass jar.[14]

---

11. Ross, Anne, *Pagan Celtic Britain*, PP. 244, 249, 257
12. Livingstone, Sheila, *Scottish Customs*, P. 133
13. Ross, Anne, *Pagan Celtic Britain*, P. 240
14. Lamb, Gregor, *Carnival of the Animals*, PP. 129-130, 133

Modern Pagans and Druids do not harm any living thing, preferring
to use vegetables, fruits or art works as fertility symbols.

Sacred Animals

Bear — The Celtic Goddess Andarta was "Powerful Bear". The name Art
means "bear", thus the God Artgenos was "Son of the Bear". A Bear
God named Matunos was worshipped north of Hadrian's Wall.[15]

Bees — If a bee flies straight towards your face expect important news.[16]

Boar — A popular Pictish symbol found on stones and carvings, the boar, is
the most common animal in Celtic iconography. It is seen on warrior's
helmets and shields and is featured on the Gundestrup Cauldron (a
first to second century BCE metal cauldron of Celtic design, found in
a Danish peat bog).

Whole pigs and pork meat were often buried with the dead. Pork
was the food of choice in Otherworldly feasts and in the courts of
kings. The boar-hunt was said to be a feature of otherworldly life, and
according to British tradition, pigs were brought to this world from
the Otherworld of Annwn. The Red Swine of Derbrenn, the magical
pigs of Mánannán and other legendary pigs are magically reborn
after being eaten. Those who partake of their flesh are said to find joy,
happiness, health, and the healing of wounds.

The "hero's portion" at a feast was often a portion of pig meat, over
which warriors hotly contended, sometimes to the death. Magical
pigs were often encountered when a hero set out on immrama voyages
(magical quests to Otherworldly islands). The Celtic trumpet known
as a Carnyx often featured a boar's head at the horn end, and the boar
is seen on Celtic coins, sometimes with three horns, implying divinity.

The Orkney Islands were once called the Orcades (little pigs). There
was a Gaulish God called Moccus (pig). The favorite food of pigs is
the acorn, and by association the oak, enhancing their sacred status.[17]

Bull — Another common symbol found on Pictish stones. A bull sacrifice
was done in thanks when gathering important medicinal plants such
as mistletoe. At Hogmanay, guizers in the Highlands and Hebrides
still dress in the hide and head of a bull.[18]

The blood of a bull was once mixed with the mortar of a new foundation
to ensure a strong building, because bulls embody strength and fertility
(see the House and Home section above).[19] The bull is often associated
with horses, stags, and swans on early Celtic iconography, and appears

15. Ross, Anne, *Pagan Celtic Britain*, P. 349
16. Livingstone, Sheila, *Scottish Customs*, P. 130
17. Ross, Anne, *Pagan Celtic Britain*, PP. 308, 317
18. McNeill, F. Marian, *The Silver Bough Vol. I*, P. 76
19. Livingstone, Sheila, *Scottish Customs*, P. 132

on the Gundestrup Cauldron (a metal cauldron of Celtic design, dated to the first to second century BCE, found in a Danish peat bog) in what may be a ritual hunt. The "bull with three cranes" motif is found in Gaulish carvings, and in Britain, the bull is sometimes depicted with three horns, implying divinity.

In Irish kingship rituals, a Tarbfeis (bull feast) was performed where a bull was ritually slaughtered, and a Druid bathed in its broth and ate of its flesh. Then, the Druid was sewn into the bull's hide and left there for the night, during which time they would dream the name of the next king.

The Táin Bó Cuálgne (The Cattle Raid of Cooley) is the oldest vernacular epic of western literature. It tells of a deadly competition between the king and queen of Ulster, both of whom coveted the magical bulls Donn Cuálgne and Findbennach (The White Horned). Both bulls ultimately killed each other in battle.[20]

Butterflies — White butterflies are very lucky when seen, while brown ones are unlucky. If a yellow butterfly flies over a coffin, the soul has passed safely to the Otherworld.[21] A blue butterfly signifies that the deceased was a healer. A white butterfly signifies a good person, a dark butterfly a bad person. Butterflies represent transformation and must never be killed.[22]

Cat — Cairbre Caitchenn (Cairbre Cat-head) is a divine ancestor of the Erainn. Imbas Forosnai was an ancient Celtic method of divination where the raw flesh of a red pig, cat, or dog, was chewed in order to see a vision (Caution: this is a very dangerous practice. Eating raw flesh can result in severe illness for anyone who tries it – not recommended!). Cath Palug (Palug's Cat) is a Welsh monster that was born to the sow Henwen (White Ancient One) who was originally a human. The Silures apparently worshipped a Cat God.[23]

Cattle — Cattle were walked between two ritual fires or washed with sea water to purify them on their way to the summer pastures. Cows were sung to, to make them easier to milk.

If the cows are restless, there is impending trouble for the family. When breeding a cow to a bull, first make a collar of rowan or ivy for the cow to wear the night before, and pass the collar three times over a ritual fire, before putting it on the cow.[24]

Chicken — An old cure for snake-bite: take a fresh warm chicken and split it in half, placing it over the wound to draw out the poison. Chicken soup is a Highland remedy for those with stomach problems, for the

20. Ross, Anne, Pagan Celtic Britain, PP. 303-307
21. Livingstone, Sheila, Scottish Customs, P. 130
22. Beith, Mary, Healing Threads, P. 166
23. Ross, Anne, Pagan Celtic Britain, P. 301
24. Livingstone, Sheila, Scottish Customs, P. 132

weak and debilitated, and the terminally ill. To help diarrhea: boil an egg in milk until hard, eat the egg and drink the milk.[25]

Cow — Otherworldly cows were white with red ears and sometimes emerged from lakes (water is a gateway to the Otherworld) such as Loch Sithgail. The Goddess Boand (She of the White Cattle) was the Mother River Goddess of the Boyne and Verbeia, also associated with cows, was the Mother River Goddess of the Wharfe in Yorkshire. The Irish Goddess Flidais had a herd of magical cattle, and the Mórrígan once turned someone into a pool of water for mating her cow with his bull. The Sea God Mánannán had magical cows that lived under the sea.[26]

When warriors were wounded by poisoned arrows, Pictish Druids would fill a hole with the milk of one hundred and fifty white-faced cows and bathe the warriors in it. Baths of cow's bone marrow were used to heal wounds, and cream was boiled, cooled, and applied to burns.

In Celtic thinking, white animals had strong Otherworldly associations. The milk of a pure white cow was especially blessed.[27]

Cows are lunar animals associated with sacred water (Sanskrit - Soma) in Indo-European tradition, because of their production of milk. Milk in turn is used to make butter, which is given as a gift to a sacred fire - another instance where fire and water are brought together to make magic.

In many ways, cows are the mothers of the human race. They have selflessly given us their milk, flesh and hides for millennia, and for this reason cows are sacred and must never be hurt or abused.

Deer — The deer or stag is another animal frequently seen on Pictish stones. They appear on the Gundestrop Cauldron where a horned figure holds two deer aloft by their hind legs. The Cornavii of Caithness were stag worshippers.

In stories, deer often lure heroes to the Otherworld and early Celtic Christians followed the tradition by wandering in the forests, sometimes for years, until they saw a white deer, because the sighting indicated where to build a monastery. Gaulish and Irish stories tell of three-antlered stags, the potent number three implying divinity.

One of Finn MacCumhail's lovers was transformed into a deer by a Druid. She gave birth to the poet Oisín (Little Deer) who was half man, half deer. The Goddess Flidais was a Forest Goddess who owned magical cattle and protected the deer. The Cailleach (Ancient Veiled Woman) of the Highlands was also protectress of the wild herds. The Lochaber Deer Goddess and other such Cailleachs were said to roam the wilds of Scotland.

25. *Beith, Mary, Healing Threads, PP. 169, 172*
26. *Ross, Anne, Pagan Celtic Britain, PP. 303-307*
27. *Beith, Mary, Healing Threads, P. 167*

The God Cernunnos was an antlered deity with deer horns who was especially connected to stags.[28] In the Highlands and Islands, sinew from a rutting stag was tied with three knots and affixed to a limb above a sprain to heal it. Stag Horn Jelly was made to be fed to invalids, especially those with chest complaints:

Stag Horn Jelly

Break up a freshly fallen antler with a hammer and boil in water and a little vinegar for 3 hours (the vinegar helps release minerals from the antler)

Strain the liquid into a pot adding candied sugar

Bring to a boil again and then allow standing and cooling until the liquid jells

Feed it to an invalid mixed with whisky, one wineglassful at a time.[29]

Dog — Dogs accompany the Gods in Celtic iconography and are often pictured as symbols of healing. The Gaulish God Sucellos (The Good Striker) is accompanied by a dog and the Goddess Epona is often depicted with a dog at Her side. The British God Nodons is also associated with dogs. The Gundestrup Cauldron features dogs in a ritual context. The temple of Sequana at the source of the Seine in Gaul had images of people holding dogs. In British iconography, hunter Gods are often accompanied by dogs. Votive images of dogs were offered to the Gods by dropping the images into ritual pits - a bronze terrier was found at Coventina's well in Northumberland. Dog bones have been found in ancient healing wells and dogs were especially connected to deities and traditions involving sacred rivers.

The ancient Irish Fili (sacred poets and Seers) chewed the raw flesh of a dog, red pig, or cat in order to perform their divinations (see a strong caution against this practice in the Cat section above). The hero Finn MacCumhail had two dogs: Bran and Sceólang who were his magically transformed nephews. Lugh's mother Ethlenn was killed while in the guise of a lap dog. Great Celtic heroes often had the preface "Cú" (dog) attached to their name: Cú Chulainn, Cú Roí, and Cunobelinus.[30] The ancient Celts placed great store in the curative effects of dog's saliva. Modern medicine is showing that dogs can help the sick in many other ways such as helping to lower blood pressure by their mere presence; guiding and assisting the lame, paralyzed, and blind; and by speeding the recovery of those with depression, autism and other mental conditions.[31]

Dolphin — Dolphins appear on the Gundestrup Cauldron (the first to second century BCE metal cauldron of Celtic provenance found in a

28. Ross, Anne, *Pagan Celtic Britain*, PP. 333, 336
29. Beith, Mary, *Healing Threads*, P. 170
30. Ross, Anne, *Pagan Celtic Britain*, P. 341
31. Beith, Mary, *Healing Threads*, P. 171

Danish peat bog), on Gaulish coins, and are associated with sacred wells such as the well of the Goddess Coventina, near Hadrian's Wall.[32]

Eel — The fat of a Conger Eel is applied to bruises and scrapes. For a sprained ankle, put the eel's skin around the affected limb and allow it to dry and it will support the ankle as it tightens. Wear the eel skin until it falls off. Eel oil is applied to arthritic parts.[33]

Goat — Goat's milk builds strength after a bout of the flu, and is taken as a cure for hangover.[34] A cosmetic face wash can be made by simmering violets in goat's milk. A common initiatory feat is for a man to ride in three concentric circles, widdershins or tuaithiuil on a goat's back. When setting out on a journey, if a goat crosses your path you must turn back and depart once again by the back door.[35] (See also the "Farming, Fertility, and Harvest Customs" chapter above)

Hare — Julius Caesar wrote that the hare, goose, and cock held religious significance for the Celts. Queen Boudicca released a hare before setting out to attack the Roman invaders of Britain, while invoking the Goddess Andraste. Hunter deities are often depicted holding hares.

Hares are associated with shape changing and Witches are said to dance as hares under the moonlight.[36] Once a Witch has shape shifted into a hare, the only way to harm them is with a pure silver bullet.

The Welsh physicians of Myddfai prescribed eating boiled or roasted hare's brains mixed with rosemary for vertigo and migraine.[37] Rabbits and hares are born with their eyes open; hence to carry the foot of the animal protects you from evil (because you can see it coming).

Horse — If a horse neighs at the door, someone inside will soon fall sick. Horse racing was once an important aspect of every large festival gathering. Place a wreath of rowan around a horse's neck to protect it from evil.

A white horse has Otherworldly associations and implies purity and goodness. To find a horseshoe and bring it home to hang over the door is very lucky. The sight of a foal before breakfast is unlucky.[38]

The horse as a sacred animal in Britain goes back to the Paleolithic era. The Pinhole Cave in Derbyshire has a drawing of a man in a horse head mask, and the Uffington White Horse is an Iron Age image cut into the turf and chalk of a hill in Oxfordshire. The association of horses with the Sun is very ancient and goes back to Vedic times:

32. Ross, Anne, *Pagan Celtic Britain*, P. 350
33. Beith, Mary, *Healing Threads*, P. 175
34. Beith, P. 176
35. Livingstone, Sheila, *Scottish Customs*, PP. 132-133
36. Ross, Anne, *Pagan Celtic Britain*, P. 349
37. Beith, Mary, *Healing Threads*, P. 177
38. Livingstone, Sheila, *Scottish Customs*, P. 131

Hymn to the Horse, Verse 1 (Rig Veda)

*"When you whinnied for the first time, as you were born
Coming from the ocean or from the celestial source..."*[39]

In some Celtic areas such as Ireland, the personification of sovereignty and the Land Goddess was a mare. For this reason, kings had to ritually mate with a mare, in effect "marrying the land" in order to claim legitimate rulership. The Gaulish Goddess Epona (Divine Horse) was personified as riding a horse. She was once worshipped from Gaul to Bulgaria and was even adopted by the Roman cavalry who built a shrine in Her honor in Rome. The wife of King Arthur, Gwenhwyfar's name means "White Mane" which is perhaps a subtle reference to the Land Goddess and to true sovereignty.

The Irish Goddess Macha, though pregnant with twins, ran against the king of Ulster's horses and won. In Wales, the last sheaf of grain is ritually "sacrificed" by first plaiting it, and then by throwing a sickle at it until it is cut. The one who succeeds in cutting the sheaf declares: "Pen medi bach caseg" (I have a little harvest mare). An ornament is made of the last sheaf called a "caseg fedi" (harvest mare). In parts of England, the last sheaf to be cut in the district is called "the mare" and the farmer who holds it must ignominiously keep it all winter (see also Farming, Fertility, and Harvest Customs above).[40]

On Celtic coins and metal objects, the horse is often associated with a crane, and sometimes the horse features wings and a beak as on the Gundestrup Cauldron. Aquatic birds such as cranes and swans have solar associations and healing powers through their relationship with sacred water. A votive bronze horse was found at Coventina's well in Northumberland (near Hadrian's Wall).

The Celtic Otherworld features beautiful, many-colored horses and endless horse racing. In Celtic belief, horses are regarded as creator-Gods: the urine of the steeds of the Gods falls on the Earth to create lochs and wells. The Sea God Manannán mac Lir rides a horse across the waves, from this world to the Otherworld.[41]

Mare's milk is a remedy for whooping cough and can be given to human infants if other milk is unavailable.[42]

Ladybug — Ladybugs are very lucky. It will bring bad luck to kill one.[43]

Limpets — The oil of limpets is placed in the ear to dissolve wax. A broth of limpets will increase breast milk in nursing mothers.[44] (See "Fishing Magic, Boats and the Lore of the Sea" above)

39. O'Flaherty, Wendy Doniger trans., *The Rig Veda*, P. 87
40. Lamb, Gregor, *Carnival of the Animals*, PP. 65-78
41. Ross, Anne, *Pagan Celtic Britain*, P. 321
42. Beith, Mary, *Healing Threads*, P. 178
43. Livingstone, Sheila, *Scottish Customs*, P. 130
44. Beith, Mary, *Healing Threads*, P. 175

Mole — An old cure for rheumatism is to take the earth from a molehill and apply it as hot as possible to the affected part. Follow with a hot seaweed poultice.[45]

Mouse — Mice are eaten fried, boiled, or roasted for whooping cough. In the Highlands, children did not place a tooth under their pillow hoping for a visit from the Tooth Fairy, instead they placed their tooth in front of a mouse's hole and asked the wee mousie to exchange the small tooth for a big one.[46]

Otter — An otter's skin is a charm against drowning and also protects women in labor.[47]

Pig — Tribes or clans that have a boar as their sacred animal totem should only eat pig meat at ritual feasts. In the Celtic Otherworld, magical pigs are killed for the daily feast, and are reborn the next day to be eaten again.[48] (See Boar above)

Ram — Ram horns are especially associated with warriors and Warrior Gods in Celtic iconography. Sacred Divine Warrior Gods were seen as healers in ancient times and sacred Tribal Protector Gods were sometimes associated with healing wells. In Bath (Aquae Sulis) in Southern Britain there is a stone carving of a horned God, a Goddess, three genii cucullati (hooded figures) and a ram. Ram horns appear on the serpent that the antlered God Cernunnos holds on the Gundestrup Cauldron. The ram also appears with a Gaulish God whom the Romans equated with Mars and with the three faced God of the Remi equated with Mercury.[49]

Rooster — If a cock crows three times and then puts its head in the door, expect a visitor. If the cock crows before sunrise, someone will die soon.[50]

Salmon — The salmon appears frequently on Pictish stones and is associated with healing wells and springs. The "Salmon of Wisdom" (éo fis) eats nuts that fall from the nine Hazels of Wisdom around Connla's Well, bestowing magical seership or poetic arts on anyone who eats the fish (see hazel above in "A Highland Herbal"). Finn gained his prophetic powers by tasting the juice of the Salmon of Linn Feic as it was cooking. By tradition the salmon is one of the oldest animals in the world.[51]

Seal — Seal oil both prevents and cures colds when taken internally. Externally, it is rubbed on the chest to cure bronchitis, massaged into

45. *Beith, P. 178*
46. *Ibid., P. 179*
47. *Ibid., P. 180*
48. *Ibid., P. 180*
49. *Ross, Anne, Pagan Celtic Britain, PP. 342-343*
50. *Livingstone, Sheila, Scottish Customs, P. 131*
51. *Ross, Anne, Pagan Celtic Britain, P. 350*

sore joints, and applied to burns.[52] "Selkies" are seal-women who shed their skin by moonlight and assume human guise. Many selkies have married fishermen from the Western Isles.[53]

Sheep — Lamb's broth made with lovage (Levisticum officinale) is given for chest complaints.[54] (See Ram above).

Snail — The juice of roasted snails (Gaelic- seilcheag) benefits lung conditions. All Celtic peoples once ate snail soup for their health, but now only the Gauls regularly consume snails.[55]

Snake (Serpent) — Snakes are often seen on Pictish stone carvings. Serpent holes are watched at Oimelc to see if the creatures emerge from their holes, predicting the end of winter. The ram-horned serpent is a religious symbol associated with Mercury and Mars (by the Romans) in Celtic areas, and with the God Cernunnos on the Gundestrup Cauldron. Serpents appear on Celtic altars and are shown being held by both Mother Goddesses and by Gods.[56] Apply baking soda to a snake bite (after you call for the ambulance!) Make a salve with serpent fat and apply it (presumably to the eyelids and the "third eye" between the eyebrows) to acquire supernatural sight.[57]

Spider — Place fresh cobwebs (not old ones) on a cut to stop bleeding.[58] To kill a spider is very bad luck.[59]

Trout — Trout are associated with sacred wells and springs. They magically appear in certain healing wells to bless them on holy days.[60]

Wolf — The Gaelic word for wolf is madadh-allaidh (wild dog). The wild wolf eventually became the family dog, the oldest domesticated animal; its relationship with humans goes back almost ten thousand years. Once domesticated, wolves were selectively bred to protect the family. They also gave their hides for clothing, and as pelts to sit upon. They were eaten, used as draught animals, and were helpers in the hunt. Neolithic chambered tombs in Orkney such as Cuween Hill Cairn and Mine Howe feature dog skulls.[61] Dogs and wolves appear on Pictish carved stones. The wolf appears on the Gundestrup Cauldron and is closely associated with the antlered God Cernunnos. Tribal Gods were said to manifest themselves as a wolf (or a horse, bull, or salmon).[62]

52. Beith, Mary, Healing Threads, P. 181
53. McNeill, F. Marian, The Silver Bough Vol. I, P. 121
54. Beith, Mary, Healing Threads, P. 181
55. Beith, P. 184
56. Ross, Anne, Pagan Celtic Britain, P. 344
57. Beith, Mary, Healing Threads, PP. 185-186
58. Beith, P. 186
59. Livingstone, Sheila, Scottish Customs, P. 130
60. Ross, Anne, Pagan Celtic Britain, P. 350
61. Lamb, Gregor, Carnival of the Animals, PP. 17-22
62. Ross, Anne, Pagan Celtic Britain, P. 341

Worm — A test of the seventh son of a seventh son's magic was to put a worm into his hand. If his claim was true, the worm would instantly die. Anglo-Saxon and Irish healers used the following charm to dispel disease (the disease was pictured as a worm):

"Gonomil, orgomil, marbumil"

(Traditional)
(Wound the worm, harass the worm, kill the worm)[63]

Once you have selected a totem animal (or once an animal has chosen you), you can dress as the animal when guizing at a festival, or shape shift into the animal to do magical work. When there is a need for a particular animal's skills and attributes, putting on an animal's skin enables you to take on the Spirit of that animal. In ancient times, sorcerers could travel across the landscape at a great speed and perform magic after taking on the Spirit of their totem animal.[64]

---

63. Beith, Mary, *Healing Threads*, P. 188
64. Lamb, Gregor, *Carnival of the Animals*, P. 129

Magical Practices

Prayers, Rituals, and Incantations

The practice of magic in Scotland and in the larger Celtic world is a long and rich tradition. Many remnants of ancient practice survive and folk traditions continue, both so closely interwoven that it is impossible to tell how old some of these practices may be. For many, the word "Druid" still carries a resonance of power and respect because of the magical abilities of the Druid caste that flourished in ancient times.

The ancient Celts distinguished between Druids and Witches. Druids were officials of the court who openly aided and advised the king and the nobles. The king or queen and their Druid were known as the "two kidneys" of a kingdom. Druids had well-defined tribal roles and functions: they were the teachers of the children of the nobility, the lawyers, doctors, ambassadors, poets, philosophers, magicians and religious professionals of the tribe. Druids engaged in battle magic and other types of magic to aid the king and the kingdom as a whole.

Witches were a different class of magical practitioner - loners who lived by their own law. They were feared as a result, because you never knew whose side they would take, or whom they would harm or help. In general, they were counselors and healers for the lower classes.

Every class of society used magic of one kind or another. In ancient Ireland and in the Gaelic areas of Scotland, when a warrior was officially recognized as such they had a geas placed upon them, a type of magical prohibition or "taboo" which human and Otherworldly enemies would do their best to make the warrior violate. Breaking the geas was a guarantee of the warrior's downfall or death.

Lay folk such as farmers and fishermen also had geasa placed upon them, for example: the necessity of always moving sunwise three times around a holy well before taking the water; to always carry a burning brand in the right hand; to circle the house, barn and fields sunwise when saining them; and other magical injunctions.[1]

There is a rich history embedded in the ancient stories of Fairy magic, battle magic, and of the magic associated with the Gods, Goddesses, and the heroes of the Celtic world. Certain objects such as cauldrons, swords, spears and stones had magical associations. The sorceress Kerridwen is said to have had a magical cauldron of inexhaustibility, regeneration and inspiration. Arthur went to Annwn, the Celtic underworld of the dead, to obtain a magical cauldron that gave forth unlimited amounts of food, but would refuse to boil the food of a coward.[2] The magical cauldron of The Daghda supplied an inexhaustible stream of food for His people.

The magical sword of the king Nuada, from which no one could escape once it was drawn, the Spear of Lugh that was so thirsty for blood it had to be kept in a vat filled with a sleeping potion made of poppy seeds when not in use, and the Stone of Fal that shrieked when the true king set his feet upon it (see The Stone of Destiny or Stone of Scone and The Old Gods above) are equally evocative and have their own powerful mythological resonances.

For most people throughout history, the aim of magic has been a practical result, such as rain for the crops, abundant fish, healthy herds, a reliable stream of milk, butter and cheese, fertile crops, protection for the house and family, success in love, and victory in battle. In the simplest terms, magic can be broken down into three principles: the utterance of a spell (or prayer), a rite to "send" the spell (to the Gods, the saints, the elements, etc.), and some kind of concrete action (sprinkling water on the ground or on a sick person or animal, leaping the fire, lighting a candle, a spell written and worn as a talisman until the paper decomposes, stones and plants worn or ingested as "elixirs" to effect a magical outcome, etc.).

"Natural magic" involves learning and using the powers of herbs, trees, stones, sun and moon, etc., and "sympathetic magic" means crafting a spell where "like cures like" or the effect resembles the cause. "Antipathy" is a type of magic where opposites are set to work on each other and "sympathetic resonance" occurs once something has been in contact with something else and the two things continue to affect each other.

"Apotropaic" magic is designed to repel or prevent evil, for example, a community rite of healing. "Purification" uses fire, water, salt, and other sacred means to drive away evil. "Blessing" magic is designed to attract good luck, healing, and love, and to find lost objects.

"Sacrifice" is an ancient form of magic where something of value is given so that the Gods and Spirits reward the giver in return. "Maleficium" or "baneful magic" is deliberate cursing or wishing ill on a person, place or thing. "Charming"

1. Ross, Anne, *Folklore of the Scottish Highlands*, PP. 98-99

2. McNeill, F. Marian, *The Silver Bough Vol. I*, P. 34

is to give help or advice regarding ailments and conditions. "Adjuration" is to command an evil power causing sickness to depart.

There are also the various forms of "divinatory magic" such as "hydromancy" or divination by water, "aeromancy" or divination by the movements of wind and air, "geomancy" or divination based on the powers of the earth, and "pyromancy" or divination by fire, etc.[3]

Quarter Days and Fire Festivals

Potent times to do magic are the Quarter Days and on the first Monday of each quarter. In Scotland the Quarter Days are: Oimelc, February 2, Old Bealltan, May 15, Lúnasdal, August 1, Old Samhuinn, November 11 (remembering that for the Celts the festival begins on the eve before the day).[4] On those days, precautions are taken to ensure that luck does not leave the house because lending fire or an item might result in your good luck leaving with the object.

Conversely, it is very good luck to bring a piece of coal or peat into the house on each Quarter Day, as it is good luck to share wine or whisky on such a day. Hospitality of all kinds always brings good luck and prosperity: to feed a visitor or a stranger, to bring a gift to a new house or to a friend when visiting, and so forth, brings luck to the doer, on any day of the year.[5]

The first person to rise on a Quarter Day should take the household pet and put it out of doors, as any lurking Spirits will follow the animal out. The first Monday of the Quarter is a good time to make a frith (divination or augury). The Frithir rises before dawn and goes fasting and barefoot to stand at the door of the house, with one hand on each door jamb. With their eyes closed they make a prayer to their Gods, and then open their eyes to perform a divination.

The first object seen determines the augury. A man standing means good health and recovery from sickness. A man lying means illness. A woman standing means an unlucky event is in the offing, and a woman passing by, or approaching, means good luck. A female with red hair is a very unlucky sign, a female with black hair is good luck, and a brown haired woman is the best luck of all. Blondes, particularly those with blue eyes, are considered very attractive to the Fairies and may draw their attention.

A bird flying by is a good omen, especially if it is a dove or a lark. A pig or a boar is good luck for everyone (especially the Campbells). To see a cat is especially good luck for the MacIntoshes, MacPhersons, and Cattenachs. To see the totem animal of your clan is always good luck.[6]

The Quarter Days are also known as "Fire Festivals" because the rituals associated with these festivals always involve sacred fire. A sacred fire, bonfire,

3. Miller, Joyce, *Magic and Witchcraft in Scotland*, PP. 3-4, 13-14
4. McNeill, F. Marian, *The Silver Bough Vol. I*, P. 18
5. Livingstone, Sheila, *Scottish Customs*, P. 78
6. McNeill, F. Marian, *The Silver Bough Vol. I*, P. 56

or "need-fire" (see Fire Magic section above in "Lore of the Elements" for how to make a need-fire) is lit and all household fires are put out and then re-lit using flame from the ritual fire. Humans and beasts are sained by being passed through or jumping through or over, or walking deiseil around the fire. Libations of milk, whisky, oil, butter, fragrant herbs and other offerings are made to the ritual fire.

The festival of Samhuinn marks the official start of the Celtic year. It is the official end of the harvest when the Spirits of the Land are thanked for their many gifts. Offerings of ale are made to Shony, the God of the Sea, in thanks for the seaweed and fish. The dead of the family are remembered and honored, disguises are put on to fool the wandering dead, and a feast is held for both the living and the dead of the family. Deep magic at the Samhuinn quarter involves going within and meditating on that which you seek to manifest for yourself and for the world in the next solar cycle.

The Winter Solstice and Yule mark the next magical interval. Fires are lit on the hills to encourage the return of the sun by sympathetic magic and divinations are made by hiding small objects in "Sowans" a type of grain pudding (see Sowans Nicht, above). Depending on the object drawn, a divination of your future fate is determined. Deep personal magic at this time focuses on the hearth and home, with gratitude felt for the warmth of friends and family and for all the ancestors, creatures and Spirits who have sacrificed their lives so that we humans may have food, clothing, warm shelter, and joy.

At Hogmanay or New Years Eve the "First Footer" or first visitor to the house will determine the luck of the house. The best possible visitor is a tall, dark man. A short, red-headed female is the worst. It is very good luck to give and receive gifts of grain, grass, water (the Waters of Life perhaps?), coal and shortbread.

A "Clavie", or tar barrel mounted on a pole, is lit and paraded around the town and finally immolated on a bonfire on top of a hill. Pieces of the burned wood are collected as good luck charms. Guizers circumambulate the house sunwise, and knock on the doors and walls for luck, receiving bread, oatmeal and whisky as payment. Deep personal magic at this time involves banishing unwanted Spirits from the house and barn, and welcoming in positive energies.

At Oimelc, candles are lit and the Goddess Bríghde is honored in many ways, hoping to attract Her blessings to the house and family (see Oimelc above). Deep magic at Oimelc involves asking Bríghde to bless and inspire your craft and that of all people of arts, and asking Bríghde to bless you with Iomas or "inspiration". A Goddess of Fire, Bríghde oversees the re-kindling of the flames of life and creation at this time, as evidenced by the melting of the ice and the appearance of the new milk from lactating sheep.

At the Spring Equinox, the Kern doll made from the last sheaf of the previous harvest is ritually burned to symbolize the death of one agricultural cycle and the start of a new one (see Spring Equinox above). Deep personal magic at this time involves visualizing that which you wish to burn away, to make way for the new.

At Bealltan, water is collected from a south-running stream or river and sprinkled on the ground, for luck. To wash your face in dew before sunrise is a magical beauty aid. Sprigs of rowan and honeysuckle are hung in the barn to protect the cattle, and the boundaries of the farm are sained with fire. It is very good luck to make love in the furrows and fields, to encourage the fertility of the crops. Deep personal magic at this time involves doing things to ensure the fertility of your projects, of your family, and the world.

At Midsummer, Saint John's Wort is gathered and smoked over the ritual fire to be hung in the house and barn as a protective charm. Thanks offerings are made to the Sun. Deep magic at this time involves taking direct action to improve your life and to aid the world.

At Lúnasdal, a "pleuch" or plow feast is given to all farm hands and family to celebrate the beginning of the harvest. A loaf made with the new grain and choice samples of fruits and vegetables from the garden are put out for the nature Spirits. The Cailleach, the last sheaf to be cut, is divided and fed to the animals for luck, baked into a ritual cake, or kept as an amulet, charm, or doll, to bless the household. Deep magic at this time involves giving thanks for the first fruits of your labors and to do whatever protective magic is necessary to ensure that your "harvest" will come safely in. It is important to thank and remember the Sacred Mother River Goddess of your bio-region at this time.

At the Fall Equinox, a bit of the grain from the year's harvest is held back to be mixed in with the next year's seed store to magically transfer the luck from one year's harvest to the next.[7] Deep personal magic at this time involves sowing the seeds of continuity and of taking steps to leave a legacy for the world, both physical and spiritual. This is a good time to contemplate the bounty of your life, and to consider which organizations and causes can use your talents. Plan how you want your legacy to be passed down.

Love Spells and Moon Magic

The phases of the Moon should be carefully kept track of, because certain types of magic will be most effective at different times. Use the Waxing Moon to initiate or grow a project, and the Waning Moon to withraw energy from something. The Dark of the Moon is a time for banishing and the Full Moon a time of powerful manifestation.

We know that the Druids did certain ceremonies on the "sixth day of the Moon", or six days after the first appearance of the New Moon (Pliny records that the sacred mistletoe was cut at that time).

A tenet of natural magic is that courtship is always most successful when carried out by moonlight. Gather nettles at Samhuinn and hide them between the blankets of your intended, to gain their love. If a pot or kettle boils over, a lover may be lost to you. To avert disaster, drop a straw or a piece of peat into the liquid.[8]

---

7. *Miller, Joyce, Magic and Witchcraft in Scotland, PP. 35-42*
8. *Marwick, Ernest, The Folklore of Orkney and Shetland, P. 86*

At Samhuinn, peel an apple and throw the peel over your shoulder to reveal the initials of a future mate, or sleep with a mirror or flowers under your pillow to dream of them. Hold an apple in your hand until it is warm and then offer it to your intended. If they take a bite, they are yours. (See the "Courtship and Marriage" section above).

The skate, a type of fish, is considered an aphrodisiac in Shetland and Orkney.

A "loving cup" is a cup passed around the table deiseil, by friends. All who drink from it are bound together by bonds of affection, but anyone who refuses to drink should be considered an enemy. In Jacobite days, a secret toast was made by passing your cup over a water jug. This showed allegiance to the "king over the water", i.e. Bonnie Prince Charlie.[9]

Magic and Luck

Lucky signs are called "rathadach" and unlucky signs are called "rosadach". To see a man with brown hair is always a good sign, but especially if the man is approaching the Seer. If the man is going away from the Seer, it is a sign of bad luck. A woman going away from the Seer is a sign of bad luck unless she has red hair, in which case it is a good thing (this fear of red heads may go back to memories of the Viking invasions).

It is good luck to see a person or an animal rising: it implies that someone will get well. But if either is seen lying down or in the act of lying down, it is a bad omen.[10]

There must always be an even number of guests at the table. If there are thirteen dinner guests it is most unlucky, because the first to rise from the table will die within a year. To see a foal or a snail, or hear a cuckoo, before breakfast means that the day will not go well. Water must not be thrown out of the house between dusk and dawn (lest you mistakenly hit a Fairy).[11]

It is bad luck if a swarm of domestic bees lands on your property and the owner does not claim them. Seeing the New Moon through glass is unlucky because the Moon should be seen out of doors and bowed to when first seen. When the head of the clan dies, a lock of their hair must be nailed to the door to keep the Fairies at bay. It is unlucky to enter a house by the rear door if you wish to occupy it. It is very unlucky if a stranger counts your children or farm animals and if anyone asks how many you have - you must always say "bless them".[12]

If honored correctly, the Moon will bring you luck. On seeing the New Moon for the first time, turn towards it, bow three times, and then turn the coins in your pocket for luck. Alternatively, a gold ring can be turned three times and a wish made. On seeing the New Moon, kiss the nearest man or woman, or kiss your own hand three times while bowing.[13]

---

9. *Livingstone, Sheila, Scottish Customs, P. 88*
10. *Ross, Anne, Folklore of the Scottish Highlands, PP. 102, 104*
11. *Ross, P. 101*
12. *Ibid, PP. 100-101*
13. *Livingstone, Sheila, Scottish Customs, PP. 96-97*

Protective Magic

If you fear you have been "Fairy led", that is if you find yourself unaccountably lost in familiar territory: turn your clothes inside out. If an article of clothing is accidentally put on backwards or inside out, it must be worn that way, or exchanged for a completely different garment.

Cheese is said to be very protective. Hold a small piece of it or carry it, on your person, to prevent being "Fairy led" or lost in a fog. Cheese may also be offered to a sacred well to prevent becoming lost (leave it nearby for the Spirits).[14]

Warrior Magic

Certain herbs and trees are protective for warriors (see "A Highland Herbal" above). The MacDonalds once wore heather (fraoch) in their caps, the Grants fir (giuthas), and the MacIntoshes holly (cuileann) when going into battle.

It is a good omen for a warrior if they meet an armed man, but if a barefooted woman crosses their path they must draw a tiny bit of blood from her forehead. If a deer, fox, hare, or other game animal is seen by warriors setting out for battle, they must kill it to ward off bad luck.

Everyone owes a cuid-oidhche (a night's portion) to the clan chief while the chief is on a raid. The tenant whose land the chief is on at nightfall must provide hospitality for the chief, the warriors, and their dogs. The blood from the first armed person encountered on enemy land must be sprinkled on the flag.[15]

Magic on the Farm

To steal your neighbor's luck, gather dew from their pasture and use it to rinse your own milking vessels. This will increase your own milk yield while lessening theirs.

To protect your own cows from being "forespoken" and to counter a similar spell, take well water before sunrise and put it into a bucket. Place a silver coin in the bucket and give the silvered water to your animals.[16]

A very simple protective spell for a cow is to tie a red thread around her tail. For a person, bind tiny rowan twigs with red thread and hide them somewhere in their clothing.

Magic and Bairns

To protect the bairns, make the cradle out of elder, rowan or oak. It is also very lucky to borrow a cradle. Place a sprig of mistletoe (gather or purchase it on the sixth day of the Moon and be sure to remove the poisonous berries!) in the cradle, under the mattress where the bairn can't get at it. Convovulus (see Hedge Bindweed above) is burned at both ends and hung over the cradle (high enough above the bairn so that it can't be reached). The father's dirk can be placed under the cradle and the bairn can wear a bracelet of coral as protection. Rattles were originally given to babies to frighten away evil Spirits.[17]

14. *Ross, Anne, Folklore of the Scottish Highlands, P. 91*
15. *Ross, Anne, Folklore of the Scottish Highlands, PP. 27-29*
16. *McNeill, F. Marian, The Silver Bough Vol. I, P. 55*
17. *Livingstone, Sheila, Scottish Customs, PP. 16-17*

The caul, a membrane covering the head of a newborn human or animal, is said to protect sailors from drowning. Those who are born with a caul are destined to be great healers.[18]

Silver Magic

To bring calm in the face of an approaching storm, "silver the water" by tossing a few silver coins into the waves. Silver coins are nailed to a ship to bring good luck in fishing and also drilled with a hole and worn for luck (see other references to this above). Silver coins are placed in the shoe to ward off evil. When selling something, be sure to hand back a piece of silver to the buyer for luck.

Place silver or other coins into an oat cake or a clootie dumpling, and the person who finds the coin will get the luck. Place a coin over a boil and cover with a bandage (please boil the coin first, to sterilize it). Place a clean copper coin over a stye.[19]

Glove Magic

If a lady proposes on a leap year and the gentleman refuses her, he must give her a gift of a pair of gloves to protect himself from bad luck. This tradition goes back to medieval times when a glove hanging from the tip of a spear was pointed towards a person who had broken a promise. Throwing down a glove (a gauntlet) is a signal that you are ready to fight. If someone returns a dropped glove it is very bad luck not to thank them.[20]

Iron Magic

Metal, especially iron, is anathema to Fairies. To avert Fairy mischief, hang a horseshoe on the house or barn, with the ends pointing up or else the luck will "run out". Nail a horse shoe to the mast to protect the ship and place one on a grave to keep the Spirit inside. Give a horseshoe to a bride for luck. Iron nails crafted by a blacksmith can be hammered into furniture, cradles, and boats as protection. Sew iron into your clothing to avert evil and to prevent wounding in battle.[21]

Of course, those who want to attract Fairies will avoid the use of iron (though it may be necessary at times to use it when the Fairies are causing a disturbance).

Spitting Magic

Spitting is very protective. You can spit for luck and to ensure the success of a project. Seal a bargain by wetting the thumbs with spit and pressing them together. Spitting on the hearth brings good luck (where fire and water come together is always good magic). Sailors and fisher folk spit on a coin for luck and throw it to the sea before setting out on a voyage. Spitting on the first coin ever earned brings luck.[22]

18. Beith, Mary, *Healing Threads*, P. 168
19. Livingstone, Sheila, *Scottish Customs*, PP. 95-96
20. Livingstone, P. 96
21. *Ibid.*, P. 94
22. *Ibid.*, PP. 93-94

Hair and Nails

Fingernail parings, toenail cuttings, and hair trimmings must always be burned, because a person of evil intent can use them to cast a spell against you. When the head of the clan dies, a lock of their hair is then nailed to the door lintel as a protective charm, and to guarantee continued prosperity for the house. If a bird steals a human hair for its nest, it can result in headaches or baldness for the person whose hair was so taken. To counter this, wear an ivy wreath.[23]

Protection from Ghosts and Spirits

Urine is protective. If you suspect that ghosts are about, have the gentlemen of the house pee on the door posts. When setting out on a journey, carry a white quartz pebble or a piece of rowan wood as protection. You can always carry fire (a lit torch, a lit peat carried in a shovel, etc.) deiseil around something to protect it: around a woman who has given birth, around a new born child, around the home and garden, around a stranger or someone who has done you a favor, etc. This is best done at dawn and again at dusk. Go around the person, place or thing three times, and give them or it your blessings.[24]

Healing Magic

"In summertime be cheerful, chaste
And early out of bed,
In winter be well capped, well shod,
And well on porridge fed".

(Advice of *The Balinaby doctors, 1550 C.E.*)[25]

When undertaking healing magic, you must first ask the patient's permission. If they say "yes" then you should ask them if they can "see" themselves perfectly healed in body, mind, and Spirit. Only if they can do this may the magic commence.

Traditional healing has survived longer in Scotland than in other parts of Europe, largely because Gaelic Scotland did not, for the most part, participate in the Witchcraft hysteria of the sixteenth and seventeenth centuries. One type of healing is simply called eólas (knowledge) and it refers to the knowledge of incantations which are sung over a potion, person, animal, or place.

Eólas charms may be recited over water to be swallowed by a sick person or animal. Persons once walked miles to obtain water from a charmer who had sung an incantation over it. The eólas charmed water was used to cure toothaches, urinary tract infections, bruises, breast swellings, epilepsy, and sprains. No money was accepted for these cures but a gift was always given in exchange.[26]

Sometimes Fairy-hammers were found – ancient stone hatchets made of green porphyry which were used to medicate or "charm" water.

---

23. *Ibid., PP. 88, 93*
24. *Ross, Anne, Folklore of the Scottish Highlands, PP. 48, 95, 96, 102-103*
25. *Beith, Mary, Healing Threads, P. 65*
26. *Beith, P. 198*

Eólas an t-snáithein (the charm of the thread) is a type of healing where three threads, usually colored red, white, and black (or blue) are wound around an affected area while an incantation is sung. Bárr á chinn (the top of the head) is a type of healing where red threads are wound around the neck of the sick person or animal, while singing or reciting a chant to drive evil Spirits out, through the top of the head.[27]

Traditional healers are often born to it. They may be deaf, dumb, a seventh son or daughter, a red head, a gardener, a blacksmith, born with a caul, born in a breech position, or the survivor of a set of twins. Seventh sons are particularly gifted at curing scrofula (tuberculosis of the cervical lymph nodes), as are kings and queens who can sometimes cure it by touch. Those born in a breach position can often cure bad backs. The deaf and dumb are particularly able to find lost or stolen objects.

The gift can be passed from a deceased relative, from an older person to a younger one, from male to female or female to male, through a whispered secret incantation, or by passing on the guardianship of a hallowed healing object.

The Fairies are known to bestow the power of healing. In 1597, Andrew Man of Aberdeen said that the Elf Queen gave him such powers after he helped her give birth. Bessie Dunlop of Ayrshire once gave the Elf Queen a drink and was rewarded by being assigned a Fairy helper named Thomas Reid who gave her advice on healing.[28]

The art of smithcraft is in and of itself magical, based on longstanding Celtic tradition. Smiths are the ones who control iron, one of the most potent substances known to repel malevolent Fairy Spirits. Smiths are also under the guidance of Bríghde, the Goddess of Smithcraft, Healing, and Poetry.

A patient puts their head on the smith's anvil and the smith (who must come from a family of traditional smith healers) raises their hammer, making as if to strike the sick person (in order for this to work the ill person must be truly terrified). The smith stops just before hitting the person in the head. Obviously the smith must be very skilled and very careful to do no harm![29]

In ancient times, smiths were also dentists and had the job of pulling out teeth. Their magic had such status that they had to be given land, making them members of the noble caste.[30]

Many are familiar with the sweat baths of Native American tradition. The Celts had their own "Sweat Houses", dating from the Bronze Age to the medieval period. Over eight hundred such sites are known in Scotland alone. Stones were heated in a fire until red hot and then dropped into a stone-lined water trough, releasing steam which would fill a small stone house or a lodge made of bent sticks covered with hides.

Another method was to build a fire on the earth inside a stone lodge, and when the ground was very hot, the coals were raked out and fresh straw placed

27. Ross, Anne, *Folklore of the Scottish Highlands* P. 21
28. Miller, Joyce, *Magic and Witchcraft in Scotland*, P. 20
29. Ross, Anne, *Folklore of the Scottish Highlands*, PP. 97-98
30. Beith, Mary, *Healing Threads*, P. 99

over the hot soil. When cold water was poured on the hot earth, the steam would rise and fill the hut and the patient could lie down on the warm straw. This type of cure was particularly good for colds, flu, cramps, rheumatism, and other cold, chilly conditions.[31]

If all else failed, the skull of an ancestor was among the most powerful of magical healing tools. The skull was dug up after dark and before dawn, and carried to a holy well. Water was collected in the skull which was then taken to the sick patient. The whole process had to be done in complete silence (such a skull was found at the Goddess Coventina's well near Hadrian's Wall).

Water from an ancestor's skull was deemed especially good for epilepsy. The patient walked to the well in the dark accompanied by a healer, and in complete silence walked three times deiseil around the well while the healer dipped the skull into the water. The healer gave the patient water from the skull three times, each time invoking the Three Worlds of Land, Sea and Sky. The healer then laid a geis (a magical prohibition or taboo) on the sufferer. The healer asked the patient if they had complete faith in the powers of sacred water. If the patient did not, then the cure would never be complete.[32]

Caution: Modern practitioners are well aware that digging up human remains is a crime and will only use bones that have been obtained from a reputable scientific supply house.

Visiting and circumambulating a holy well, drinking or bathing in the source of a river or a sacred loch are also well attested healing methods involving water. And as we have seen in many examples throughout this text, sacred fire is also one of the most powerful agents of magic and healing. A circle of fire can be constructed, consisting of a ring of flaming peat or logs or a large burning hoop suspended in the air. The patient is handed from person to person and passed through the flames.[33]

Herbs and trees also play their part (as described in "A Highland Herbal" section above). Circumambulating an old oak tree three times to effect a cure is an old custom. An all-purpose herbal healing spell is to cut woodbine at the waxing March Moon and make a wreath out of it. The wreath is passed over a sick person three times or they can step through it, pull it down over their head, and so forth.[34]

Some Specific Magical Cures For Ailments and Conditions

Depression — A sickly child or a "melancholy" adult may have been "forespoken". When praising an animal or a child you must always add the phrase "bless your heart" or "the Gods protect you" otherwise the child or animal might be "forespoken" and attract the attentions of evil Spirits.

To cure this condition, gather three pebbles from the seaside: one black, one white, and one that is red, blue or green. Place the stones in water. A healer utters the word "sain" over the water while inscribing a solar, equal armed cross on the surface of the water. The patient should

31. Beith, PP. 136-137
32. Ross, Anne, Folklore of the Scottish Highlands, P. 92
33. Beith, Mary, Healing Threads, P. 99
34. McNeill, F. Marian, The Silver Bough Vol. I, P. 58

drink a few sips, after which the healer sprinkles the rest of the water over them. It is also a good idea for the sufferer to visit holy wells and sacred springs and to eat dulse (a type of sea weed).

A person suffering from wasting disease or lethargy may be "in the hill", or under the influence of Trows or Fairies,, or the sick person's spirit may have been "taken" by someone recently dead (understandable since grief is known to weaken the immune system). A healer must determine if the cause of the affliction is a Hill Spirit, a recently deceased friend or enemy, or a Water Spirit.

Sheep and cattle may also be "taken" and some Trowie breed substituted.

Fairy Doctors are called in if the cause of the illness is Otherworldly. Fairy Doctors get their training by intimate contact with the Trows and the Hill Folk, by dancing with the Fairies under the Moon and by bringing them gifts.

If it is determined that the patient has been afflicted by the newly dead, earth from that person's grave is mixed with the patient's food (and first thoroughly cooked to sterilize it!) or rubbed on the patient's afflicted part, or placed in their stocking.

The earth must be gathered from the graveyard at midnight and none must fall on the ground after it is collected. It should be gathered by a person of the opposite sex to the patient in complete silence.

A decoction of earth (sterilize the earth by baking or boiling it before use) collected from the grave of the recently dead and tormentil root (Potentilla tormentilla) can be made and then placed in a ceramic vessel for twelve hours to steep. Strain it and feed it to the patient.[35]

Toothache — The Cailleach Chearc (Hen Wife) of a village was the midwife for the community who, along with the local blacksmith, was consulted for toothache. She was mistress of charms, love spells, incantations, and advice about travel.[36] A simple charm for toothache was to hold a stone while touching the patient and reciting the following:

> "Three Finnmen* came from their home in the sea
> From the weary worm the folk for to free
> And they shall be paid with the white money
> Out of the flesh and out of the bone;
> Out of the sinew, and out of the skin;
> Out of the skin and into the stone.
> And there may you remain!
> And there may you remain!
> And there may you remain!
> (Traditional charm for tooth ache from Shetland)[37]

*Literally Finns, who were known to have great healing powers. The stone was cast away after the charm was recited.

35. Marwick, Ernest, *The Folklore of Orkney and Shetland, PP. 130, 134*

36. Beith, Mary, *Healing Threads, P. 95*

37. Marwick, Ernest, *The Folklore of Orkney and Shetland, P. 48*

Whooping Cough — To cure a child of whooping cough, bring it to a married couple who were of the same name before they married, as they will be able nurse it to health.[38] Or, put the cuttings of the child's hair into a bread and butter sandwich, and feed the sandwich to a dog. When the dog coughs the child will be cured.[39]

Styes – Draw a hair from a cat's tail across the stye during the Full Moon. Or stand on your head in the ocean until nine waves pass over you.[40]

Jaundice – Boil nine stones in water skimmed off the tops of nine waves. Soak the patient's shirt in the water and have them put it on wet. Or, take water from nine streams where cresses grow (watercress is a sovereign remedy for all kinds of liver ailments which may be where this cure originated) and soak the patient's shirt as above.[41]

Scrofula — A seventh son of a seventh son or a seventh daughter of a seventh daughter will have special healing powers. Their powers will be greatest when healing a member of the opposite sex, and they will have the ability to cure scrofula (chronic discharges and glandular eruptions caused by the tuberculosis bacillus).[42]

Sciatica — In the Hebrides, girdles of sealskin were used to help both sciatica and back pain.

Swollen Glands — to cure swollen glands, the healer should say a magical invocation over a knife blade, on a Friday, while holding the blade close to their mouth. Then, the healer should gently, and without cutting, place the blade on the swelling which is symbolically "divided" into nine sections.

Each time the blade very gently and softly touches one of the nine sections, the blade is then pointed towards a hill, so that the swelling may be transferred to the hill. Finally, the blade is pointed to the ground saying: "the pain be in the ground and the affliction in the earth".[43]

Snake Bite — Apply the severed head of a rabbit or a snake to a snake bite. Or, place the dried head of a snake into water and then wash the bite with the water.[44] Highland healers once made a charm bag called a pocan cheann (bag of heads) which was carried by a medicine woman. It contained the head of a toad, a newt and an adder. When someone was bitten, the bag was immersed in a stream that flowed between two crofts. The water that dripped off the bag was then applied to the snake bite (and also to wounds).[45]

38. Beith, Mary, *Healing Threads, P. 92*

39. Livingstone, Sheila, *Scottish Customs, P. 93*

40. Beith, Mary, *Healing Threads, P. 135*

41. Beith, *P. 135*

42. *Ibid. P. 93*

43. Ross, Anne, *Folklore of the Scottish Highlands, P. 108*

44. Ross, *P. 100*

45. Beith, Mary, *Healing Threads, P. 27*

Boils — Beeswax, lard, and pine resin harvested from the outer bark of a
    pine tree, are heated to simmering, cooled slightly, and spread onto a
    clean cloth. One inch of margin should be left at the edges where there
    is no wax or oil. Apply the cloth to the boil and leave it on for twelve
    hours. After removing the plaster it should be burned and discarded.
    Bathe the area and repeat.[46]

Warts — Wash the wart with rain water or the blood of a recently
    butchered pig.[47]

Sore Eyes — To heal sore eyes, wear golden earrings or rub the eyes with
    gold.[48]

Small Pox — Fried mice are a cure for small pox when eaten.[49]

Colds, Fevers and Chills — To treat a cold with fever and chill, keep the
    patient warm in bed and feed them oatmeal with butter, salt and
    pepper. Give them Spruce Beer to drink (beer made from Spruce tips
    and molasses), or make a tea of Spruce tips sweetened with molasses.
    Another traditional cure is to run fully clad into the sea, allow the
    water to cover you, and then run straight home to bed, keeping the wet
    clothes on (place a plastic tarp under the sheets before you try this, or
    use a plastic air mattress). Sea bathing is a traditional cure for many
    conditions such as bone diseases and rheumatism. Drinking a cup of
    sea water at the same time is most effective (sea water is a powerful
    purgative).[50]

Sprain — Take a long thread and fold it several times, then lay it on the
    knee. Spit on the palm of the right hand, twist the thread a few times,
    and then tie a knot. Continue doing this until there are twelve knots.
    Chant a healing spell over the thread and then tie it to the injury or
    tie nine knots into a thread of natural, black wool and tie the knotted
    thread around the affected part.[51] The healer should sing or chant the
    following charm as they tie the knots:

> *Sinew to sinew*
> *Vein to vein*
> *Joint to joint*
> *Bone to bone.*
> (Traditional)

Each day after that, one knot is undone, the healer blowing on the
    knot as they undo it. By the time the last knot is undone, the sprain
    will be healed.[52]

---

46. Beith, P. 233

47. Ross, Anne, *Folklore of the Scottish Highlands*, P. 101

48. Ross, P. 101

49. Ibid., P. 101

50. Beith, Mary, *Healing Threads*, PP. 135, 224

51. Livingstone, Sheila, *Scottish Customs*, P. 93

52. Marwick, Ernest, *The Folklore of Orkney and Shetland*, P. 132

Blister — A blister on the tongue is caused by someone telling lies about you.[53]

Bones and Joints — Bone-setters were specialists who treated bone and joint injuries. The males usually dealt with fractures while the women performed massage and manipulation. Their fee was most often butter which was used to massage the lungs in cases of tuberculosis, and the legs in cases of rickets.[54]

Sick Children — The best cure for a sick child is "nine mothers meat". Collect food from nine mothers whose first borns are sons and feed it to the child.[55]

Abortifacients — Women of the Highlands once took a strong purgative at the "change of the season" (in spring and fall) to prevent sickness. It is interesting that these herbs were strong abortifacients.[56]

CURSES

"What is the sharpest of points?
A satire or a curse".
(From Bretha Nemed Dédenach, an Old Irish tract
on the privileges and responsibilities of poets)[57]

Cursing and "baneful magic" are sad but traditional aspects of Celtic culture. They speak of a tragic human frailty, which is the need to express revenge. It is also a fact that all magic returns to the sender, so engaging in this kind of destructive magic is generally a sign of low intelligence and lack of sense. That said, it is sometimes necessary to protect yourself from a bully or an aggressor. But the only completely ethical uses of magic are for healing, protection and guidance.

The Evil Eye

The "Evil Eye" or droch shúil results from jealousy and can interfere with crops, childbirth, the herds, and milking. The person giving someone or something "The Eye" may not even realize they are doing it, and the ability to do so is often genetic or hereditary (Those who fall victim to it may also have done something to attract the envy and or resentment of others).

To protect yourself from the droch shúil, place gold, silver, and copper coins or jewelry into water taken from a place where both the dead and the living cross over, for example, a bridge near a burial ground over which coffins are transported. Sprinkle some of the water onto an affected person or animal while reciting a healing charm. The rest of the water should be poured into the fire or onto a rock in the front of the house.[58]

---

53. *Marwick, P. 132*
54. *Beith, Mary, Healing Threads, P. 96*
55. *Marwick, Ernest, The Folklore of Orkney and Shetland, P. 134*
56. *Beith, Mary, Healing Threads, P. 96*
57. *Gwynn, ed., "An Old Irish Tract on the Privileges and Responsibilities of Poets", Bretha Nemed Dédenach, Eriu xiii.*
58. *Ross, Anne, Folklore of the Scottish Highlands, P. 87*

Rowan wood: ashes, crosses made from the twigs, sprays hung in the house and barn, or placed in the cradle, are especially powerful to counteract the droch shúil.

Envy Spell

Whoso made thee the envy,
Swarthy man or woman fair,
Thee I will send to thwart it:
Land, Sea, and Sky.

(Based on Carmina Gadelica 156,
Envy Spell, and slightly re-Paganized)[59]

"The Eye" of a man is less dangerous than "The Eye" of a woman, but also more difficult to cure.[60] To counteract "The Eye", carry a clay pot to a stream over which the living and the dead pass (find a bridge over which coffins are transported, for example) in silence. Go down on your right knee, take one palmful of water, and place it into the clay vessel saying:

"I am lifting a little drop of water
In the name of all the Gods
I am lifting a little drop of water
In the name of the Spirits."

(Based on a traditional saying from
Inverness-shire and slightly re-Paganized)[61]

Rub the water on the ears of an afflicted person or down the spine of an afflicted animal saying:

Shake from thee thy harm
Shake from thee thy jealousy
Shake from thee thy illness,
In the name of the Land,
In the name of the Sea,
In the name of the Sky.

(Traditional saying from Inverness-shire, slightly re-Paganized)[62]

Pour the rest of the water onto a rock that is fixed in the earth while uttering the name of the person or animal.

Another way to undo "The Eye" is to rise before dawn and go to a stream over which the living and the dead pass over, and which marks a boundary, in complete silence. Take a palm full of water in the name of The Three (for Pagans that means: Land, Sea, and Sky, while for Christians it may mean The Trinity). Pour the water into a wooden bowl, and go back the same way you came. Sprinkle some of the water on the back of the afflicted person or animal and sprinkle the rest on the hearth-fire flag stone, in the name of The Three.

---

59. Ross, P. 86
60. Beith, Mary, *Healing Threads*, P. 133
61. Carmichael, Alexander, *Carmina Gadelica – Hymns and Incantations*, P. 147
62. Ross, Anne, *Folklore of the Scottish Highlands*, P. 87

You can also take three swallows of silvered water (water into which a silver coin has been placed after first sterilizing it in boiling water for twenty minutes or so). The first swallow is taken in the name of the Land, the second in the name of the Sea and the third in the name of the Sky.[63] An exceptionally pretty child should be sprinkled with silvered water to protect it from "The Eye".

The first Monday of any quarter is an especially vulnerable day. Here is a traditional warning:

> *The first Monday of the quarter,*
> *Take care that luck leave not thy dwelling.*
> *The first Monday of the spring quarter,*
> *Leave not thy cattle neglected.*
>
> *(Traditional)*[64]

On the first Monday of the quarter some farmers would leave their cows inside the barn all day and would only let them out at night, because the only person who could safely set eyes on the cattle was their owner. Anyone else might put "The Eye" on them.

If a farmer suspects that Witchcraft is harming his herd, he should dig a pit at the entrance to the farm and bury a foal in the pit while reciting a charm and horse shoes should be nailed to all buildings on the farm.[65] The farmer should also walk three times deiseil around each affected animal while chanting a prayer to undo the damage.[66]

Salt or silver can be placed in the churn or a red ember flung after a departing guest if "The Eye" is suspected. One who can confidently counteract "The Eye" is said to have eólas or secret wisdom.

A "Canny Woman" (Cunning Woman) or "Skeely Woman" (Skilled Woman) can counteract "The Eye" with a blessing. Such a woman might tie a red thread with knots, uttering a blessing on each knot, and tie it around a child's neck. She might also pass a child through a fiery circle to sain it.[67]

Molluka Nuts (see "A Highland Herbal" chapter above) that wash up on the Western beaches are powerful charms against "The Eye". The white ones are especially prized, because when worn they will turn black if sorcery is used against the wearer. These nuts can also be placed in the milk pail if the cows are ailing and will cause the cows to gradually get better.[68]

Cursing Threads

In the Highlands, threads were used to both activate a curse and to remove a curse. To make a cursing thread, take three threads of three colors (usually black, red, and white) and tie three knots in each thread while uttering a curse

---

63. *Ross., P. 85*
64. *Ibid., P. 84*
65. *Lamb, Gregor, Carnival of the Animals, P. 110*
66. *Ross, Anne, Folklore of the Scottish Highlands, P. 85*
67. *McNeill, F. Marian, The Silver Bough Vol. I, PP. 154-155*
68. *Ross, Anne, Folklore of the Scottish Highlands, P. 84*

on your foe.[69] To undo a curse, knot the threads in the name of the Three Worlds and twist the threads three times around the tail of an afflicted animal, and tie them with a triple knot.[70]

A sorcerer or ill intentioned Witch can delay the birth of a child, even for years, by using a ball of cursed black thread which they keep in a bag behind the loom. When the ball is destroyed the sorcerer's power is undone.[71]

An unrequited or rejected suitor can braid threads of three colors, tying three knots in each, while cursing the bridal bed of his lover. This curse can be countered by the groom putting a silver coin under his foot inside his shoe, and by leaving his shoe untied.[72]

Earth Curses

In Glen Lyon, Perthshire, river stones were blackened in a fire and spells sung over them to cause harm. Alternatively a circle of blackened stones was made in the Waning Moon and a chant sung over them.[73]

Carve your curse and a prophecy onto a stone using an ancient alphabet such as Ogham and place it at the doorstep of your intended victim. Or carve your curse into the smooth turf of a field using an ancient alphabet.[74]

Fasting Against

In ancient times, a person could "fast against" a more powerful person such as a lord or a king who had wronged them by sitting before their door and refusing to eat. If the faster died, it meant utter disgrace and loss of face to the person being "fasted against" and was thus a powerful way to get redress for a grievance, because causing someone to die of starvation at your door was seen as a gross violation of the law of hospitality. Four generations of the faster's family would be the beneficiaries of their sacrifice.

Fasting was also a method of cursing someone. For three days the faster abstained from both food and water. Then, they bathed in a holy well in the dark and kindled a fire, walking nine times around it repeating a curse. At the ninth circuit they said the curse nine times.[75]

Weather Magic

To conjure a storm thrash a stone with a knotted rag while chanting the following:

> *I knot this ragg upon this stane* (stone)
> *To raise the wind in the Cailleach's name;*
> *It shall not lye till I please againe.* (Traditional)[76]
> *The Corpse Creathe* (Clay Body)

---

69. Beith, Mary, *Healing Threads*, P. 21

70. Ross, Anne, *Folklore of the Scottish Highlands*, P. 87

71. Ross, P. 82

72. Livingstone, Sheila, *Scottish Customs*, P. 92

73. Ross, Anne, *Folklore of the Scottish Highlands*, P. 90

74. Marwick, Ernest, *The Folklore of Orkney and Shetland*, P. 56

75. Marwick, P. 56

76. Livingstone, Sheila, *Scottish Customs*, P. 92

Make a body of clay representing a person and pierce it with thorns from a Hawthorn tree, then place the image in a running stream. As the clay dissolves the targeted person will wither away.[77]

Protection from Evil

To escape from any evil thing that is coming after you, go to the "Black Shore", that is, below the line of seaweed, between the seaweed and the water's edge. Nor can evil cross a running stream.[78] You can draw a "ring pass not" of magical protection around yourself by extending your dirk, a flaming brand, a tree branch or a sapling, or even your finger, and inscribing a circle around yourself while saying a protective spell such as this one:

> *Whatever evil comes to me,*
> *May it be returned three times three,*
> *To whoever sent it, so mote it be,*
> *In the name of the Greatest Goddess.*[79]

A more ancient method might be to chant out loud the name of an Ogham letter of protection such as Luis (rowan), inscribing the letter in the air with your finger or a lit branch as you turn.

---

77. *Livingstone, P. 92*

78. *McNeill, F. Marian, The Silver Bough Vol. I, PP. 96-97*

79. *This charm of protection was given to me by my mentor Lord Theodore Mills*

Elves, Spirits, Witches, and Monsters

Banshee — *Bean sidh* (Fairy Woman), a dead ancestress who becomes the guardian Spirit of a particular family. She is known as a Glaistig in the Highlands (see Glaistig below). In Aberdeenshire, the local Banshee is offered barley cakes at wells near hills. The Banshee is called a Hill Goddess when she is of the type that favors wild places. Banshees wander through the woods at twilight, or along the bank of a river, or near a ravine or a waterfall. Occasionally they will lure a traveler to their death or misfortune.[1]

Bean-nighe — (The Washer at the Ford). This female Spirit is seen at midnight, washing the clothing of those who are about to die. She sings a dirge associated with the clan of the one who will die, and if the clothing she is washing is blood stained it means that the person will die in battle.[2]

Blue Men of the Minch — Ocean Spirits that cause rough seas between the Shiant Islands and the Isle of Lewis where they seek to sink ships. They are excellent poets and will spare the life of anyone who can finish a verse that they shout at them.[3]

Bogie — A type of Urisk. (See Urisk below)

Brigdi — A sea monster with huge, sail-like fins with which it can destroy a boat or drag it under the sea. The best protection against it is a "Lammer" - an amber bead. If the monster appears, the "Lammer" is thrown into the sea and the monster disappears.[4]

1. McNeill, F. Marian, *The Silver Bough Vol. I, P. 117*
2. McNeill, P. 117
3. Ibid, P. 120
4. Marwick, Ernest, *The Folklore of Orkney and Shetland, P. 21*

Brownie — A friendly, domesticated Fairy that helps farmers, fishermen and their wives at their work. The Brownie is a human sized, dark skinned fellow who lurks hidden in the house by day and emerges at night to do tasks for the benefit of the household. The bodachan sabhaill (little old man of the grain) is a Brownie that helps with the threshing and tying up of straw bundles. A Brownie may also help with spinning, weaving and the upkeep of boats. He works at night and feeds on warm milk left out for him.

Easily offended, the Brownie may leave the family if he is not allowed to help, if he is given an unsuitable present, or if a servant criticizes his work. If given a gift of new clothes, he disappears and is never seen again. A portion of food and a libation of milk should be poured onto a "Brownie Stone" for his use.[5]

Búcan — A type of Urisk. (See Urisk below)

Caoineag — (The Weeping One) a Fairy who weeps and wails in the dark before a death or a massacre.[6]

Cailleach — (Old Veiled One) Many mountains have their own Cailleach or "Storm Hag" who when angry, creates whirlwinds and tempests.[7]

Cuachag — A river-sprite or river–hag.[8]

Cubbie Roo, Cobbie Row, Coppie Row — A giant who lives in Orkney and is responsible for flinging large stones around the landscape. His finger prints can still be seen on the stones.

> *Hush thee bairn*
> *An' dinna fret thee*
> *Cobbie Row*
> *Will never git thee.*
> *(Traditional rhyme from the Island of Westray)*[9]

Each-Uisge — (Water-Horse) If a young maiden sits in a wild place by a lake or a river, a beautiful man may come and sit beside her. He will to talk with her, and she, being thoroughly charmed, will welcome his amorous embraces. She will find herself stroking his head and singing sweet love songs to him until he dozes off, at which point she finally, but probably too late, notices the water weeds in his hair and his feet shaped like horse's hooves. If she can escape without rousing him her life will be spared, but more usually the beautiful young man convinces the maiden to climb onto his back and he carries her off to his home under the water.[10]

---

5. *McNeill, F. Marian, The Silver Bough Vol. I, P. 123*

6. *McNeill, P. 117*

7. *Ibid, P. 119*

8. *Ibid, P. 119*

9. *Lamb, Gregor, Carnival of the Animals, P. 125*

10. *Ross, Anne, Folklore of the Scottish Highlands, PP. 95-96*

Elf — An ugly little man who likes to harass humans. Elves are short with yellow skin, red eyes, and green teeth and dress in grey but wear brown wool mittens. A sickly cow may have been "elf-shot" with a stone, flint, or wooden arrow. Humans may be "elf-shot" as well, though less often. Anyone who finds a tiny elf arrow is ever after immune from attack. [11]

Elf-Wind — The breath of elves which raises blisters on their victim. [12]

Fairy — Fairies engage in fierce battles with their own kind while dressed in beautiful armor. These are not the tiny cute Disneyesque creatures of modern cartoons. They are a tall, ancient and noble race who can be seen at midnight galloping madly by on their white horses. Sometimes they will replace one of their own sickly cows or children with a healthy one from a human farm. The Fairies are said to be fallen angels who fell into the land. (Those that fell into the Sea became seals). (See the chapter on Fairies below) [13]

Fairy-Ring — A circle where the grain has been worn away by the dancing feet of the Fey (Fairy) Folk. [14] In a forest, such rings are made of circles of mushrooms.

Fin-Folk — A Fin-man looks like a human with a dark, sad face, but with fins tightly formed around his body. The Fin-folk have farms under the ocean and will sometimes pursue fishing boats. To repel them, just throw a silver coin to them because they love silver. They are consummate magicians and can travel many miles with but one stroke of an oar. (Mermaids are a type of Fin-folk, see Mermaid below). [15]

Finfolkaheem — The home of the Fin-folk under the sea which is filled with gardens, colorful seaweeds, and giant pearls. Mermaids grind the pearls in giant querns (stones used to mill grain) and use the powder to add luster to their tails. They have a huge ballroom there which is made of crystal and lit with sea phosphorus and the glow of the Northern Lights. [16]

Furl O' Fairies Ween — A Whirl of Fairies Wind, a whirlwind caused by Fairies that raises dust on the road on a calm summer day. To stop them from "taking" people or animals you must throw your left shoe, your hat, a knife, or earth from a molehill at them saying: *"This is yours that is mine!"* [17] I myself have experienced a Fairy Wind, right in my backyard in Massachusetts. After it spun by, one of my cats went completely mad and never fully recovered.

Giants — These are quarrelsome Land Spirits who throw boulders at each other and place huge rocks close to the shore so they can sit on them and

11. Marwick, Ernest, *The Folklore of Orkney and Shetland*, PP. 42-45

12. Marwick, PP. 42-45

13. Ibid, PP., 42, 45-46

14. Ibid., P. 45

15. Ibid, P. 25

16. Ibid, P. 25

17. McNeill, F. Marian, *The Silver Bough Vol. I, P. 117*

fish because they hate to get their feet wet. They also build clumsy bridges of stepping stones from island to island, and often stay out too long at night with the result that they are turned into stone by the light of the sun.[18]

Giantesses — Their querns (stones for grinding grain) create whirlpools in the ocean as they grind salt for the sea.[19]

Glaistig — In the Highlands, the Glaistig is sometimes called Maighdeann Uaine, the Green Clad Maiden or The Green Lady. She can be seen at twilight moving around the grounds of her former home, often a castle or mansion, or moving through the rooms. If a favorable or unfavorable event is about to affect the family, she is heard to wail. Another type of Glaistig frequents the barn and the herds. If a herder forgets to finish his work, she does it for him and in return expects a daily offering of milk.[20]

Gobar-Bachach — (The Lame Goat) A Spirit that wanders the landscape and gives enough milk to supply a host of warriors. In Skye the last sheaf of the harvest is named after her.[21] (See the chapter Farming, Fertility, and Harvest Customs above for more on this topic.)

Gruagach — The Gruagach is the wandering Spirit of a mother who has died in childbirth or the Spirit of a woman who had been "stolen" by the Fairies. She is tied to a particular piece of land rather than to a family and helps in the home and dairy, especially if offerings of milk are left for her regularly. She is easily offended if not given her due, and will retaliate by letting loose the cows, spilling or spoiling the milk, or ruining the grain. Offerings of milk should be left for her on a Clach na Gruagach (Gruagach stone). She will appear happy when a family is about to get good news and appears sad and weepy if bad news is coming.[22]

In Tiree and Skye, the Glaistig is called a Gruagach.[23] (See Glaistig above)

Gyre, Gyro — An Ogress with many tails and multiple horns.[24] The Gyre-Carline is the name of the Queen of the Fairies in Fife who is the Patron Spirit of spinners.

Hildaland — The summer home of the Fin-Folk - a green island with white houses, babbling streams, lush cornfields, and vast herds of cattle which appears only sporadically to mortal eyes.[25]

Hogboon, Hogboy, Hugboy — From the Old Norse haug-búi a mound-dwarf or guardian Spirit that inhabits a burial mound. While these Spirits are helpful to those who offer them gifts such as wine, ale, or milk, they resent interference with their mounds, for example, children

18. Marwick, Ernest, *The Folklore of Orkney and Shetland*, P. 32
19. Marwick, P. 32
20. McNeill, F. Marian, *The Silver Bough Vol. I*, P. 116
21. McNeill, P. 127
22. Miller, Joyce, *Magic and Witchcraft in Scotland*, P. 24
23. McNeill, F. Marian, *The Silver Bough Vol. I*, P. 116
24. Marwick, Ernest, *The Folklore of Orkney and Shetland*, P. 32
25. Ibid, P. 26

playing on them, or cows grazing on them (not to mention the intrusions of archaeologists and tourists!). They especially resent those who come to steal treasure from a mound.

The very best offerings for a Hogboon are the first milk when a cow calves, the first jug of new ale, or the offering of a rooster or a cow from the farmstead. It is very good luck to set up housekeeping near a burial mound, provided the proper offerings are made on a regular basis. Neglect of the local Hogboon can lead to sickness in the cattle, loss of possessions, or a haunted house. A Hogboon that is well respected and cared for will help with the farm chores and even follow the family if they move house.[26]

Kelpie (From the Gaelic colpach – a colt) — A Kelpie is a magical horse-like creature that lives in water.[27] Known as a Njuggle in Orkney and Shetland, a Water Kelpie inhabits lochs and streams and can take any shape, but most often appears as a horse or a pony. If you ride on its back it will drag you under, but when defeated it turns into a quivering, jelly-like mass.[28]

In its horse form, it strikes the water three times with its tail making a loud noise before it disappears into the water. It has a magic bridle, and if you look through the holes in its bridle you will be able to see Fairies and Spirits. A Kelpie can be seen when a sudden wind ripples over a lake, raising a wave.[29] (See also Each-Uisge above)

Kilmoullach, Kiln-carle — A type of Brownie that works with millers.[30]

Merfolk — (See Mermaid below)

Mermaid — Mermaids hunger for the love of human males whom they pursue and then take to the sea bottom. Their song can lull a man to sleep after which they will entrap him. If a Mermaid marries a human she will drop her tail, but if she marries one of the Fin-folk (her own kind) she becomes uglier and uglier until she becomes a Fin-wife.

The Merfolk are said to live in coastal caves and are known as Sea-Trows in Shetland.[31] (See Fin-folk above).

Njuggle — also Nyuggle or Shoupiltin - See Kelpie above.

Nuckelavee — A sea monster with a head that is three feet in diameter containing one red eye and a mouth like a whale's. It has a profound odor, arms that almost drag the ground, and a lower body that resembles a horse but with fins attached to its legs. It has no proper skin, just raw, red flesh and black veins. Its breath can blight the crops or infect the animals and humans with disease. To escape it you must cross a stream because it detests fresh water.[32]

26. *Ibid, PP. 39-42*
27. *Lamb, Gregor, Carnival of the Animals, P. 67*
28. *Marwick, Ernest, The Folklore of Orkney and Shetland, P. 23*
29. *McNeill, F. Marian, The Silver Bough Vol. I, P. 124*
30. *McNeill, P. 124*
31. *Marwick, Ernest, The Folklore of Orkney and Shetland, P. 24*
32. *Marwick, P. 22*

Sea-Trows — These are clumsy Land-Trows who were banished to the sea by their kin for some unknown (to humans anyway) offense. They live by stealing fish off fishermen's hooks. (See Trows below and Mermaids above)[33]

Seefer — A type of whale whose leaping in the water is prophetic: if it leaps the "right way" it means good fishing and death to the fish. If it leaps the wrong way it means death to men.[34]

Selchie, Selkie, Seal Women — Large grey seals that take the form of beautiful humans in the moonlight: on Midsummer's Eve, at the Spring Tide, or every ninth night. They can be trapped and kept on shore by hiding their sealskins without which they cannot get back to their ocean home.

Selkies often marry fishermen of the islands. Children born of these unions will have horn-thick skin on their palms and on the soles of their feet. If a human woman seeks to contact a Selchie she should weep seven tears into the sea at High Tide[35]

Shelly-Coat — A type of Urisk covered with shells that can be heard clattering as it approaches. (See Urisk below)

Sifan — A large whale-like creature with humps and a long neck. If seen at Bealltan it means a good fishing season.[36]

Sighean — A Highland word for Trow or Fairy

Skekil — A type of Troll, an amalgam of horse and rider with fifteen tails.[37]

The Sluagh – These are aerial hosts of the Spirits of dead mortals. They travel at night, especially around midnight, like a flock of birds, visiting the scenes of their transgressions and may attack any person working at night in a home over which they fly.[38]

Stoor Worm — A creature from Orkney also known as the World Serpent, whose breath could kill any living thing. It was defeated by a young lad who threw burning peat down its throat as it yawned, setting fire to its liver.[39]

Trolls — Ill tempered creatures with gross bodies that are disproportionate in regards to length and width and features, who ride through the air between dusk and midnight (the "Fairy-hours") on bulrushes. If they are still about at sunrise, they are day-bound and visible to mortals until the next sunset.

Their high festivals are Midsummer Eve and the seven days before Yule. At Yule-tide they will attempt to do mischief to humans who have not protected themselves and at the end of the Yule festivities they retreat back into the Underworld.[40]

---

33. *Ibid, P. 30*
34. *Ibid, P. 21*
35. *Marwick, Ernest, The Folklore of Orkney and Shetland, PP. 27-28*
36. *Marwick, P. 21*
37. *Ibid, PP. 32-33*
38. *McNeill, F. Marian, The Silver Bough Vol. I, P. 17*
39. *Marwick, Ernest, The Folklore of Orkney and Shetland, P. 20*
40. *McNeill, F. Marian, The Silver Bough Vol. I, P. 115*

Trow (from Old Norse Troll), Hill-Trows, Hill-Folk, Peerie-Folk —
Smaller than a human and often dressed in grey, these beings live in
social groups inside of hills. They are usually invisible and not seen
except at night. They can ride through the air using a stem of docken
for a steed. They are very ugly by human standards, have sickly children
and often seek to exchange their children and animals for human ones.

The Trows love music and will try to lure human fiddlers to their
home under a hill. If they succeed in this, the fiddler passes a year
and a day with them and retains no memory of the encounter. They
reward fiddlers well by keeping their pockets full of money so long as
the fiddler never speaks of the experience (if they have any recollection
of it). Trows also steal brides and women in labor, and sometimes
will inflict disease. They especially like to kidnap girls and midwives,
and when they steal a woman, a man, a cow, or a child, they leave an
incredibly life-like likeness in its place.

Trows hate steel and love fire and will disappear in a flash of sparks
if the word "Trow" is spoken in their presence. Trows are especially
active at Yuletide. Seven days before Yule, the farm should be sained by
placing an equal armed Solar Cross made of the year's reaping, at the
stile leading to the place where the grain and straw are stored.

To protect the house and land from enchantment by Trows, take hair
from every animal on the farm and make a plait. Fasten the plait to the
barn door, and then carry a blazing peat in and through all the farm
buildings. Banging pots and pans or keeping a dog with double back
claws (dew claws) is also considered effective. To repel them, brandish
a knife or a pair of scissors or any other metal object, and draw a circle
in the air around you.[41]

Urisk, Uruisg — This Spirit is half human and half goat, with long hair,
teeth, and claws. It is found in watery, forested areas and may be seen
at twilight sitting on a rock. It stays in the high places all summer
and descends to the farmlands in winter, sometimes haunting a mill
or a waterfall. Depending upon how it is treated it is capable of loyal
service to humans, or butchery and arson. It is very easily offended but
also craves human kindness.[42]

The Washer at the Ford — See Bean-nighe above.

Water Bull and Water Cow — Magical kine that live in a loch and can only
be killed with a silver bullet.[43]

Water-Horse — See Each-Uisge above

Witch — One who has learned their craft from the Trows. To become a
Witch, go to a lonely beach at midnight on the day of the Full Moon,

---

41. Marwick, Ernest, *The Folklore of Orkney and Shetland*, PP. 33-39
42. McNeill, F. Marian, *The Silver Bough Vol. I, P. 121*
43. McNeill, P. 127

turn three times deiseil and then lie down on the Black Shore (between the line of seaweed and the sea) with legs and arms stretched out like a star. Place a stone beside each hand, foot, at the head, on the heart, and on the loins saying:

> *Powers of the sea and hill*
> *Fill me with the Witch's skill,*
> *And I shall serve with all my will.*
> *Come take me now,*
> *Take me away*
> *Take me; take me, now I say,*
> *From the top of my head*
> *To the tip of my toe*
> *Take all that's out and in me.*
> *Take hide and hair,*
> *Flesh, blood, and bone,*
> *Take all between the seven stones.*
> *In the name of the Gods I love!*
> (*Traditional incantation from Orkney, slightly re-Paganized*)

Lie quietly for a while and then turn onto the right side, rise and throw the stones, one at a time, into the sea. Utter a blessing as each stone is thrown. A simpler version of this rite is to place one hand at the crown of the head and one at the soles of the feet saying:

> *Take all that is between my two hands.*[44]

---

44. Marwick, Ernest, *The Folklore of Orkney and Shetland*, P. 50

The Fairies

According to those who know, the typical Fairy is slender and dressed in green, with golden combs in her yellow hair. She can change clear water into wine, weave spider webs into tartan cloth, and make music from a stalk of reed that brings peace to the listener if they need it, and rouses others to joyful dancing.

Fairy bows are made from the ribs of a man buried where three laird's lands meet. Their arrows are made of reeds tipped with white flint points that they dip into the dew of a hemlock tree. They ride on silent steeds that would not disturb a flower, and take their milk from the red deer who are their "cattle".[1]

It has been said that the Fairies were once proud angels who rebelled, demanding their own kingdom. They stepped out of heaven and fell to earth and ever since have dwelt underground.[2] There are different sorts of Fairies, the "good" ones, or at least the ones that are kindly disposed to the human race, are called "Gude Wichts" or "The Seely Court". Those that are less well disposed to humanity are known as "Wicked Wichts" or "The Unseely Court". The "good" Fairies help humans in the house and barn. The "wicked" ones are always ready to inflict injury on mortals.[3]

Some of the damage that Fairies may inflict on humans is to steal a bairn, a sheep or other animal, and substitute one of their own bairns for the wean (from wee ane, little one). They will sometimes abduct a nursing mother and keep her hostage to feed their Fairy children, and if a bairn falls suddenly ill or if its behavior dramatically changes it may be a "changeling". Purification by fire is the prescribed method to restore it, by passing the bairn over red hot coals and then placing some of the cinders into a cup of water which is given it to the bairn to drink (this method also cures Fairy Stroke).[4]

1. McNeill, F. Marian, *The Silver Bough Vol. I*, PP. 107-108
2. Evans-Wentz, W.Y., *The Fairy Faith in Celtic Countries*, P. 84
3. McNeill, F. Marian, *The Silver Bough Vol. I*, P. 108
4. Evans-Wentz, W.Y., *The Fairy Faith in Celtic Countries*, P. 91

Another way to cause a changeling to return is to place the sick child on the cold hearth after the fire has been removed, or to pass the bairn very quickly through a fire (taking extreme care not to burn the child!). Newborn babies can be protected from Fairy abduction by the use of silver such as a silver coin, a silver ornament, or a rattle - one reason babies were traditionally given a silver rattle.[5] Another method is to place a knitting needle or an iron object in the cradle, under the mattress where the bairn can't get at it.

Burning a scrap of leather in the fire is said to dissuade Fairies. The father's pants can be hung over the cradle at night as protection, and Rowan twigs, leaves and berries are a sure safeguard when placed in the child's bed.

Be sure not to cut a child's hair or nails until it is one year old, and be careful to burn any clippings after that, because such parings and cuttings can be used to cast spells.[6] Iron may also be hung over the bed and Móthan fed to the cow that provides milk for the newborn (see Móthan in the Highland Herbal chapter above).[7] A "Trowist" is a woman with particular knowledge of how to deal with such Fairy problems.

Teine Sith is Fairy Fire, which may be seen on nights when the Fairy Mounds are open and their lamps are lit to illuminate their singing and dancing. Breaca Sith are Fairy Marks, spots that appear on a dead or dying person. Marcachd Shith is Fairy Riding, a spinal paralysis in an animal caused by a Fairy mouse riding on their back. A Piob Shith is a Fairy Pipe or Elfin Pipe, sometimes found in underground houses.

Miaran na Mna Sithe is "The Thimble of the Fairy Woman" or Foxglove (Digitalis) and Lion na Mna Sithe is "The Lint of the Fairy Woman" or Fairy Flax (Linum catharticum), a medicinal herb. Curachan na Mna Sithe is "The Coracle of the Fairy Woman", a type of blue shell called the Blue Valilla.[8] Saighead Shidh are Fairy arrows, tiny flint arrowheads said to have been shot at a cow or a person by the Fairies (sometimes known as "Elf Shot").[9]

Those who have visited the Fairy realms of Avalon (Emain Abhlach, Emain of the Apples) or Tir-Na-N'Og (The Land of Youth or The Land of the Ever Young), report that these are places of eternal youth and eternal spring, of clear waters, sunshine, flowers, fruits, honey and birds. It is a country ruled by Aengus, the young God of Love, who plays his golden harp with its silver strings.

To enter the Land of Heart's Desire, a silver apple branch or a single apple is needed, given from the hand of a Fairy woman. The Fairy Land is also called Tir nam Béo (The Land of the Living) because there all the joys of life: hunting, feasting, and love making, reign supreme.[10] The Tuatha dé Danann are the gentry who come from the Land of Promise and the Sea God Manannan Mac Lir is actually a Fairy Chieftain.[11]

5. *Miller, Joyce, Magic and Witchcraft in Scotland, P. 28*
6. *Livingstone, Sheila, Scottish Customs, P. 17*
7. *McNeill, F. Marian, The Silver Bough Vol. I, P. 111*
8. *Evans-Wentz, W.Y., The Fairy Faith in Celtic Countries, P. 86*
9. *Evans-Wentz, W.Y., P. 88*
10. *McNeill, F. Marian, The Silver Bough Vol. I, PP. 103-104*
11. *McNeill PP. 34-35*

The Fairy Hills (Cnoc an t-Suidhe)

Fairies live in Fairy Hills, in scattered communities usually ruled by a queen, where they dwell inside bee-hive structures covered with turf that look like ordinary grass hills to human eyes. Another term for such a Hill is trowie knowe, or a knoll inhabited by trolls.

Fairies have their own herds and flocks, but they do not grow crops and have a great horror of iron (though they do work bronze). Their main weapon of choice is the Saighead Shidh (Elf Bolt or Fairy Arrow).

They are consummate masters of poetry and music and are most often seen at twilight. I have not seen them but I have heard the Fairy music and I can report that they sing in a beautiful ancient language in perfect, razor-sharp, three-part harmony.

The "Queen of Elfame" rides a beautiful milk-white steed upon which she carries off mortals who have taken her fancy. Sometimes Fairy women come in magic boats from a green island in the west, to capture mortals whom they love, and take them into the hills.[12]

A number of such Fairy Hills are known to the race of humans – places where the Fairies gather on the eve of the Fire Festivals. Tom-na-hurich in Inverness (now a churchyard) is one such place. Others are The Fairy Hill of Aberfoyle, Calton Hill in Edinburgh, Eildon hills in the Borders, and the greatest hill of all, Schiehallion (Sídh Chailleann) a mountain in the Grampians that is the home of the Fairy queen, which overlooks the Fortingall Yew, the oldest tree in Europe.

Above Lochcon near the source of the Forth is Coir-shian (Cove of the Women of Peace) and in Eigg is Cnoc-na-Piobaireachd (The Hill of Piping), where you can hear tunes on a Full Moon night.[13]

Sightings

Fairies used to be more plentiful and easily seen in the Highlands, but when the land was given over to sheep, and when deer and grouse shooting became common, they retreated from human eyes. Glenshee, Perthshire, was once full of Fairies but the sound of the train whistle scared them underground.

Sometimes a "Fairy Hunt" can still be heard – the barking of dogs and the bleating of sheep when there are no sheep to be seen, and bagpipes can still sometimes be heard when there is no piper about.[14] In my own experience, the most powerful places to hear Fairies are Old Growth forests and abandoned stone circles, yet another reason why we humans must do all in our power to preserve the last vestiges of untouched wilderness.

At one time, Highland women were careful to not take a newborn out at night for fear the Fairies would "take" the child. No one would dare step inside a Fairy Ring for fear of being "taken" and folk were known to disappear for twenty years or more, into the hills.[15]

12. *Ibid, PP. 101-102*
13. *Ibid, PP. 108-110*
14. *Evans-Wentz, W.Y., The Fairy Faith in Celtic Countries, PP. 86, 94-95*
15. *Evans-Wentz, W.Y., PP. 91, 94-95*

Fairy Rings reveal where the Fairies dance. They can be detected when the green sward of an old heath forms a circle that is darker than the surrounding grasses, or when mushrooms grow in a perfect circle.

The best time to see Fairies is on the eve of a Fire Festival when they move house, from Fairy mound to Fairy mound. It is particularly important to leave offerings on your Fairy Altar at those times (a wooden or stone construction in the garden where food and drink offerings are left), for their refreshment.[16] Fairies appreciate gifts of milk and ale on these nights, and milk and ale are offered to the Fairies at Samhuinn by pouring libations into tombs.

On Samhuinn, the Fairies get into fights and mischief, just like humans do. You will know there has been a Fairy Battle in your area if you examine the lichen on the rocks. After a frost, the lichen on the rocks turns yellowish, and when it thaws, red spots will appear on the stones which are actually Fairy blood.[17]

In the summer sheiling (grazing), when one is milking the cows at twilight, Fairy dancers may appear, dancing their reels. But if anyone hears the Fairy music and sees the dancing they must leave a bit of iron at the entrance to the bower, or else the Fairies will close the door on the watcher and they themselves will end up dancing for years. The person who has been "Fairy led" will think they have been gone for a day but their human family will mourn their death.[18]

The Color Green

In Britain and Ireland the Fairies wear green, the color of rebirth and of the force of nature as it emerges from the seeming death of winter. Green implies immortality, eternal life, truth and victory. In British stories, when queen Guinevere decided to go a-Maying, she commanded her retinue to dress in green, the color of spring and of re-birth. Green is the favorite color of the Tuatha dé Danann (Tribe of the Goddess Danu) and of all the Fairy tribes who will dwell under Earth until the end of creation.[19]

Fairies and Hosts

Fairies are Spirits that live without material food, are "good" (by human standards) and help humanity. "Hosts" are evil (at least from the human perspective) and live on that which they can steal. "Hosts" will pick up a person and deposit them miles away. Some say that "Hosts" are a different type of Fairy that lives in the high places. Also called "Fairies of the Air", they are distinct from the Fairies who live in the hills. These "Fairies of the Air" are most active at midnight.[20]

Fairy Gifts

In Barra, a carpenter's apprentice was building a boat and went to work one morning only to discover that he had forgotten one of his tools. He went home briefly to fetch it and on returning to the carpenter's shed, found it filled with Fairy men and women.

16. McNeill, F. Marian, *The Silver Bough Vol. I, P. 57*
17. Evans-Wentz, W.Y., *The Fairy Faith in Celtic Countries, PP. 91-92*
18. Evans-Wentz, W.Y., *PP. 88, 116*
19. *Ibid., P. 313*
20. *Ibid, PP. 104-106*

The Fairies were frightened at the sight of him and ran away so fast that one of the Fairy women left her belt behind. The apprentice picked it up and when the Fairy woman came back to claim it, he refused to give it back to her. She then said that if he would give it back she would bestow on him such skill that he would instantly become a master carpenter with no further need of apprenticeship.

The next morning when the master came to view the boat, he was amazed at the fine quality of workmanship. The apprentice then told the master how he had acquired his sudden skill. This story is from the early 1800's in Barra.[21]

One time when the heir of the Macleods was born, a beautiful Fairy woman (a Banshee) appeared at the castle and sang a series of verses over the bairn as a protective charm, and then disappeared. For generations afterwards the nurse of the Macleod heir always sang those verses.[22]

The Macleods of Dunvegan have a Fairy Flag (Am Bratach Sith) that once belonged to the Fairy wife of a clan chief. Some say it is a cloth that the Fairy was using to wrap the chief's son as she sought to abduct him from his human mother. Others say the fabric belonged to a Macleod who brought it back from the Crusades (the fabric is silk dating to the fourth to seventh century CE).

In any case, the flag has special powers to protect the Macleods. Draped over the marriage bed it ensures fertility, and it has been carried to guarantee success in battle. Macleod airmen serving in World War II carried it for their protection.[23]

The Mackays also have such a flag, gifted to their clan by a Fairy.[24]

Fairy Music

The Macleods had chanters gifted to them by Fairy women and The Black Chanter of Clan Chattan was given to a talented MacPherson piper by a Fairy lover. The MacCrimmons have a silver chanter given to them by a Fairy woman. Mairi Nic Iain Fhin, Bard to the MacNeill of Barra, received her gift of song from a Fairy lover.[25]

On Cnoc-na-Piobaireachd (The Hill of Piping) on the Isle of Eigg, musicians can hear tunes emanating from under the ground.[26] On the Isle of Skye, Fairies have been heard singing a "waulking song" of the type heard when tartan cloth is processed. This song is heard at two locations, the Dun-Osdale round tower and also near two hills called Heléval Mhor (the greater) and Heléval Bheag (the lesser).

In Perthshire, a member of clan Campbell married a beautiful woman who was "taken" on her wedding day. The Fairies put a cloak of invisibility upon her for a year and a day. She could be heard singing to the cows of her husband every day when she came to do the milking, but he could not see her in physical form until a year had passed.[27]

21. *Ibid, PP. 106-107*
22. *Ibid, P. 99*
23. *Miller, Joyce, Magic and Witchcraft in Scotland, P. 21*
24. *McNeill, F. Marian, The Silver Bough Vol. I, P. 110*
25. *McNeill, P. 110*
26. *Miller, Joyce, Magic and Witchcraft in Scotland, P. 20*
27. *Evans-Wentz, W.Y., The Fairy Faith in Celtic Countries, P. 98*

Some Fairy Lore

Fairy women will sometimes appear, dressed in green, to help a woman with her carding and spinning.[28] In an account from Barra, a newly married couple was on the way to the bride's father's house when the groom fell behind. He had seen a Fairy mound along the side of the road and entered it and was not seen again for two generations. When he finally reappeared he was the same age as the day he married.[29]

Donald MacAlastair of Arran reported that the Fairies used to travel to Ireland and back, riding a stalk of ragwort.[30]

A fiddler of my acquaintance was traveling and playing for his supper in local pubs. His style was very lively and fast. An old man approached him at the bar one evening and warned him to stop playing that way, lest he be "taken" by the Fairies.

A day when the weather alternates between sun and rain is known as "The gueede folk's bakin day" or "the fairies' bakin day." The rain supplies water to make the leaven and the sun's fire bakes the bread.[31]

28. *Evans-Wentz, W.Y., P. 110*

29. *Ibid, P. 113*

30. *Ibid, P. 87*

31. *Dictionary of the Scots Language, http://www.dsl.ac.uk/dsl/*

In Conclusion

*O*ne might well ask if the traditions and practices of the Picts, Celts, Norse and Anglo-Saxon ancestors that make up Scottish folk ways have any relevance for the people of today. We live in the era of disappearing oil reserves and there will soon come a time when long distance travel will again be the luxury and adventure that it has been for most of human history. As is already happening in places like Oregon, family farms and local, community based agriculture will once again flourish. It will be too expensive, both in cash and in globally warming carbon emissions, to ship food half way around the planet in all seasons (the only possible solution will be if we embrace alternative energy solutions).

As people's lives become once more agriculturally based, folk will look to the old ways for inspiration as they seek to honor the Land Sprits and the seasons. It is for these future generations that I offer this book, in hopes that they will tend the Earth and Her creatures, the seen and the unseen, with loving care.

A note about Witches: some of the kindest, most helpful and altruistic people I know are Witches. If I am ever sick or in need they are often the ones I turn to for support.

Appendix
Pronunciation Guide

A

Abaris	Ah-BAH-riss
achlasan chaluim chille	AKH-luss-un KHAl-UM hill-YUH
Aedh	EETH (ancient) EE (modern)
Aengus	EN-gus
Aidan mac Gabhrán	EE-thawn mak GOW-rawn
ainis	ANN-ish
áiridhean	AH-ree-yun
Airmidh, Airmidh	AR-VEY or AR-vee } variants of the same name
áirneag	AHR-nyug
Airts	(English word)
aiteann	AHH-chunn
aladh	AH-lugh
Alator	ah-LAH-tor
Alfadir	Al-fah-theer (Norse)
Allt Eireann	AWLT Ey-ryun
am beárnan Bríghde	um BYAHR-nun BREE-juh
Am Bratach Sith	um BRAH-Tokh SHEE
am bualan	un BOO-u-lun
am maraiche	um MAR-ih-hyuh
An Daghda	un DAGH-thuh (ancient); un DEYE-duh (modern)
an neónan mór	un NYAW-nun MAWR
Ana	AH-nuh
Andarta	ahn-DAHR-tuh
Andraste	ahn-DRAHSS-the
Angus Og	EN-gus AWG
Annwn	AHN-noon

Antenociticus	ahn-the-no-KEE-tee-kooss (Latin or possibly Latinized)
Anu	AH-nuh (older spelling of Ana)
Aquae Sulis	AH-kweye-SOO-lis (Latin)
Arecurius	ah-reh-KOOR-yoos (Latin)
Ard-gael	ahrd-gehl
Artogenos	ahr-to-GEH-noss
Atecotti	ah-teh-KOT-tee
Ath Fodhla	AH FOW-luh

B

Badb	BAH-thur (ancient); BOYV (modern)
Balder	BAHL-der (probably originally from Frisia or Denmark area)
Ball Mo-Luidhe	BAWL mo-LWEE-yuh
Banba	BAHN-vuh
Bara Brith	BAH-rah BREETH
Barmbrack	(English)
Bárr á chin	BAHR uh HEEN
barr brisgein	BAHR BRISH-kin
Barrecis	bahr-EH-kiss
Barrex	BAH-rex
bealaidh	BYAL-ee
Bealltan	BYAL-tun
Bean sidh	BAN SHEE / BAHN-she
bean-tuirim	BAN-TIHR-im
Beannachadh na Cuairte	BYAN-nuh-khuh nuh KOOR-chuh
Bean-nighe	BAN-NEE
bean-tuirim	BAN-TIHR-im
beith	BEY
Belatucadros	Beh-lah-too-KAHD-ross
Belinus / Belenos	Beh-LEY-noss or BEY-leh-noss
Bestla	BEST-lah (Norse)
bhán	VAWN or WAWN
biolair	BEE-lur
biolair ghriagain	BEE-lur GHREE-gih
bioras	BEE-rus
Blodeuwedd	Blo-DEYE-weth
Boand	BO-awn
Bodach	BO-dukh
bodachan sabhaill	BO-dukh-un SAH-vil
bodan coille	BOD-un KOL-lyuh
Bonnach	BON-nukh
Bor	BOR
borrach	BOR-rukh
Boudicca	boo-DEEK-kah
Braciaca	brak-YAH-kah

Bran	BRAHN
Branwen	BRAHN-wen
braoileag	BRUH-il-yug
Breaca Sith	BRYAHH-kuh SHEE
Brehon	(English)
Bretha Nemed Dédenach	BRETH-uh NEV-uth THEY-thun-ukh
Brideag	BREE-jug
Bríghde (Brighid, Brigantia, Bride)	BREE-juh
brisgean	BRISH-gyun
bróg na cuthaid	BRAWG nuh KOO-hij
Broichan	BRIH-khun
buaghallan	BOO-khul-lun
Búcan	BOO-kun
buidhe	BWEE
buntáta	bun-TAH-tuh
burmaid	BUR-mij

C

Caelestis	keye-less-tiss (Latin)
Caereni	keye-REY-nee
Cailleach	KAL-lyukh
Cailleach an Dúdain	KAL-lyukh un DOO-din
Cailleach an Teampuill	KAL-lyukh un CHAM-pull
Cailleach Bhéara	KAL-lyukh VYEY-ruh
Cailleach Bheur	KAL-lyukh VYEYR
Cailleach Chearc	KAL-lyukh HYARK
Cailleach Oidhche	KAL-lyukh UH-ee-hyuh
Cairbre Caitchenn	KAR-ub-ryuh KACH-hyan
cairgein	KAR-uh-gin
cál deanntaig	KAWL JAWN-tigh
Caledonia	(Possibly Old Norse – from the Latin)
Caledonii	Kah-leh-DO-nee-ee
Callanish	(English)
calltainn	KAWL-tin
camobhaidh	KOM-ov-ee
camobhil	KOM-o-veel
Camulos	Kah-moo-loss
caochag	KUH-oo-khug
Caoilte	KUH-il-chuh (Scottish); KWEEL-chuh (Irish)
Caoineag	KUH-in-yug
caorann	KUH-run
carra	KAW-ruh
carrachan	KAH-ruh-khun
carra-meille	KAW-ruh MEYL-yuh
caseg fedi	KAHSS-eg VEH-dee

cas-on-uain	KAHSS un OO-in
Cath Palug	KAHTH PAH-loog
ceílidh	KEY-lee
Cernennus	Kehr-NEH-noss
Cernunnos	Kehr–NOON-noss
ceud-bhileach	kyeyd VEEL-yukh
chaochail e	KHUH-u-khul eh
ciar	Kee-ar
Cináed mac Ailpín	KIN-eeth mak AL-pin
Clach Bhuaidh	KLAKH VOO-ee
Clach Dearg	KLAKH JAIR-ug
Clach na Gruagach	KLAKH nuh GROO-u-gukh
Clach na h-Iobairte	KLAKH nuh HEE-bur-chuh
Clach Nathrach	KLACH NAHH-rukh
clach raineach	KLACH RAN-yukh
Clachan	KLAH-khun
Clachan nan Gilleadha Cráigein	KLAH-khun nun GEEL-yuh KRAH-gin
Clachan-glúin a' choilich	KLAH-khun GLOOIN uh HUL-ikh
Clach-bhan	KLAHKH-vahn
cliabh	KLEE-UV
clois	KLOSH
cluaran	KLOO-u-run
cluas an fleidh	KLOO-uss un FLEY
cluas liath	KLOO-uss LEE-uh
Cnaipein Seilcheig	KRAH-pin SHEL-u-heg
Cnó Mhoire	KROE VWOIR-ruh
Cnoc an t-Suidhe	KROHK un TEE
Cnoc-na-piobaireachd	KROHK nuh PEE-bur-yukhk
Cocidius	Ko-KEED-yooss
cóinneach dhearg	KAWN-yukh YAIR-ug
Coinneach Odhar Fiosaiche	KON-yukh OW-ur FEESS-uh-hyuh
Coir-shian	KOR HEE-un
Coligny	ko-lee-NYEE
colpach	KOL-u-pukh
copag	KOLP-ug
copan an driúchd	KOH-pun un DRYOOKH
coranach	KOR-un-ukh
corc	KOR-uk
corcur	KOR-u-kur
Cornavii	Kor-NAH-wee-ee
Corrgainecht	KOR-ghin-yukt
Coventina	ko-wen-TEE-nuh
Craig Choinnich	KRAG HON-yikh
craobh uinnsinn	KRUH-uv UN-shin
creamh	KREV

creamh na muice fiadhaich	KREV nuh MUK-yuh FEE-uh-ikh
Creathe	KREYTH (from mediaeval Irish créide but adopted into an English-language context)
Crios Bríghde	KREES BREE-juh
Crios Chu-chulainn	KREES KHOO KHUL-in
crioslachan	KREESslukh-un
crosphuing	KROSS-fing
Cú Chulainn	KOO KHUL-in
cuach	KOO-ukh
cuach Phádraig	KOO-ukh FAH-rig
Cuachag	KOO-u-khug
Cuan	KOO-un
cuid-oidhche	KIJ UH-ee-hyuh
Cuileann	KUL- yun
Curachan na Mna Sithe	KUR-u-khun nuh MRAH SHEE
curran	KUR-run

D

dá-dhuilleach	DAH-GHUL-yukh
Daghda	DAHG-duh
Dál Riata	DAHL REE-uh-tuh
Danu	DAH-nuh
darach	DAH-rukh
Dá-Shealladh	DAH-HYELL-ugh
Deagh Dia	JA yee-uh
deanntag	JAWN-tug
dearg	JAIR-ug
Decantae	Deh- KAHN-teye
deiseil	JEH-shel
Dewar	(a family name in Scotland)
Dian Cécht	JEE-un KYEKHT
dian stane	(Orcadian, possibly from the Norwegian "Dyne stein" or "din-stone", the core of a supernaturally generated thunder bolt)
Domnall Brecc	DOW-nul BREK
Donn Cuálgne	DOWN KOOL-nyuh
Draighionn	dry-un
dreas	DRESS
droch shúil	DROKH HOOIL
druidh-lus	DROOY-luss
Druim Brecc	DRUM BREK
dubh	DOO (Scottish) DUV (Irish)
Dubhan ceann-cósach	DUV-un (or DOO-in) Kyawn-KHOSS-ukh
Dubhan Pcean-dubh	DUV-un (or DOO-in) KYAWN-duv (or doo)
dubhchasach	DOO-khass ukh

Dúil Mhail	DOOIL VWIL
duileasg	DOOL-yusk
duilleag bháite	DUL-yug VAH-chuh
duilleag-bháite bhán	DUL-yug VAH-chuh VAHN
Dun-Shi	DOON HEE

E

Eachdhonn Mór	AKH-un MAWR
Each-Uisge	AKH USH-kyuh
earr-thalmhainn	AR-HAL-vin
Eastre	EH-os-truh
eidheann	EY-un
eileabor geal	EL-yu-bor GYEL
eileabor leathann	EL-yu-bor LYEH-hun
Eire, Ériu	EY-ryuh
Elen	Eh-len
Eliwlod	eh-LEEW-lod
Emain Abhlach	EH-vwin OW-lukh
éo fis	EH-o FISH
Eochaid Ollathair	O-khee OLL-a-hur (modern),
	yo-khith OL-lath-ur (ancient)
Eólas	O-luss
Eólas an t-snáithein	O-luss un TRAH-hin
eórna	OR-nuh
Epona	eh-PO-nah
Erainn	Ey-ran
Ethlenn	ETH-lyen

F

Fal	FAHL
faochag	FUW-u-khug
fealladh-bog	FYEL-lugh BOG
feamainn	FYEH-mun
feamainn chírean	FYEH-mun HEER-yun
feanntag	FYAWN-tug
fearn	FYARN
féithlean	FEYH-lun
Fid na ndruad	FEE-nahr-rue
Fili	FIH-luh
Findbennach	FIN-vyawn-ukh
Finn MacCumhail	FIN mak KOO-il
Flidais	FLEE-thush
fliodh	FLEE-ugh
Fodla	FOW-luh

Follasgain	FOLL-as-kin
fraoch	FRUH-ukh
Frayja , Freya or Freyja	FREY-ah (Norse)
Frigg	FRIGG (Germanic, Odin's wife)
frith	FREE (from Old Norse)
Frithir	FREE-hir
fuath a' mhadaidh	FOO-uh uh VAD-ee
fuinnseag	FWIN-shug

G

gallan mór	GAL-un MAWR
gaoth a deas	GUH-uh uh JESS
gaoth a deas ear-dheas	GUH-uh JESS AR-YESS
gaoth a deas iar-dheas	GUH-uh JESS EE-ur YESS
gaoth a tuath	GUH-uh TOO-uh
gaoth a tuath ear-thuath	GUH-uh TOO-uh AR-HOO-uh
gaoth an ear	GUH-uh un AR
gaoth an ear ear-dheas	GUH-uh un AR AR-YESS
gaoth an ear ear-thuath	GUH-uh un AR AR-HOO-uh
gaoth an iar	GUH-uh un EE-ur
gaoth an iar iar-dheas	GUH-uh un EE-ur EE-urYESS
gaoth an iar iar-thuath	GUH-uh un EE-ur EE-ur HOO-uh
garbhag an t-sléibhe	GAR-u-vug un TLAIV-yuh
geal	GYEL
geanais	GYEN-ush
geas	GYASS
geasa	GYASS-uh
genii cucullati	GAIN-ee-ee KOO-kool-LAH-tee
genius loci	GAIN-yooss LO-kee (Latin)
gíogan	GEE-gun
giuthas	GYOO-uss
giuthas lochlannach	GYOO-uss LOKH-lun-nukh
Glaine Nathrach	GLAN-yuh NAHH-rukh
Glaistig	GLASH-chig
glan ruis	GLAHN RUSH
glas	GLAHSS
glas-leum	GLAHSS-LYAIM
glúineach an uisge	GLOON-yukh un USH-kyuh
glúineag dhearg	GLOON-yug YAIRG
gobar-bachach	GOV-ur BAK-ukh
Gododdin	go-DOTH-een (Brythonic)
grábhan bán	GRAH-vun BAHN
grábhan nan clach	gRAH-vun nun GLAHKH
grádh is fuadh	GRAH iss FOO-uh
grán	GRAHN

Grannos	GRAHN-oss
greim saighdeir	GRAIM SEYE-jer
Gronw	GRO-noo
grósaid Gruagach	GRAW-sij GROO-u-gukh
gruth	GROO
Guid Nychburris	(Good Neighbors – Scots)
Gwenhwyfar	gwen-HOOY-rahr
Gwernabwy	GWAIRN AH-boo-ee
Gwydion	GWID-yon

H

haug-búi	haawg-booee (Old Norse)
Heléval Bheag	HEY-val BYEG
Heléval Mhor	HEY-val VAWR

I

iadhshlat thalmhainn	EE-uh HLAHT HAL-vin
Iasg Sianta	EE-usk HEE-un-tuh
Imbas Forosnai	IM-uss For-oss-nee
immrama	IM-rahv-uh
iogh	EE-ugh
ioghar	EE-ghur
Iona	(English)
ioua	EE-OO-AH
iubhar	YOO-wur

K

Kerridwen	Ker-ID-wen
kirn	(English)

L

lasair-theine	LAHSS-ur HAIN-yuh
Latis	LAH-tiss
leamhnach	LYAW-nukh
Léigheagan	LYAY-u-gun
Lenus	LAIN-ooss
Lia Faill	LEE-uh FAHL
liath	LEE-uh
liathus	LEE-uh-huss
lili bhan	LEE-lee VAHN
Linn Feic	LIN FAIK
lion na mná (or ban) síthe	LEEN nuh MRAH SHEE (or BON SHEE)
Lir	LEER
LLeu	LHUH-ee

Llyr	LHEER
loch	LOKH
Loch Eireann	LOKH AIR-yun
Loch Sithgail	LOKH SHEE-gal
Lludd	LHEETH
Lug, Lugh	LOO
Lugi	LOO-ee
Lugudunum	LOO-goo-DOO-noom (Latinized)
Lugus	LOO-gooss
luibh bhán	LIV VAHN
luibh na purgaid	LIV nuh PUR-gij
lúireach	LOOR-yukh
Lúnasdal	LOON-uss-tal
Lunastain	LOON-us-tin
lus a' chraois	LUSS uh KHRUH-ish
lus a' chrúbain	LUSS uh KHROO-pin
lus an easbaig	LUSS uh ASS-pig
lus an ellain	LUSS uh AL-lin
lus an rígh	LUSS uh REE
lus an róis	LUSS uh RAWSH
Lus an Tálaidh	LUSS uh TAHL-ee
lus an torranain	LUSS uh TORR-u-nin
lus an t-saoidh	LUSS uh TUH-ee
lus beathaig	LUSS BAH-ig
lus caolach	LUSS KUH-u-lukh
lus chasgadh na fala	LUSS KHASS-kugh nuh FOL-uh
lus Ghlinne Bhrácadail	LUSS GHLIN-lnyuh VRAH-ku-dul
lus Máiri	LUSS MAH-ree
lus míosach	LUSS MEESS-ukh
lus na caithimh	LUSS nuh KAH-hiv
lus na fala	LUSS nuh FOL-uh
lus na Frainge	LUSS nuh FRANG-yuh
lus na Spainnte	LUSS nuh SPAN-chuh
lus nam bansíth	LUSS num MON-SHEE
lus nan cluas	LUSS nung GLOO-uss
lus nan cnapan	LUSS nung GRAH-pun
lus nan grán dubh	LUSS nung GRAHN DOO
lus nan laugh	LUSS nan LAH
lus nan leac	LUSS nun LYEHK
lus-leíghis	LUSS-LYAY-ish

M

Mabon vab Modron	MAH-bon vahb MOD-ron
Macha	MAH-khuh
madadh-allaidh	MAH-tuh AL-lee

Madog	MAH-dok
Maetae	meye-AH-teye (Latin)
Maighdeann Uaine	MEYE-jun OO-in-yuh
Manannán	MON-un-awn
Manannán Mac Lir	MON-un-awn MAK LEER
Manawyddan Ap Llyr	Mahn-ah-WUTH-an ap LHEER
Maponos	mah-PO-noss
Marag Dubh	MAH-rug DOO
Marcachd Shith	MAR-kakhg HEE
Marc-raineach	MARK-ran-yukh
Matres	MAH-tress
Matunos, Matunus	mah-TOON-oss
meacan dubh	MECK-un DOO
meant	MANT
meilbheag	MELV-yug
meóir Mhoire	MYAWR VOIR-yuh
Miach	MEE-ukh
Miadhach	MEE-ukh
Miaran na Mna Sithe	MEER-un nuh MRAH SHEE
mílsean monaidh	MEEL-shun MON-ee
Mither	(Scots)
Moccus	MOK-kooss
Modron	MOD-ron
Mogons	MOG-onss
Morrigan	MOR-ree-un
Móthan	MAW-hun
muir-droighinn, múr-dhroigheann, mur-druidheann	MWIR– DREYE-in
múisean	MOOSH-un
Myddfai	MUTH-veye

N

Nantosuelta	nahn-to-SWEL-tah
násad	NAH-suth (Old Irish)
Neimheadh	NEV-yuh
Nemain	NYEV-in
neóinean	NYAW-nun
Nighean	NEE-un
nion	NEE-un
Njuggle	Nyuggle
Nodons	NO-donss
Nuada	NOO-uh-thuh (ancient); NOO-uh (modern)
nuallach	NOO-u-lukh
Nuckelavee	(Scots)
Nudd	NEETH

O

Ocelus	O-KEL-ooss
odhar	OW-ur
Odin, Odínn	OH-thin (import from Continental Germanic lands)
Oenach Tailten	EEn-ukh TAL-chun
Oengus	EN-gus
Oengus Og	EN-gus AWG
Ogham	OW-um
Ogma	OGH-muh (ancient) OW-muh (modern)
Oimelc	EE-myelk
Oisín	OSH-een
oragan	OR-u-gun
Owein	O-wine

P

peabar	PEB-ur
pearsal	PER-sul
peighinn pisich	PEY-in PEESH-ikh
peighinn ríoghail	PEY-in REE-yil
Pen medi bach caseg	PEN meh-dee bakh kahsegh (Welsh)
Picts	(English, from the Latin "Picti")
pin-chrann	PEEN-Khrawn
Piob Shith	PEEB HEE
pláigh na carra	PLEYE nuh KAWR-uh
pocan cheann	POK-un HYAWN
pónair chapaill	PAWN-ur KHOP-ul
praiseach gharbh	PRASH-ukh GHAR-uv
preas nan airneag	Press nun AR-nyug
preas súbh chraobh	PRESS SOO KHRUH-uv
puinneag	PUN-yug
puinneagan	PUN-yug-un

Q

quern	kwern (Scots)

R

raineach ríoghail	RAN-yukh REE-yil
Rata	RAH-tuh
rathadach	RAH-u-dukh
Ratis	RAH-tiss
Remi	RAIM-ee
rideag	REE-jug
Rigisamus	ree-gee-SAH-mooss

Ro-ech	RO-ekh
rós	RAWS
rosadach	ROSS–ud-ukh
rú beag	ROO-byeg
Ruad Rofhéssa	ROO-uth RO-ess-uh
ruamalach	ROO-mul-ukh
ruis	RUSH

S

Saighead Shith, Saighead Sith	SEYE-ud HEE (Irish, arrows of the Sidhe, usually flint arrowheads carried as amulets)
sail chuach	SAL KHOO-ukh
Saille	SAHL-yeh
sáiste	SAHSH-chuh
samh	sawv
samhan	SAHV-un
samhnag	SOW-nug
Samhuinn, Samthain	SAHV-in
saoghal thall	SUH-ul HAWL
Sceólang	SKYAW-lung
Scotti	Scotty
sealbhad	SHEL-vud
sealbhag nam fiadh	SHEL-uh-vug num VEE-uh
sealbhag nan con	SHEL-uh-vug nung gon
seamrag	SHAM-rug
Segais	SHEH-ghush
seilcheag	SHEL-khug
seilistear	SHEL-ish-chur
Selkies	sell-keys (Scots)
Sennachie	SHEN-na-kie (Gaelic)
Sequana	Seh-KWAHN – ah
searraiche	SHER-rikh-yuh
Setlocenia	Set-lo KAIN-yah
sgeallag	SKYEL-lug
sgiach, sgitheach	SKEE-ukh
sheiling	Shee-ling (Scots)
Shiehallion	Shee-halyon (from the Gaelic) Mountain of the Hag
shiubhaile	HYOO-vul-yuh
Sídh Chailleann	SHEE KHAL-lyun
Silures	See-LOO-ress
Silvanus	Sil-WAH-nooss (Roman, the God of Forests)
saunas	Sow-nuh (a Finnish/ northern Slavic style bath house heated by a wood stove)
slachdan	slakh-kun
Slachdan Druidheachd	Slakh-kun DROO-yukhk

Slachdan Geasachd	Slakh-kun GYASS-ukhk
slánlus	SLAHN-luss
slócan	SLAW-kun
Sluagh	SLOO-ugh
Smáladh	SMAH-luh
Smertae	SMER-teye
sneud	snyayd
sóbhrag	SAWV-rug
Sowans	Soo-ans (Scots) double meaning of thin oatmeal or semen
sporran na fala	SPOR-run nuh FOL-uh
stamh	STAV
stang	(from the Norse, a pole or staff)
Strath Eireann	SRAH AIR-yun
struan	STROO-un
Sucellos	Soo-KEL-loss (Celtic, "Good Striker")
súgh dharaichsunais	soo-GHAR-ikh soo-nish

T

Taezali	tie-SAL-ee
Taghairm	TO-ghur-um
Taibhsear	TAV-sheer
Taibnsearachd	TAV-shur-urhk
Tailtiu	TAL-chuh
Táin Bó Cuálgne	TAHN BOE KOOL-nyuh
Tanarus	tah-NAHR-oss
Taran	TAH-rahn
Taranis	tah-RAHN-iss (also called Tarann; Celtic thunderbolt God)
Tarbfeis	TAR-uv-aish
Tarnach	TAR-nukh
teimheil	CHEV-el
Teine	CHEN-yuh
Tein-eigin	CHEN-yegin
Teran	TEHR-ran
Teuchter	Too-(soft ch)-ter (Scots)
Teutates	The-oo-TAH-tess
tí	CHEE
Tigh na Cailliche	cHEE nuh KAL-lee-hyuh
Tir nam Béo	CHEER nuh MYAW
Tir-Na-N'Og	CHEER nun AWG
tombaca	tom-BAK-uh
torranan	TOR-run-un
tríbhileach	tree-veel-yukh
Trinouxtion Samonii	tree-NOOKH-tyon Sah-MON-ee-ee
trusgan	TRUSS-gun

tuaithiuil	TOO-heil
Tuatha dé Danann	TOO-u-huh JAY DON-un

U

ubhall	oo-ul
uil'- íoc	ool-yee-uk
uinnean	oon-yun
uisge-beatha	USH-kyuh BA-huh
Up Helly Aa	OOP-helly-oh (Shetland and Orkney)
ura bhallach, úrach bhallach	OO-ruh VAL-lukh
Uruisg	OR-ishk

V

Vates	WAH-tess
Verbeia	wair-BAY-yah
Vinotonus	win-TOH-noos (Latin)
Vitris	Wee-TEE-ris (Latin)

W

Wee ane	wee ain (Scots)

Bibliography

Bartram, Thomas, Bartram's Encyclopedia of Herbal Medicine, Marlowe and Company, New York, 1998

Beith, Mary, Healing Threads, Polygon, Edinburgh, 1995

Bord, Colin and Janet, Sacred Waters, Paladin Grafton books, London, 1986

Carmichael, Alexander, Carmina Gadelica – Hymns and Incantations, Lindisfarne Press, NY, 1992

Davies, Norman, The Isles – A History, Oxford University Press, New York, 1999

Evans-Wentz, W.Y., The Fairy Faith in Celtic Countries, Citadel Press, Carol Publishing Group, New York, N Y, 1990

Foster, Steven and James A. Duke, Eastern/Central Medicinal Plants, Houghton Mifflin, New York and Boston, 1990

Fraser, Iain and J.N.G. Ritchie, Royal Commission on the Ancient and Historical Monuments of Scotland, Pictish Symbol Stones, an Illustrated Gazetteer, Edinburgh, 1999

Grieve, M. A Modern Herbal, Vol. I, II, Dover Publications, New York, 1971

Gruenwald J et al, PDR for Herbal Medicines, Medical Economics Company, Inc. Montvale, NJ , 1998

Gwynn, ed., "An Old Irish Tract on the Privileges and Responsibilities of Poets", Bretha Nemed Dédenach, Eriu xiii.

Hoffmann, David: Medical Herbalism. Rochester, VT: Healing Arts Press, 2003

Hopman, Ellen Evert, A Druids Herbal – For the Sacred Earth Year, Destiny Books, Rochester, VT, 1995

Hopman, Ellen Evert, A Druid's Herbal of Sacred Tree Medicine, Destiny Books, Rochester, VT, 2008

Hopman, Ellen Evert, Grow a Harry Potter Garden, class for the Grey School of Wizardry, www.greyschool.com , 2005-2007

Hopman, Ellen Evert, Tree Medicine-Tree Magic, Phoenix Publishing Inc., Custer, WA, 1991

Hunter, John, A Persona for the Northern Picts, Groam House Museum Trust, Rosmarkie, Scotland, 1997

Kelly, Fergus, A Guide to Early Irish Law, Dublin Institute for Advanced Studies, Dublin, Ireland, 1991

Lamb, Gregor, Carnival of the Animals, Capall Bann Publishing, Somerset, 2005

Livingstone, Sheila, Scottish Customs, Barnes and Noble Books, New York, 1997

Lust, John, The Herb Book, Bantam Books, New York, 1974

Marwick, Ernest, The Folklore of Orkney and Shetland, Birlinn Limited, Edinburgh, 2005

McNeill, F. Marian, The Silver Bough Vol. I, MacLellan, Glasgow, 1977

Miller, Joyce, Magic and Witchcraft in Scotland, Goblinshead, Musselburgh, Scotland, 2005

O'Flaherty, Wendy Doniger trans., The Rig Veda, Penguin Books, London, 1981

Potterton, David, ed., Culpepper's Color Herbal, Sterling Publishing Co. Inc., New York, 1983

Ross, Anne, Folklore of the Scottish Highlands, Tempus Publishing Ltd., Gloustershire, UK, 2000

Ross, Anne, Pagan Celtic Britain, Columbia University Press, New York, 1967

Smith-Twiddy, Helen, Celtic Cookbook, Y Lolfa Cyf, Talybont, Ceredigion, Wales, 2002

Tabraham, Chris, ed. The Brochs of Gurness and Midhowe, Historic Scotland, Edinburgh, 2001

Thoms, Penelope Ann, Thin the Veil, Book Surge, LLC, Charleston SC, 2006

Websites consulted

Bendis, Cailleach Bheara, The Blue Roebuck, http://www.blueroebuck.com/ cailleach_bera.htm, February, 2008

Niafer, Flidas, The Cailleach: Hag of Samhain, AncientWorlds LLC, Celtia, http://www.ancientworlds.net/aw/HomesiteRoom/10548 , February 2008

Mannies an Horses, Electricscotland.com, http://www.electricscotland.com/ newsletter/070105, January 2007

Nicholson, Francine, et al., Land Sea and Sky http://homepage.eircom. net/~shae/ Chapters 14-15 March 2007

www.treesforlife.org.uk March 2007

Traditional Scottish Festivals, Up-Helly-aa, Rampantscotland.com, http:// www.rampantscotland.com/features/festivals.htm, April 2007

Traditional Scottish Festivals, Hunt the Gowk – 1st April, Rampantscotland. com, http://www.rampantscotland.com/features/festivals.htm, April 2007

Traditional Scottish Festivals, Glasgow Fair, Rampantscotland.com, http://www.rampantscotland.com/features/festivals.htm, April 2007

Traditional Scottish Festivals, Braemar Gathering, Rampantscotland.com, http://www.rampantscotland.com/features/festivals.htm, April 2007

Doutré, Martin, The Calendar of Coligny, http://www.celticnz.co.nz/Coligny/ColignyPart1.htm, April 2007

(Personal communications)   www.tvscots.com April 2007

Sagina procumbens, Floral Images, http://www.floralimages.co.uk/psaginprocu1.htm, May 2007

Sagina procumberns, Birdseye pearlwort, E*vue, Emergent Vegetation of the Urban Ecosystem, http://www.gsd.harvard.edu/loeb_library/information_systems/projects/E_vue/plants/sagina_procumbens.htm   May 2007

Scottish Plant Uses, Pinguicula vulgaris, Flora Celtica, http://193.62.154.38/cgi-bin/nph- readbtree.pl/parent=/filename=usedata/firstval=11/SID=182.1174013887?SPECIES_XR EF=Pinguicula May 2007

L., Pinguicula vulgaris-L., Plants For a Future, http://www.pfaf.org/database/plants.php?Pinguicula+vulgaris May 2007

O'God, Heather: Calluna vulgaris & the ericas, Druidry.org, http://druidry.org/obod/trees/Heather.htm May 2007

L., Sonchus oleraceus - L., Sow Thistle, Plants For a Future, http://www.pfaf.org/database/plants.php?Sonchus+oleraceus May 2007

McAlister, Neil Harding, The Stone of Destiny, Brigadoonery Canada http://www.durham.net/~neilmac/stone.htm May 2007

Filmer-Davies, Cath, Celtic Recipes, http://cathf.addr.com/recipe1.htm May 2007

Kreitzberg, Tom, Haggis Recipes, http://www.smart.net/~tak/haggis.html#four May 2007

Porridge, Carrbridge Community Council, http://www.goldenspurtle.com/porridge.htm May 2007

Wilkie, George Scott, Understanding Robert Burns, Electricscotland.com, www.electricscotland.com/burns/understanding June 2007

Clavie Burning, Hopeman F.C., www.hopemanfc.com/clavie_burning.htm June 2007

Lindemans, Micha F., Odin, Encyclopedia Mythica, http://www.pantheon.org/articles/o/odin.html June 2007

Lindemans, Micha F., Odin, Encyclopedia Mythica, http://www.pantheon.org/articles/b/balder.html June 2007

Article by "Mac", The Burns Supper, The World Burns Club, The Robert Burns World Federation, http://www.worldburnsclub.com/supper/burns_supper_1.htm June 2007

Recipe for Cooking Hot Cross Buns, Fabulous Foods, http://www.

fabulousfoods.com:80/recipes/breads/yeast/hotcrossbun.html June 2007

Black Pudding, FoodDownUnder, http://fooddownunder.com/cgi-bin/recipe.
cgi?r=28464 June 2007

London, Anna, Oatmeal Bannock (Scones part 1), Baking for Britain, http://
bakingforbritain.blogspot.com/2006/06/oatmeal-bannock-scones-part-1.
html June 2007

Caudle recipe, http://theskirmish.com/seren/?page_id=53 June 2007

O'God, Heather: Calluna vulgaris & the ericas, Druidry.org,

http://druidry.org/obod/trees/Heather.htm June, 2007

L., Onopordum acanthium – L., Plants For a Future, http://pfaf.org/database/
plants.php?Onopordum+acanthium June, 2007

Carmina Gadelica Vol 2, Am Mothan, Sacred-texts.com, http://www.sacred-
texts.com/neu/celt/cg2/cg2055.htm July, 2007

Scottish Plant Uses, Flora Celtica, Alphabetical Listing of Genera, http://rbg-
web2.rbge.org.uk/celtica/dbase/genera/GENERA.HTM July, 2007

Scottish Plant Uses, Senecio vulgaris, Flora Celtica, http://193.62.154.38/
cgi-bin/nph-readbtree.pl/parent=/filename=usedata/firstval=11/
SID=440.1185305064?SPECIES_XREF=Senecio+vulgaris July, 2007

Scottish Plant Uses, Taxus baccata, Flora Celtica, http://193.62.154.38/
cgi-bin/nph-readbtree.pl/usedata/maxvals=10/firstval=1?SPECIES_
XREF=Taxus+baccata August, 2007

Scottish Plant Uses, Nymphaea alba, Flora Celtica, http://193.62.154.38/
cgi-bin/nph-readbtree.pl/usedata/maxvals=10/firstval=1?SPECIES_
XREF=Nymphaea+alba August, 2007

Ní Dhoireann, Kym, The Problem of the Woad, http://www.cyberpict.net/
sgathan/essays/woad.htm June, 2004

Traditional Scottish Recipes, Atholl Brose, Rampantscotland.com,

www.rampantscotland.com/recipies/blrecipe_brose.htm June, 2007

Atholl Brose, The Original One and Only Recipe, Cabarfeidh.com, www.
cabarfeidh.com/atholl_brose.htm December, 2006

Dictionary of the Scots Language, http://www.dsl.ac.uk/dsl/ January, 2008

For further information on Druids and Druidism please see
www.whiteoakdruids.org

Index

A

A. alpina, 152
A Highland Herbal, 11, 113, 215, 225, 229, 235
Abaris, 21, 255
Abduction by Fairies, 100, 155, 170
Aberdeenshire, 57, 239
Aberfoyle, 110-111, 249
Abhalloch, 65, 208
Abortifacients, 233
abortive, 145, 154, 162, 177
abscesses, 128, 130, 141, 144
Achillea armica, 175
Achillea millefolium, 144, 154, 186
achlasan chalium chille, 170
Aconite, 155
acorn, 209
adder, 232
Adder-Stanes, 51
Address to A Haggis, 74
Aedh, 27, 255
Aegopodium podagraria, 136
Aengus, 31, 248, 255
aeromancy, 221
Agaric, 45
agricultural calendar, 63
Agrimonia eupatoria, 118
Agrimonia spp, 178

Agrimony, 118, 178
ague, 118, 120, 124
Aidan mac Gabhrán, 17, 255
ainis, 119, 255
áiridhean, 80, 255
Airmidh, 24, 27, 255
Airts, 11, 37, 255
aiteal, 151
aiteann, 151, 255
aladh, 38, 255
Alator, 24, 255
Albatross, 205
Alchemilla vulgaris, 152
alcoholism, 179
alder, 46, 118, 176
ale, 70-72, 81, 83, 96, 100-102, 105, 147, 181, 192, 195, 203, 222, 243, 250
Alexander III, 61
Alexanders, 119
Alfadir, 30, 255
alga, 172
alkaloids, 115, 132-133
All Saints Day, 65
All Souls Day, 67
All-Heal, 119, 143, 154
Allium cepa, 159
Allium ursinum, 142

Allt Eireann, 31, 255
Alnus glutinosa, 118, 176
altar, 21, 23, 26, 44, 56-57, 61, 74, 83-84, 198, 250
am beárnan Bríghde, 134, 255
Am Bratach Sith, 251, 255
am bualan, 145, 255
am maraiche, 171, 255
Amber, 27, 50, 53, 99, 239
amenorrhea, 161
American Mountain Ash, 168
amulet, 50, 125, 131, 223
An Daghda, 26-27, 255
an neónan mór, 134, 255
Ana, 24, 31, 255-256
anaphrodisiac, 183
ancestors, 16, 34, 38, 40, 47, 59, 65, 101, 115, 222, 253
Andarta, 209, 255
Andrasta, 24
Andraste, 24, 213, 255
anemia, 142, 150, 170, 179
angelica, 164
Angelica archangelica, 164
angina, 164
Angles, 13, 17
Anglo-Saxon, 13, 186, 217, 253
Angus Og, 30, 255
animal totem, 205, 215
Anise, 119, 202
Annwn, 209, 220, 255
anorexia, 156
Antenociticus, 24, 256
Anthemis nobilis, 129, 144, 158, 174
Anthemis pyrethrum, 161
Anthyllis vulneraria, 181
anti-bacterial, 142, 155, 162
anti-biotic, 147
anti-depressant, 178
anti-fungal, 117, 147, 155, 186
anti-microbial, 147
antiseptic, 15, 151, 157, 162-163, 176, 179, 183, 186
anti-spasmodic, 124, 149
anti-tumor, 155, 178
anti-tussive, 124
anti-viral, 142, 147, 153, 155, 163

antlered deity, 212
antlered Goddess, 27
antlers, 16, 24, 26, 28
Antonine Wall, 13, 26-27
Anu, 24, 31, 256
anvil, 98, 228
aphrodisiac, 153, 160, 224
Aphrodite, 25
Apollo, 24, 28-29
Apotropaic magic, 220
appetite, 119, 123-124, 130, 135-136, 139, 156, 167, 173, 179, 185-186
Apple, 46, 108, 120, 155, 208, 224, 248
apple cider, 120
apprentice, 201, 250-251
Aquae Sulis, 215, 256
Arbroath Abbey, 61
Ard-gael, 17, 256
Arecurius, 24, 256
Argyll, 17
Arran, 14, 58-59, 252
arrows, 52, 187, 211, 247-248, 266
Artemesia absinthum, 185
Artemisia vulgaris, 156
arterial degeneration, 179
arteries, 142, 160
Artgenos, 209
arthritis, 143, 147-148, 151, 155, 166
ascarids, 179
Ash, 41, 46, 60, 104, 120-121, 145, 159, 168
Asperula odorata, 151, 184
Asplenium scolopendrium, 139
Asplenium spp, 140
assemblies, 86
asthma, 59, 121, 124, 126-127, 132, 134, 137, 143-144, 149, 157, 161-162, 164
Atecotti, 14, 256
Ath Fodhla, 31, 256
Athena, 24
athlete's foot, 186
Atholl Brose, 202, 272
augurer, 109
augury, 76, 109, 221
Auk, 16
Austria, 14, 69
Avalon, 65, 120, 208, 248
Avena sativa, 159

B

baby, 29, 56, 101
back pain, 231
bad breath, 175
bad dreams, 50
bad luck, 38, 40, 63, 70, 75, 84, 88, 91, 93, 95, 102, 104-105, 137, 193-194, 197, 203, 214, 216, 224-226
bad vision, 50
Badb, 207, 256
bag of heads, 232
bagpipes, 249
bairn, 46, 49, 92, 97, 99-102, 129, 155, 164, 180, 226, 240, 247-248, 251
Balder, 27, 30, 69, 155, 256, 271
Ball Mo-Luidhe, 53, 256
ball playing, 39
Ballochyle Brooch, 52
Banba, 27, 31, 256
baneful magic, 40, 220, 233
banishing, 222-223
bannock, 39, 64, 66, 77, 80-81, 84, 87-88, 96, 101, 107, 272
Bannock Bread, 64
Bannock Night, 77
Banshee, 239, 251
baptism, 110
baptismal fonts, 55
Barberry, 130
Bards, 20-21, 75
Barley, 15, 38, 121, 133, 139, 192, 202, 239
barn, 43, 45, 60, 70, 72, 76, 88, 95, 102, 106, 137, 151, 168-169, 198, 220, 222-223, 226, 234-235, 242, 245, 247
Bárr á chinn, 228
barr brisgein, 174, 256
Barra, 88, 250-252
Barrecis, 24, 256
Barrex, 24, 256
Barrow, 58, 93
basket, 46, 68, 73, 94, 97, 100, 194, 196
battle, 17, 19, 24-25, 27, 29, 31, 37-38, 53, 68, 87, 143, 155, 178, 202, 205-208, 210, 219-220, 225-226, 239, 250-251
battle magic, 19, 38, 219-220
Battle of Dunnichen, 17
Battle of Moytura, 27, 87
Battle of Nechtansmere, 17

Bayberry, 125
bealaidh, 127, 256
Bealltan, 20-21, 24, 38-39, 42, 44, 57, 60, 63-64, 72, 80-83, 85, 91, 118, 122, 137, 146, 151, 184, 221, 223, 244, 256
Bean sidh, 239, 256
Beannachadh na Cuairte, 46, 256
Bean-nighe, 239, 245, 256
Bear, 26, 29, 33, 41, 142, 209
Bear God, 29, 209
Bear's Garlic, 142
Beating the bounds, 83
Beating the house, 203
beauty, 27-28, 35, 38, 44, 69, 80, 223
bedwetting, 159
bee stings, 135, 150
Beef Brose, 77
beer, 28, 39, 124-125, 129, 143, 158, 176, 192, 203, 232
Bees, 46, 105, 117, 129-130, 132-133, 135, 151, 163, 165, 209, 224
bees wax, 46, 117, 129-130, 132-133, 135, 163
Behavior of Your Mate, 107
beith, 31, 122, 188, 256, 269
Bel, 24
Belatucadros,, 24, 256
Belenos, 24, 256
Belinus, 24, 83, 256
bell-branch, 104
Bellis perennis, 134
Ben Nevis, 89
Benshi, 104
Berberis vulgaris, 130
best man, 92-94, 96-97
Best Man, 92-94, 96-97
Bestla, 30, 256
Betonica officinalis, 121
Betonica pauli, 121, 170
Betony, 121, 154, 178
Betula alba, 122
bhán, bioras, 152
Bigswell, 58
bikko, 84, 197
Bilberry, 59, 123
Bilberry Sunday, 59
Bindweed, 122, 226

biolair, 134, 182, 256
biolair ghriagain, 134, 256
Birch, 15, 41, 45-46, 75, 122
bird feathers, 206
birthing, 54, 99, 102
Birthing, 54, 99, 102
births, 20, 105
Bistort, 122
bitch, 69, 84, 197-198
bites, 120, 128, 132, 144, 163, 169
black cock, 99
black currant, 164
black eye, 164
black he-goats, 69
black hounds, 69
Black Lovage, 119
Black Pepper, 67, 162
Black Pudding, 67-68, 272
Black Shore, 106, 237, 246
Black Spleenwort, 140
black steeds, 69
Black Tea, 138, 178
Blackberry, 126
Blackthorn,, 123
bladder, 121-123, 127, 134-135, 139, 143-144, 148-149, 151, 157, 159, 161, 164, 166, 170, 184, 186
bladder problems, 122, 134, 164
Blaeberry, 123
bleeding, 51, 123, 131-132, 152, 154, 157-158, 162-163, 165, 170, 174-175, 179, 183-186, 216
blessing, 33, 41, 45-46, 77, 81-82, 85, 91, 96, 100, 105, 195, 203, 220, 235, 246
Blessing magic, 220
blight, 37, 64, 81, 87, 243
blister on the tongue, 233
blisters, 128, 135, 141, 175, 177, 241
Blithe-Feast, 101
Blodeuwedd, 207, 256
blood, 30, 36, 39, 47, 51, 55, 67-68, 95, 115, 127, 130, 137, 142-143, 145, 147, 150, 154, 157, 160, 167, 170-171, 174, 177, 182, 185-187, 203, 206-207, 209, 212, 220, 225, 232, 239, 246, 250
blood circulation, 185
blood pressure, 115, 127, 142, 145, 147, 154, 160, 174, 177, 212
bloody cough, 186

blue cohosh, 154
Blue Men of the Minch, 239
blueberries, 86
Blueberry, 123
Boand, 211, 256
Boann, 75
boar, 16, 31, 198, 201, 209, 215, 221
Boats, 12, 15, 33, 43, 46, 63, 106, 168, 191-193, 214, 226, 240-241, 249
Bodach, 56, 256
bodachan sabhaill, 240, 256
bodan coille, 184, 256
bog, 26, 60, 124-125, 176, 180, 186, 209-210, 213, 260
bog body, 186
Bog Moss, 176
Bog Myrtle, 125
Bog Violet, 124, 180
Bogbean, 124, 153, 166
Bogie, 239
Boils, 128, 142, 150, 152, 159, 163, 165-166, 171, 183, 223, 232
Bonduc Bean, 126
Bonduc Beans, 51
bone, 11, 16, 25, 27, 53-55, 98, 109, 115, 211, 230, 232-233, 246
Bone Magic, 11, 54
Bones, 11, 16, 36, 47, 49, 54-55, 58, 83, 95, 102, 121, 132, 193, 212, 229, 233
boneset, 154
Bone-setters, 233
bonfire, 33, 66, 74, 83, 221-222
Bonfires, 21, 44-45, 80, 88
Bonnach, 64, 256
Booking Night, 91
Bor, 30, 256
Borage, 126
Borago officinalis, 126
borrach, 126, 256
Borrowing Day, 80
Boudicca, 213, 256
Boundary Stones, 60
Bourtree, 137
Bovista nigrescens, 15, 165
bowels, 122, 137, 160, 179, 185-186
Boxing Day, 70
Braciaca, 25, 256
Braemar Gathering, 87, 271
Brahan Seer, 52, 59, 111-112

Brahmins, 19
Brakeroot, 139
Bramble, 126, 151
Bran, 207, 212, 257
Branwen, 25, 257
braoileag, 123, 257
Breaca Sith, 248, 257
bread, 29, 40, 42-43, 46, 59, 64, 71, 76, 82, 84, 86, 100, 105, 110, 131, 135, 160, 192, 195, 202-203, 222, 231, 252
Breadalbane, 104
breast lumps, 130
breast milk, 100, 116, 119, 126, 139, 147, 161, 169, 174, 214
breast swellings, 130, 228
breasts, 42, 56, 100, 131, 145, 161, 166, 182
Brehons, 47
Bretha Nemed Dédenach, 233, 257, 269
brewing, 124
Bride, 23-25, 41, 64, 74-76, 89, 91-98, 226, 252, 257
Bride's Garter, 96
Bride's Maid, 92
Brideag, 75, 257
Brigantia, 23-25, 29, 257
Brigdi, 239
Bríghde, 23-25, 27, 41, 50, 58, 64, 66-67, 74-77, 89, 98, 134-135, 195, 222, 228, 255, 257, 259
Brighid, 24, 41, 77, 257
Briochan the Druid, 52
brisgean, 174, 257
Britons, 8, 13, 15
bróg na cuthaid, 181, 257
Broichan, 21, 257
Brón Trogain, 86
bronchial afflictions, 139
bronchitis, 121, 126, 132-133, 137, 139, 142, 144, 148-149, 157, 162, 164, 176, 215
bronze, 14, 20, 57-58, 65, 102, 208, 212, 214, 229, 249
Broom, 94, 96, 127

Brownie, 59, 198, 240, 243
Brownie Stone, 59, 240
Bruide, son of Bili, 17
bruises, 128, 132, 134, 140-141, 144-145, 148, 152, 165, 169, 175, 177, 179, 181, 185, 213, 228
buaghallan, 166, 257
Búcan, 240, 257
Buckbean, 124
buckwheat, 116, 157
buidhe, 37, 257
Bull, 16, 44, 82, 104, 110, 198, 203, 206, 209-211, 216, 245
bull feast, 210
bull sacrifice, 209
Bulls, 21, 209-210
Bundling, 90
buntáta, 164, 257
Burghead, 73
Burial, 43, 58, 60, 105-106, 109, 111, 234, 242-243
Burial cairns, 58, 60
burial mound, 58, 242-243
burmaid, 185, 257
burn, 15, 31, 77, 81, 93, 103, 108, 116, 133, 137, 139, 149-151, 157, 164-165, 222, 248
Burning O' The Sneud, 93
Burning Of the Clavie, 73
burns, 69, 73-74, 93, 108, 126, 128, 132-133, 135, 137, 150, 157, 159-160, 165, 170, 184, 211, 216, 271
butter, 34, 40, 43-44, 50, 60, 64-65, 68, 71, 75-76, 78-79, 81-83, 85, 95, 100, 104, 116-117, 121, 127, 129, 135, 142-144, 150, 159-160, 166-167, 170, 172-173, 195, 199, 203, 211, 220, 222, 231-233
Butterbur, 127
Buttercup, 128
Butterflies, 210
butterfly, 103, 210
Butterwort, 124-125, 151, 180

C

cabbage, 36, 199
Caelestis, 25, 257
Caelestis Brigantia, 25

Caereni, 14, 257
Cailleach, 23-25, 31, 37, 56, 67, 88, 196, 206-207, 211, 223, 230, 237, 240, 257, 270

Cailleach an Dúdain, 88, 257
Cailleach an Teampuill, 206, 257
Cailleach Bhéara, 206, 257
Cailleach Bheur, 25, 37, 257
Cailleach Chearc, 230, 257
Cailleach Oidhche, 207, 257
Cairbre Caitchenn, 210, 257
Cairbre Cat-head, 210
cairgein, 172, 257
Cairn, 21, 33, 60, 106, 216
Caithness, 14, 58, 211
cál deanntaig, 157, 257
Caledonia, 11, 13-15, 17, 257
Caledonii, 13-14, 257
Calendula, 125, 128, 136, 151, 153, 160, 198
Calendula arvensis, 128
Calendula officinalis, 125, 128, 136, 151, 198
calf, 44, 110, 180
Calistegia, 122
call up a wind, 193
Callanish, 21, 58, 257
calltainn, 146, 257
Calluna vulgaris, 147, 188, 271-272
calm the waves, 192-193
Calton Hill, 8, 80, 249
Camellia sinensis, 178
Camellia thea, 178
camobhaidh, 129, 257
camobhil, 129, 257
Campbells, 52, 125, 221
Camulos, 26, 257
cancer, 104, 148, 160, 162, 177, 179, 187
cancerous tumors, 129, 154
candida, 152
candles, 69, 75, 77, 104, 222
Candlemas, 74-75
Canisbay, 72
Canny Woman, 235
caochag, 165, 257
Caoilte, 208, 257
Caoineag, 240, 257
caorann, 168, 257
Capsella bursa-pastoris, 174
Capsicum frutescens, 127, 162
caraway seed, 178
carbohydrates, 146
Cardamine pretense, 134
cardiac edema, 127, 142

cardiac irregularities, 179
cardiac tonic, 142
carding, 69, 141, 252
Carduus heterophyllus, 178
carminative, 138
carnelian, 52
Carnyx, 209
carra, 171, 257, 265
carrachan, 181, 257
Carrageen, 172
carra-meille, 181, 257
Carrot, 66, 129-130, 161, 202
Carrot Sunday, 66
Carrots, 36, 66-67, 86, 88, 129-130
Carum petroselinum, 161, 164
Caryophyllus aromaticus, 178
caseg fedi, 214, 257
cas-on-uain, 181, 258
Cassia acutifolia, 173
Cassia angustifolia, 173
Cassia fistula, 173-174
Cassia spp, 154
Cat, 104, 192-193, 203-204, 210, 212, 221, 231
Cat God, 210
catarrh, 139, 143, 151, 164, 185
Cath Palug, 210, 258
cats, 15, 28, 110, 241
Cattle, 16, 24-25, 28, 31, 36, 38, 40, 44, 46, 51, 58, 65, 67-68, 80, 83, 88, 91, 111, 148, 151, 187, 201, 210-211, 223, 230, 235, 242-243, 247
Caudle, 81, 272
caul, 100, 193, 226, 228
Cauldron of Plenty, 26, 89
Cauldrons, 102, 220
Caulophyllum thalictroides, 154
cavalry, 27, 214
cayenne pepper, 67, 127, 162
ceílidh, 66, 258
celandine, 15, 130, 164
Celandine, 15, 130, 164
Celtic Christians, 211
Celts, 13-14, 19-20, 23, 54, 56, 65, 108, 135, 170, 187, 212-213, 219, 221, 229, 253
Centaurium erythraea, 130
Centaury, 130
cereal, 133

Cernennus, 26, 258
Cernunnos, 26, 212, 215-216, 258
cervical ulceration, 152
ceud-bhileach, 130, 258
chafing, 133
Chambered Tombs, 58, 216
Chamomile, 129, 144, 158, 164, 174
Channelled Fucus, 173
chaochail e, 103, 258
chapped hands, 124, 145, 153, 186
chariots, 102
charms, 21, 51, 54, 168, 222, 227, 230, 235
charm bag, 232
Charm of the Thread, 54, 228
Charm stones, 52
Charming, 220
cheese, 38, 42, 46, 59, 71-72, 95, 100-101, 105, 192, 195, 202, 220, 225
Chelidonium majus, 15, 164
chest complaints, 119-120, 124, 153, 157, 159, 165, 212, 216
chest congestion, 134, 151, 155, 158, 170
Chicken, 55, 75, 108, 158, 210
Chickweed, 131, 136
Chickens, 64, 80
chilblains, 147
child, 33, 43, 45-46, 50, 52-53, 59, 66, 76, 93, 96-103, 109-110, 112, 116, 120-122, 129, 144, 154, 174, 185, 193, 227, 229-231, 233, 235-236, 245, 248-249
Childbirth, 11, 51, 58-59, 89, 98, 119, 159, 167, 173, 233, 242
chives, 160
cholera, 158, 177
Christening Feast, 101
Christian, 13, 20, 29, 38, 56, 65, 74, 77, 110
Christmas, 69
Christmas Eve, 69
Chrysanthemum leucanthemum, 134
church, 21, 39, 56, 65-66, 74, 77, 193
Church of Scotland, 21
churn, 43, 50, 75-76, 82, 125, 169, 199, 235
churning butter, 199
Cicuta virosa, 148
cigarettes, 156
Cináed mac Ailpín, 18, 258
Cinnamomum cassia, 180
Cinnamomum zeylandicum, 173
cinnamon, 79, 157, 159, 173-174, 180

Cinquefoil, 174
circulatory system, 128
Clach Bhuaidh, 52, 258
Clach Dearg, 52, 258
Clach na Gruagach, 242, 258
Clach na h-Iobairte, 59, 258
Clach Nathrach, 51, 258
clach raineach, 139, 258
Clachan, 39, 51, 258
Clachan nan Gilleadha Cráigein, 51, 258
Clachan-glúin a' choilich, 51, 258
Clach-bhan, 58, 258
Clan Chattan, 59, 251
Clan Chief, 52, 59, 225, 251
Clava Cairns, 58
Clavie, 73-74, 222, 271
cliabh, 73, 258
clois, 149, 258
cloot, 39
clootie dumpling, 226
Clootie Well, 41
cloth, 15-16, 39-40, 52, 79, 84, 95, 105-106, 110, 116, 121, 132, 136, 145, 157-159, 163, 167, 185, 193, 195-196, 203, 232, 247, 251
Cloutie's Croft, 47
clove, 122, 157, 208
cluaran, 178, 258
cluas an fleidh, 178, 258
cluas liath, 132, 258
Club Moss, 131
Cnaipein Seilcheig, 51, 258
Cnó Mhoire, 51, 126, 258
Cnoc an t-Suidhe, 249, 258
Cnoc-na-Piobaireachd, 249, 251, 258
coal, 63, 71, 102-103, 146, 193, 221-222
coastal caves, 243
Cobbie Row, 240
cobwebs, 110, 216
Cochlearia officinalis, 171
Cocidius, 26, 258
cock, 51, 99, 103, 198, 213, 215
Cock's Knee Stones, 51
coffee, 119, 135, 138-139, 144, 148, 159, 166, 183
Coffins, 33, 43, 169, 234
cog, 72, 96
coin, 34, 38-40, 49, 70, 72, 92, 102, 191-193, 198-199, 225-227, 235-236, 241, 248

cóinneach dhearg, 176, 258
Coinneach Odhar, 59, 111, 258
Coinneach Odhar Fiosaiche, 111, 258
Coir-shian, 249, 258
Cold Stones, 51
Colds, 127, 132, 134, 137-138, 141, 147, 159, 168, 176, 186-187, 202, 215, 229, 232
colic, 119, 134, 139, 141-142, 153, 159, 161-162, 173
Coligny Calendar, 20, 65
colitis, 128, 152, 163
colpach, 243, 258
colt, 243
Coltsfoot, 132, 156
Columba, 21, 170, 187
Comfrey, 132, 135
Common Fern, 139
Conception and Childbirth, 11, 98
Conger Eel, 213
conjunctivitis, 138
conjure a storm, 237
Connla's Well, 146, 215
constipation, 122, 124, 131, 135, 142, 162, 173, 180
consumption, 59
Contract Night, 91
contracts, 60, 67, 74, 86
Convovulus, 226
copag, 135, 258
copan an driúchd, 152, 258
Copper, 16, 146, 186, 226, 234
Coppie Row, 240
coracles, 15
coral, 53, 99, 226
coranach, 103, 258
corc, 159, 258
corcur, 37, 258
coriander, 173-174
Coriandrum sativum, 173
Cormorant, 16
Corn, 12, 37, 73, 81, 84, 87, 133, 152, 164, 196-197
Corn Dolly, 197
Corn Poppy, 164
Cornavii, 211, 258
corns, 150, 152, 183
cornucopia, 8, 29, 197
Cornus suecica, 136
corpse, 50, 104-105, 237

Corpse Creathe, 237
Corrgainecht, 206, 258
Coryllus avellana, 135
coughs, 120, 124, 132, 134, 139-141, 143-144, 146-149, 153, 157, 159-161, 163-164, 171, 176, 179, 182, 184, 231
Courtship, 11, 89, 223-224
Courtship and Marriage, 11, 89, 224
courtship customs, 89
Cove of the Women of Peace, 249
Coventina, 26, 212-214, 229, 258
cow, 25, 36, 39, 44-45, 50-52, 70, 75, 110, 125, 146, 170, 180, 198, 210-211, 225, 241, 243, 245, 248
co-walker, 103, 109
Cowbane, 148
cowrie shell, 193
Cows, 20, 24, 65, 70, 83, 85, 110, 204, 210-211, 225, 235-236, 241-243, 250-251
Cowslip, 133
crab apple, 120
cradles, 168, 226
Craig Choinnich, 87, 258
cramps, 119, 123, 128-129, 139, 154, 162, 167, 170-171, 174, 186, 229
cranberries, 202
Crane, 29, 205-206, 214
Crane Bag, 29, 206
crane's stance, 206
cranes, 205-206, 210, 214
craobh uinnsinn, 120, 258
Craobh-fhearn, 118
Crataegus monogyna, 145
Crataegus oxyacantha, 142, 145, 154
cravings for sweets, 169
cream of tartar, 174
creamh, 139, 142, 258-259
creamh na muice fiadhaich, 139, 259
creator deity, 67
Creeling the Groom, 97
Crios Bríghde, 76, 259
Crios Chu-chulainn, 166, 259
crioslachan, 66, 259
cripple goat, 197
Cromlechs, 58
Crone, 42, 196
crosphuing, 126, 259
cross-beam in the chimney, 169
Crow, 27, 81, 90, 99, 103, 206-207

crowdie, 202
Crowfoot, 128
Cry the Kern, 87
Cryin' Bannock, 101
Cryin' Cheese and Groaning Malt, 101
Crystals, 11, 49, 52, 203
Cú Chulainn, 207, 212, 259
cuach, 125, 163, 259
cuach Phádraig, 163, 259
Cuachag, 240, 259
Cuan, 29, 86, 259
Cubbie Roo, 240
CuChulainn, 166
Cuckoo, 134, 205, 224
Cuckoo Flower, 134
cuid-oidhche, 225, 259
cuileann, 148, 225, 259

Cuileann, 148, 225, 259
Cumberland, 30
cumin, 202
Cupid, 30
cup-reading, 85
Curachan na Mna Sithe, 248, 259
Curlews, 191
curran, 129, 259
Curses, 12, 78, 233, 236
Cursing bones, 55
Cursing Threads, 236
Cursing Wells, 40
Cuttin' Butter, 85
cutting wood, 36
cystitis, 147, 151
Cyanide, 120
Cytisus scoparius, 127

D

Dá – Shealladh, 111
dá-dhuilleach, 160, 259
Daghda, 25-27, 30, 75, 89, 207, 220, 255, 259
Dairy Magic, 12, 198
Daisy, 134
Dál Riata, 17, 259
Dalriada, 17-18, 86
Dálriadans, 17
Damiana, 170
dance, 33, 66, 69, 71, 76, 88, 96-97, 105, 195, 197, 213, 250
dancing, 39, 68, 75-76, 84, 91, 93, 96, 105, 107, 193, 196, 230, 241, 247-248, 250
Dandelion, 82, 125, 127, 134-135, 151, 178
dandruff, 150, 171
Danu, 27, 29, 250, 259
darach, 158, 259
Dark of the Moon, 35-36, 223
Dá-Shealladh, 108, 259
dawn, 39, 55, 57, 60, 63, 70, 75, 82-83, 94, 105, 109, 147, 187, 221, 224, 227, 229, 235
Day of the Dead, 65
deafness, 111, 202
Deagh Dia, 75, 259
deanntag, 157, 259
dearg, 37, 52, 258-259
Death Omens, 103
Death Rites, 11, 102

deaths, 20
Decantae, 14, 259
Deer, 15-16, 25-26, 28, 55, 67, 175, 211-212, 225, 247, 249
Deer sorrel, 175
deid-claes, 105
deid-drap, 103
Deid-lights, 103
deiseil, 33, 38, 40-42, 52-53, 55-56, 59, 66, 74, 83, 86, 90, 94, 98-100, 102, 155, 192-193, 196, 198, 203, 222, 224, 227, 229, 235, 246, 259
Demons, 49, 74
dentists, 228
depression, 58, 126, 147, 155, 170, 178, 212, 229
destructive magic, 233
Devil's Bit, 171
dew, 44, 80, 82, 152, 223, 225, 245, 247
Dewar, 54, 259
diabetes, 115
Dian Cécht, 24, 27, 29, 54, 259
dian stane, 195, 259
Diana, 28
diaper rash, 133, 135
diarrhea, 119-120, 122-123, 125-126, 128-129, 132, 141-144, 146-148, 152, 154, 158, 162-164, 166-168, 170, 174, 177, 179-180, 183, 185, 211

dieters, 169

digestion, 119-120, 124, 129, 139, 143-144, 151, 153, 156, 162

digestive aid, 15, 130

Digitalis purpurea, 142, 160

dill, 170

diphtheria, 142, 160

Dipping the Sark, 107

dirk, 72, 110, 155, 226, 237

distaff of the loom, 169

distance healing, 52

diuretic, 15, 126-127, 136-137, 141, 147, 149, 161, 175, 178, 184

Divination, 8, 11, 66, 107-109, 120, 210, 221-222

Divination Practices, 11, 107

divinations, 19, 63, 65-66, 85-86, 90, 107, 212, 222

divinatory magic, 221

Divine Bear, 29

Divine Horse, 27, 214

Divine Mother, 24, 29

Divine Smith, 27-28

Divine Son, 29

Divine Youth, 29

diviners, 8, 20

Dock, 44, 135

Docken, 135-136, 245

Dog, 27, 84, 103-105, 136, 175, 181, 197, 204, 206, 210, 212, 216, 231, 245

Dog bones, 212

Dog Sorrel, 175

Dog violet, 181

Dog's Mercury, 136

dogs, 15, 30, 110, 212, 216, 225, 249

doll, 75, 78, 84, 87, 98, 222-223

Dolmen, 58

Dolphin, 212

Domestic life, 12, 201

Domnall Brecc, 17, 259

Don, 26, 39, 116-117

Donn Cuálgne, 210, 259

dove, 30, 207, 221

draighionn, 123, 259

dream of a future lover, 187

dreas, 126, 259

droch shúil, 233-234, 259

drought, 38, 81

drowning, 52, 125, 193, 215, 226

Druid's Wand, 88

druidh-lus, 154, 259

Druidical Fields, 21

Druids, 8, 11, 14, 19-21, 26-27, 31, 35, 44, 59, 65, 74-75, 121, 131, 155, 158, 187-188, 208-209, 211, 219, 223, 269, 272

Druim Brecc, 206, 259

drums, 82

drunkenness, 25, 181

Dryopteris felix-mas, 140

dubh, 38, 68, 119, 132, 259, 263-264

Dubhan ceann-cósach, 119, 259

Dubhan Pcean–dubh, 119

dubhchasach, 140, 259

ducks, 64

Dúil Mhail, 122, 260

duileasg, 173, 260

duilleag bháite, 152, 260

duilleag-bháite bhán, 183, 260

Dulse, 15, 173, 230

Dumézil, 19

Dun Eidyn, 17

Dunkeld hill, 14

Dun-Osdale round tower, 251

Dun-Shi, 110, 260

dusk, 60, 63, 110, 224, 227, 244

Dwarf Cornel, 136

Dwarf Elder, 136

dye, 183-184

dysentery, 122-123, 126, 158, 174, 177, 180

E

Eachdhonn Mór, 206, 260

Each-Uisge, 240, 243, 246, 260

eagle, 206-208

Eagle, 206-208

ear, 37-38, 130, 150, 160, 167, 170, 214, 261

ear ache, 160

ear plant, 150

Earl of Atholl, 202

earr-thalmhainn, 186, 260

Earth Curses, 236

Earth Magic, 11, 46

Earth Mother, 86
Earth Spirits, 47
Earthen mounds, 47
earth-fast stane, 203
Easter Monday, 78
Eastre, 27, 78, 260
echinacea, 160
eczema, 133, 141-143, 159, 167, 182
edema, 120, 123, 126-127, 134-135, 137, 142, 149, 151, 157, 161, 166, 171, 177
Edinburgh, 8, 17, 61, 80, 188, 249, 269-270
Edward I, 61
Eel, 30, 213
eel's skin, 213
Eels, 16
egg, 27, 52-53, 66, 78-79, 108, 121, 129, 158, 193, 196, 211
Eggs, 16, 27, 36, 68, 78-79, 81, 96, 199, 206
eidheann, 150, 260
Eigg, 249, 251
Eildon Hills, 112, 249
eileabor geal, 147, 260
eileabor leathann, 147, 260
Eire, 27, 260
Elder, 93, 130, 136-137, 154, 164, 177, 179, 186, 225
elder flowers, 137, 154, 186
Elen, 27, 260
Elf, 52, 60, 228, 241, 248-249
elf arrow, 241
Elf Bolt, 249
Elf Cups, 60
Elf Queen, 228
Elf Shot, 52, 248
Elfin Pipe, 248
Elf-shot, 52, 241
Elf-Wind, 241
Eliwlod, 206, 260
Elm, 46, 116, 129, 132, 140, 152, 183
Elopement, 97
Elves, 12, 52, 110, 239, 241
Emain Abhlach, 248, 260
Emain of the Apples, 248
Emerald Heart of the Earth, 55
emetic, 127, 136-137, 145, 150, 177, 182
emmenagogue, 119, 125, 131, 145, 151, 156

emphysema, 142, 179
Enbarr of the Flowing Mane, 29
engagement ring, 50, 94
English Holly, 148
English Ivy, 150
enteritis, 148, 186
éo fis, 215, 260
Eochaid Ollathair, 27, 260
Eólas, 54, 227-228, 235, 260
Eólas an t-snáithein, 54, 228, 260
eórna, 121, 260
epilepsy, 99, 154, 182, 228-229
epileptic fits, 134
Epipactis helleborine, 147
Epipactis latifolia, 147
Epona, 27, 206-207, 212, 214, 260
Equinoxes, 192
Equisetum arvense, 149
Erainn, 210, 260
Erica cinerea, 147
Erica tetralix, 147
Eros, 30
erysipelas, 120, 126, 142, 148, 167, 177
erythema, 142
Ethlenn, 212, 260
Eupatorium perfoliatum, 154
Euphorbia peplus, 177
Euphrasia officinalis, 138
European Holly, 148
European Mistletoe, 154
European Mountain Ash, 168
European Ragwort, 166
European Sanicle, 184
European Water Hemlock, 148
Evil Eye, 43, 141, 151, 169, 191, 233
evil Spirits, 44, 74, 78, 82, 94-95, 104, 137, 203, 226, 228, 230
ewes, 20, 75, 86
exhaustion, 29, 126, 167, 179
expectorant, 133-134, 143, 149, 153, 163, 182
eye diseases, 50
eye infections, 138
eye irritations, 166
eye strain, 138-139
eye wash, 138-139, 148, 183
Eyebright, 138
eyewash, 119, 138-139

F

Fairies, 12, 21, 33-34, 37-38, 40, 44, 47, 50-52, 58, 70, 81, 84, 87, 92, 98-102, 110-112, 115, 120, 125, 137, 141-142, 146, 155, 159, 166, 169-170, 180, 197-198, 201, 203, 221, 224, 226, 228, 230, 241-243, 247-252

Fairies of the Air, 250

Fairy, 1, 3-4, 7-8, 11, 13, 21, 38-40, 43-44, 47, 49, 51-52, 55, 60, 66, 81, 98, 103-104, 109-112, 120, 125, 138, 142, 146-147, 180, 183, 185, 191, 215, 220, 224-226, 228, 230, 239-241, 244, 247-252, 269

Fairy abduction, 49, 248

Fairy Arrow, 249

Fairy Arrows, 52, 248

Fairy blood, 250

Fairy dancers, 250

Fairy Doctors, 230

Fairy double, 103, 109

Fairy Fire, 248

Fairy Flag, 251

Fairy Flax, 125, 138, 248

Fairy Gifts, 250

Fairy Hills, 21, 249

Fairy Hunt, 249

Fairy led, 225, 250

Fairy lover, 251

Fairy Marks, 248

Fairy Mound, 13, 21, 39, 52, 111, 250, 252

Fairy mouse, 248

Fairy music, 249-251

Fairy Pipe, 248

Fairy Queen, 13, 112, 249

Fairy Riding, 248

Fairy Ring, 249

Fairy Spring, 52

Fairy Stroke, 247

Fairy struck, 183

Fairy track, 98

Fairy Wind, 241

Fairy woman, 104, 142, 239, 248, 251

Fairy women, 138, 180, 249, 251-252

Fairy-hours, 244

Fairy-Ring, 241

Fal, 220, 260

Falcon, 206

Fall Equinox, 78, 87, 223

fallen angels, 241

falling hair, 122

famine food, 174

Famous Seers, 11, 110

faochag, 162, 260

farmers, 19, 35-36, 43, 87, 187, 192, 220, 235, 240

Farming, 11-12, 35, 87, 195, 213-214, 242

Farming by the Moon, 11, 35

Fastern's E'en, 77

Fasting Against, 236

Father God, 26-27

Father Nature, 26, 89

fatty acids, 146

fealladh-bog, 148, 260

feamainn, 172-173, 260

feamainn chírean, 173, 260

feanntag, 157, 260

fearn, 260

feasts, 20, 23, 63, 209, 215

febrifuge, 162

féithlean, 149, 260

female complaints, 150

Female Fern, 139

Fennel, 139, 202

Ferns, 139, 141

Fertility, 12, 24-29, 42, 44, 58, 66-67, 69, 76, 78, 80, 87, 89, 92, 96, 98, 155, 195, 209, 213-214, 223, 242, 251

fetal development, 179

Fever Stones, 51

fevers, 53, 82, 118, 120, 128, 137, 149, 153-155, 158-159, 161, 163, 166-167, 170-171, 175-176, 182-187, 232

Fianna, 56

fibroids, 152

fid na ndruad, 168, 260

fiddler, 69, 94, 245, 252

fiddles, 88

Field Gentian, 143

Fife, 202, 242

Figwort, 141, 198

Fili, 108, 206, 212, 260

Filipendula ulmaria, 166

Findbennach, 210, 260

Fin-Folk, 241-243

Finfolkaheem, 241
Fin-man, 241
Finn MacCumhail, 206, 211-212, 260
Fin-wife, 243
Fionn MacCumhail, 56
Fire Altar, 21, 83
Fire Blessing, 100
Fire Festivals, 11-12, 20, 23, 33, 42, 45, 63-64, 107, 169, 192, 221, 249
Fire Goddess, 24, 27, 75
Fire Magic, 11, 44, 222
Fires of Life, 66, 69, 75
First Footer, 222
First footing, 71
first fruits, 20, 84-86, 88, 223
first plowing, 20, 195
first sheaf, 84, 86
Fish, 29, 37, 41-42, 44, 50-51, 72, 92, 107, 191-194, 198, 202, 215, 220, 222, 224, 242, 244, 260
Fishermen, 29, 52, 59, 74, 84-85, 98, 106, 171, 192, 216, 220, 240, 244
fishing, 12, 16, 33, 37-38, 46, 72, 84-85, 94, 191-194, 214, 226, 241, 244
fishing boats, 33, 46, 241
Fishing Ends, 85
Fishing lines, 194
Fishing Magic, 12, 191, 193, 214
fishing tackle, 191
fishnets, 158
fistulas, 148
Fittin' Feast, 101
Fit-Washin', 91
Flag, 98, 141, 225, 235, 251
Flammula jovis, 175
flatulence, 129
Flax, 15, 89, 125, 138, 197, 248
fleas, 125
Flidais, 28, 211, 260
flint, 52, 115, 203, 241, 247-248, 266
fliodh, 131, 260

flu, 137, 153, 166, 176, 186, 202, 213, 229
Flummery, 70
foal, 84, 213, 224, 235
Fodla, 27, 31, 260
Foeniculum vulgare, 139, 202
Follasgain, 128, 261
Fomoire, 87
Food and Whisky, 12, 201
fool, 65, 79, 82, 94, 96, 222
forespoken, 225, 230
Forest Goddess, 211
Fortingall Yew, 8, 56, 187, 249
fortune teller, 108
foundation stone, 203
four leafed clover, 84
fox, 64, 81, 193, 225
Foxglove, 142, 159, 248
fractures, 132, 140, 233
fraoch, 147, 225, 261
Fraxinus excelsior, 120
Frayja, 28, 261
Frazers, 187
freckles, 133
Freya, 28, 91, 261
Freyja, 206, 261
Frigg, 27, 30, 261
frith, 109, 221, 261
frithir, 109, 221, 261
frog, 51, 55
Frog or Toad-Stones, 51
frost bite, 159
fuath a' mhadaidh, 155, 261
Fucus canaliculatus, 173
fuinnseag, 143, 261
Full Moon, 35-36, 57, 223, 231, 246, 249
funeral, 86, 102, 104-106, 109-110
funeral games, 86, 102
funerals, 30, 102
fungal infection, 162
Furl O' Fairies Ween, 241

G

Gaelic, 6, 14, 17-18, 26, 28, 51, 54, 73, 117- 187, 202, 207, 216, 219, 227, 243, 266
Gaels, 14, 17, 27, 31
gall, 135, 161, 185-186
gall bladder, 135, 161, 186
gallan mór, 127, 261

gallows tree, 54, 60
gallstones, 161
gambling, 39
gangrene, 141, 160
Gannet, 16
gaoth a deas, 37, 261

gaoth a deas ear-dheas, 37, 261
gaoth a deas iar-dheas, 37, 261
gaoth a tuath, 38, 261
gaoth a tuath ear-thuath, 38, 261
gaoth an ear, 37-38, 261
gaoth an ear ear-dheas, 37, 261
gaoth an ear ear-thuath, 38, 261
gaoth an iar, 37, 261
gaoth an iar iar-dheas, 37, 261
gaoth an iar iar-thuath, 37, 261
garbhag an t-sléibhe, 131, 261
Garden violet, 181-182
gargle, 15, 118-119, 123, 125, 128, 149, 152-153, 158, 161, 163, 167-168, 170-171, 174, 179-180, 182-183, 185
garlic, 139, 142, 159-160, 176
Garlic wild, 142
garnet, 52
gas, 119, 139, 143, 151-153, 155, 160, 162, 185
gastritis, 148, 179, 186
gastro-intestinal problems, 164
Gaul, 14, 26, 28-30, 88, 206-207, 212, 214
Gaulish, 14, 20, 24, 26, 29-30, 65, 108, 205-207, 209-215
geal, 37, 147, 260-261
Gean, 142
geanais, 142, 261
Geasa, 55, 220, 261
geis, 229
geld animals, 36
genealogy, 20, 106, 205
Genii Cucullati, 28, 215, 261
genius loci, 28, 261
Gentian, 143
Gentiana campestris, 143
Gentle Annis, 37
geomancy, 221
Geranium Rrobertianum, 167
germander, 121, 143, 170
Germander Speedwell, 121, 143
Ghosts, 100, 137, 227
Giantesses, 242
Giants, 25, 241
ginger, 73, 122, 157, 165, 173-174
gingivitis, 175
gíogan, 178, 261
giuthas, 163, 176, 225, 261
giuthas lochlannach, 176, 261

Glaine Nathrach, 51, 261
Glaistig, 239, 242, 261
glan ruis, 138, 261
glands, 49, 128, 149, 231
glas, 37, 261
Glasgow Fair, 84, 271
glas-leum, 175, 261
Glen Lyon, 56, 236
Glenshee, 249
glúineach an uisge, 122, 261
glúineag dhearg, 122, 261
Goat, 69, 125, 181, 197-198, 213, 242, 245
Goat's milk, 181, 213
Gobar-Bachach, 242, 261
gobhar bacach, 197
God of eloquence, 30
God of light, 27
God of Love, 30, 155, 248
God of medicine, 27
God of soldiers, 26
God of the people, 26
God of the Sea, 192, 222
God of the Vines, 31
God of War, 24, 26, 206
God of wild animals, 26
Goddess of Beer, 28
Goddess of Fertility, 26, 29
Goddess of Fire, 222
Goddess of grief, 30
Goddess of Horses, 29
Goddess of Long Life, 30
Goddess of Love, 28, 91
Goddess of Motherhood, 75, 135
Goddess of Smithcraft, Healing, and Poetry, 228
Goddess of Sovereignty, 24
Goddess of spring, 27, 78
Goddess of the Hearth, 24
Goddess of the Pool, 28
Goddess of War, 29
Goddess of wild animals, 28
Goddess of Winter, 24-25
Goddess of wisdom, 24
Goddesses, 23-25, 31, 34, 146, 207, 216, 220
Goddesses of War, 207
Gododdin, 17, 261
Godparent, 102
Gods, 11, 21, 23-25, 27-28, 30-31, 34, 44, 69, 82, 86, 105, 109, 146, 159, 192, 195, 197,

202, 212, 214-216, 220-221, 230, 234, 246
Gods of the Harvest, 86
Gods of the Sea, 192
Gods of thunder, 146
Goibniu, 28, 50
goiter, 172-173
Gold, 26, 49, 92, 100, 146, 191, 199,
   207-208, 224, 232, 234
Goldenrod, 119, 121, 143, 170
Goldenseal, 138
goldsmith, 85
Good God, 30, 75
good luck, 38, 50, 59, 73-74, 76, 86, 92,
   96, 100, 102, 120, 147, 155, 194-195,
   198, 204, 220-224, 226-227, 243
good luck charms, 222
goose, 28, 30, 53, 206, 208, 213
Gooseberry, 144
Gorse, 67, 208
gout, 118, 120, 135-136, 143, 145, 148,
   150, 155-156, 159-161, 165-166, 182
Goutweed, 136
Govannon, 28
Gowan, 134
grábhan bán, 149, 261
grábhan nan clach, 177, 261
grádh is fuadh, 160, 261
Grain, 12, 15, 28, 55, 60, 66, 68-69, 72-73,
   75, 78, 84-88, 96, 105, 133, 194-196,
   198, 203, 214, 222-223, 240-242, 245
Grain Goddess, 69, 87
grán, 119, 133, 261, 263
Grannos, 28, 262
graves, 36, 102, 111, 187
Gravesite, 106
gravestone, 50
graveyards, 187
Great Bear, 33
Great Glen, 13
Great Horse Father, 27

Great Mother, 25, 29, 43
Greeks, 15
Green, 25, 27, 37, 52-53, 70, 78, 92, 115, 117,
   121, 146, 156, 161, 172, 176, 178, 180, 186,
   228, 230, 241-242, 247, 249-250, 252
Green Clad Maiden, 242
Gregorian calendar, 39, 80
greim saighdeir, 185, 262
Gronw, 207, 262
groom, 72, 89-98, 236, 252
grósaid, 144, 262
Ground Elder, 136
Ground Hog Day, 75
Ground Ivy, 144
Groundsel, 145
groundsel root, 145
Gruagach, 58-59, 242, 258, 262
Gruagach stone, 242
gruth, 202, 262
Guardian of the Well, 41
guardian Spirit, 239, 242
Gude Wichts, 247
Gudeman's Croft, 47, 197
Guid Nychburris, 83, 262
Guilandina bonduc, 126
Guildandia bonduc, 51
Guinevere, 250
Guizers, 68, 71, 74, 96, 209, 222
gum, 122, 149, 202
gum infections, 202
gums, 120, 153, 158, 164
Gundestrup Cauldron, 26, 209-210,
   212, 214-216
Guy Fawkes, 68
Gwenhwyfar, 214, 262
Gwernabwy, 206, 262
Gwydion, 207, 262
Gyre, 242
Gyre-Carline, 242
Gyro, 242

H

Hadrian's Wall, 14-15, 24, 26, 28-30,
   209, 213-214, 229
Hag, 25, 31, 56, 67, 88, 206-207, 240,
   266, 270
Hag of the Mill-Dust, 88
Hag of Winter, 67

Haggis, 67-68, 74, 271
Hags, 30, 67, 168
hair, 28, 54, 71, 76, 83-84, 93, 122, 161- 162,
   182, 221, 224, 227, 231, 240, 245-248
haley stones, 203
Halloween, 66, 108

Hallowmass Foy, 67
Hallstatt Celts, 14
haltadans, 197
Halyman's Rig, 47
hame-fare, 97
Hand-fasting, 33, 93, 108
Handsel, 73, 96-97
Handsel Monday, 73
handsel-money, 96
hang over, 179, 213
Hare, 27, 78, 193, 196, 198, 213, 225
harp, 30, 248
harper, 85
Hart's Tongue Fern, 139
Harvest, 12, 20, 35-37, 65-66, 75, 78, 84-88, 115-117, 195-198, 213-214, 222-223, 242
Harvest Customs, 12, 87, 195, 213-214, 242
Harvest Goddess, 78
Harvest Home, 12, 198
Harvest knots, 84
Harvest Suppers, 85
Harvest-home, 85
haug-búi, 242, 262
Hawthorn, 40-41, 80, 116, 142, 145-146, 154, 159, 237
hay-fever, 147
Hazel, 15, 35, 45, 135, 137, 146, 215
hazelnut milk, 100
hazelnuts, 66, 202
Hazels of Wisdom, 215
headache, 121, 124, 142, 147, 150, 153, 163, 165, 170, 173, 179, 202
Healing, 8, 11-12, 20, 24, 26-28, 30-31, 37, 39-40, 44-45, 51-56, 60, 75, 77, 82, 86, 115, 118, 121, 124, 131-134, 137, 140, 155-156, 159, 164-165, 177, 180, 188, 202, 208-209, 212, 214-216, 220, 227-229, 231-234, 269
Healing Charms, 54
Healing Magic, 12, 45, 227
healing objects, 52
healing salves, 118, 131-134, 140, 164-165, 180
Healing Stones, 51, 55-56
Healing Threads, 11, 31, 53, 77, 188, 269
Healing Threads and Knots, 11, 53
healing wands, 121
Healing Wells, 39, 54, 86, 212, 215-216

hearse, 105, 137
heart, 7, 50, 55-56, 67, 86, 88, 124, 127, 142, 145, 147, 149, 151, 154-156, 160, 167, 174, 178-179, 184, 230, 246, 248
heart conditions, 124, 154, 184
heart palpitations, 154-156
heart problems, 155
heartburn, 121, 143, 185
hearth, 24, 30, 44-46, 69, 71, 73, 75, 80, 97, 207, 222, 227, 248
hearth fire, 44, 46
hearths, 66
heather, 15, 81, 83, 94, 147, 157, 181, 188, 202, 225, 271-272
Heather, 15, 81, 83, 94, 147, 157, 181, 188, 202, 225, 271-272
heather ale, 81, 181
Hebrides, 9, 15, 34, 61, 126, 209, 231
Hedeoma pulegioides, 126
Hedera helix, 150, 154
Hedge Bindweed, 122, 226
Hedge Mustard, 156
heifer, 30, 83
Heléval Bheag, 251, 262
Heléval Mhor, 251, 262
Helleborine, 147
Hemlock, 148, 247
hemorrhage, 125, 144, 150, 186
hemorrhoids, 158, 163, 174
Hen Night, 93
Hen Wife, 230
Henwen, 210
Hera, 24
herb of gluttony, 136
herb of the Fairy woman, 142
Herb Robert, 148, 167
Herbal Healers, 24
herbal tobacco, 124, 156
Herbalists, 27, 29, 142
Herding bannocks, 85
heroes, 211-212, 220
heron, 206
hiccoughs, 149
High Tide, 244
Highland Games, 87
Hildaland, 242
Hill Folk, 92, 230
Hill Goddess, 239
Hill o' Many Stanes, 58

Hill Spirit, 230
Hill-Folk, 245
Hill-Trows, 245
Hindu, 19
hoarseness, 132, 141, 202
hobby horse, 69, 82, 95
Hogboon, 242-243
Hogboy, 242
Hogmanay, 70-73, 193, 203, 209, 222
Holed Stones, 59
Holey Stones, 59
Holly, 41, 67, 69, 82, 148, 151, 208, 225
Holly King, 82
Holy Days, 11, 21, 23, 41, 44, 63, 169, 192, 216
holy stones, 203
Holy Wells, 25, 38-39, 41-42, 76, 82, 86, 230
honey, 34, 56, 70, 81, 86, 100, 116, 118, 120, 129, 134, 140, 143-144, 146-147, 149-150, 154, 157, 159-160, 163-165, 167-168, 179, 182, 202-203, 248
Honeysuckle, 149, 184, 223
Honoring the Sun and Moon, 11, 34
Hooded One, 67
hops, 124-125, 129, 143, 147
Hordeum distichon, 121
Hordeum vulgare, 121
Horehound, 149
horned God, 24, 26, 28, 30, 215
horns, 24, 26, 36, 39, 69, 209-210, 212, 215, 242

horse, 24, 27-29, 37, 66-67, 69, 73, 82, 86, 88-89, 95, 99, 120, 170, 194-195, 197, 203, 206, 213-214, 216, 226, 235, 240, 243-244
Horse Goddess, 206
Horse Goddesses, 24
Horse Racing, 66, 82, 86, 88, 213-214
horse radish, 120
horse shoes, 235
horses, 27-29, 67, 69, 73, 81, 83, 85, 95, 110, 145, 153, 158, 209, 213-214, 241, 270
horseshoe, 50, 191-192, 213, 226
Horsetail, 149
Hosts, 97, 244, 250
Hot Cross Buns, 78, 271
hot toddy, 156-157
House and Home, 12, 203, 209
House Blessing, 203
Houseleek, 130, 150, 164, 177
Hugboy, 242
Humulus lupulus, 124, 129, 143, 147
Hunt the Gowk, 79, 270
hunter God, 26
hunting, 24, 29-31, 56, 72, 103, 248
Hydrastis Canadensis, 138
hydromancy, 221
Hypericum perforatum, 43, 121, 143, 170
Hypericum pulchrum, 170
hypertension, 154

I

iadhshlat thalmhainn, 144, 262
Iasg Sianta, 41, 262
Iberia, 14
Iceni, 24
Ilex aquifolium, 148
Imbas Forosnai, 210, 262
immortality, 187, 250
immrama, 209, 262
immune system, 142, 154, 182, 230
In Conclusion, 253
incantation, 56, 126, 199, 228, 246
Incantations, 12, 20, 219, 227, 230, 269
incense, 163
incoming tide, 44, 100, 141, 198
indigestion, 135, 143, 147, 153, 185

Indo-European, 19, 34, 85, 197, 211
infections, 128-129, 138, 142, 159, 184, 202, 228
inflamed eyes, 120
inflamed prostate, 161
inflamed tendons, 132
inflammations, 118, 122-123, 126, 136, 148-150, 152, 170, 175, 180, 182-183, 185
initiation, 146
insecticidal, 162
insects, 115, 125, 158
insomnia, 122, 129, 131, 133, 135, 140, 147, 150, 153, 164, 170, 178, 182-184
insulin, 124

Insults to Wells, 42
intermittent fever, 120, 158, 161, 177
internal bleeding, 154, 157-158, 183-185
intestinal colic, 159
intestinal irritations, 137
intestines, 134
invalids, 135, 157, 212
Inverness, 58, 111, 249
invocations, 54
Invocation of Bríghde, 41, 98
iogh, 187, 262
ioghar, 187, 262
Iomas, 222
Iona, 15, 21, 52, 187, 262
ioua, 187, 262
Ireland, 7, 14, 17, 25-26, 28-29, 31, 42, 58, 61, 85-86, 208, 214, 219, 250, 252, 270
Iris pseudoacorus, 141

Iron, 14, 16, 39, 46, 50-51, 95, 97, 99, 101, 103, 115, 131, 137, 157, 161, 169, 172, 176, 178, 182, 193, 196, 198, 203, 213, 226, 228, 248-250
Iron Age, 14, 51, 103, 213
Isatis tinctoria, 14, 186
Iscador, 154
Island of Apples, 65
Island of Stroma, 73
Island of Westray, 240
Isle of Lewis, 21, 111, 239
Isle of Man, 15
Isle of Skye, 52, 147, 197, 251
Isle of Troda, 52
Isles of the Blessed, 106
itching, 143, 167, 171
iubhar, 187, 262
Ivy, 144, 150-151, 154, 210, 227

J

James VI, 68
Jaundice, 118, 120, 124, 128, 130, 135, 138-140, 153, 161, 170, 180, 182, 184, 231
jelly, 123, 147, 172, 182, 212
Jesus, 110
John O'Groats, 72
Joint, 53, 165, 233
joint injuries, 233
Joints, 129, 135-136, 216, 233

journey, 35, 37, 39, 63, 106, 175, 213, 227
judges, 20
Judgments, 60
Juice of the Oak, 154
jump the flames, 80, 196
Juniper, 15, 127, 151, 202
Juniperus communis, 15, 127, 151, 202
Juno, 24
Jupiter, 27

K

karma, 55
Kava-Kava, 170
Keel-Stane, 60
keening woman, 105
Kelpie, 243
Kenneth MacAlpine, 18, 61
Kenneth MacKenzie, Earl of Seaforth, 111
Keppoch stone, 52
Kern Doll, 78, 84, 222
Kerridwen, 220, 262
Kettling, 95
kidney, 121, 123, 127, 143-144, 151, 157, 159, 161, 166, 175, 181-182
kidney stones, 123
Kidney Vetch, 181
kidneys, 20, 119, 121, 130, 134, 144, 151, 157, 182, 185, 219

Kilmoullach, 243
Kiln-carle, 243
king, 13, 15, 17-18, 20-21, 28, 37, 61, 68, 74, 82, 85, 87, 95, 158, 202, 206, 208, 210, 214, 219-220, 224, 236
king Malcolm III, 87
king of the trees, 158
King of Winter, 82
kirn, 198, 262
knee injuries, 140
Knights Templar, 61
knitting needle, 248
knockin-stane, 203
Knots, 11, 53-54, 84, 92, 191, 212, 232, 235-236
knots in the wood, 191

L

La Téne, 14

labor, 33, 50-51, 54, 58, 75, 86, 99-100, 110, 125-126, 174, 180, 185, 187, 215, 245

Lad's Love, 89

Lady's Mantle, 152

Ladybug, 214

laird, 95, 106, 247

lakes, 40, 56, 88, 211

Lakelander Spruce, 176

lamb, 66-67, 80, 82-83, 91, 119, 152, 216, 270

lambs, 64, 86, 89

Laminaria digitata, 173

Lammas "Brother and Sister, 85

Lammas Fair, 84-85

Lammer, 50, 53, 239

Lanark, 78

Land Goddess, 24, 27, 31, 56, 196, 198, 214

Land of Fairy, 38, 120

Land of Heart's Desire, 248

Land of Promise, 248

Land-Trows, 244

Larch, 58

Lark, 206, 221

lasair-theine, 175, 262

Lathyrus montanus, 181

Latis, 28, 262

Lavandula vera, 136

lavender, 136

Laver, 172, 202

lawyers, 20, 219

laxative, 120, 123, 137-138, 149, 163, 167-168, 173, 179, 182

Lead, 50, 94, 137, 146, 150, 178-179, 182, 243

leamhnach, 180, 262

leaping the fire, 66, 220

leather, 195, 248

Lee Penny, 53

leeks, 160

Léigheagan, 262

lemon balm, 153, 174, 178

Lenus, 28, 262

Lesser Celandine, 15

Lesser Periwinkle, 162

lethargy, 230

leucorrhea, 149, 158, 163, 177, 180, 183, 186

Levisticum officinale, 216

Lewis, 21, 58, 111, 239

Lia Faill, 61, 262

liath, 37, 132, 258, 262

liathus, 156, 262

lice, 118

life after death, 102

Life Passages, 11, 89

lightning, 30, 146, 150, 159, 195

lili bhan, 183, 262

lime flowers, 154

liminal space, 60, 208

Limpets, 16, 193, 214

Linarich, 172

Lindow Man, 186

linen, 46, 100, 104-105, 125, 157, 163, 203

linens, 91, 179

Linum catharticum, 125, 138, 248

Lion na Mna Sithe, 248

lions, 26

Lir, 28-29, 214, 248, 262, 264

Listera ovata, 160

little old man of the grain, 240

liver, 67, 118-120, 124, 127, 129-130, 134-135, 138-139, 141-142, 144-145, 151, 159, 161, 166, 182, 185-186, 231, 244

liver complaints, 129, 135, 185

LLeu, 206-207, 262

Lludd, 28, 263

Llyr, 28-29, 263-264

loch, 8, 25, 31, 40-41, 56, 187, 206, 211, 229, 245, 263

Loch Eireann, 31, 263

Loch Lomond, 206

Loch Lyon, 56

Loch Sithgail, 211, 263

Loch Tay, 8, 187

Lochaber, 52, 211

Lochaber Deer Goddess, 211

Lochcon, 249

lochs, 40, 214, 243

Lockharts, 53

Loki, 206

long life, 30, 38, 103

Lonicera periclymenum, 149

Lord Lyon, 21

Lord of Winter, 82

Lore of the Elements, 11, 33, 222

Lore of the Sea, 12, 191, 214

Lovage, 119, 152, 216
love, 12, 28, 30, 55, 85-86, 89-92, 107-
   108, 112, 125, 155, 160, 180, 220, 223,
   230, 240-241, 243, 245-246, 248-249
love charm, 180
love magic, 55
Love Potion, 55
love spells, 12, 160, 223, 230
Love Spells and Moon Magic, 12, 223
lover's quarrel, 55
Lover's vows, 43
lovers, 30, 43, 84-85, 89-90, 208, 211
loving cup, 224
Luck, 12, 33, 37-38, 40, 49-50, 55, 59-60,
   63-64, 69-70, 73-76, 78, 82-84, 86, 88,
   91-96, 100, 102, 104-105, 120, 137,
   147, 155, 168-169, 180, 191-198, 203-
   204, 208, 214, 216, 220-227, 235, 243
Lucky Bonnet, 100
Lug, 29, 263
Lugh, 23, 29, 66, 85-87, 206-207, 212, 220, 263
Lughnasad, 85
Lugi, 14, 263
Lugudunum, 207, 263
Lugus, 206-207, 263
luibh bhán, 175, 263
luibh na purgaid, 167, 263
lúireach, 172, 263
lumbago, 159, 165
Lúnasdal, 20, 29, 39-40, 42-43, 63-64,
   84-88, 91, 93, 151, 221, 223, 263
Lunastain, 64, 263
lung, 59, 139, 149, 153, 157, 163-166, 170,
   179, 216

lung conditions, 59, 139, 149, 153, 164,
   166, 170, 216
lus a' chraois, 136, 263
lus a' chrúbain, 143, 263
lus an easbaig, 136, 263
lus an ellain, 148, 263
lus an rígh, 179, 263
Lus an rócais, 128
lus an róis, 148, 263
Lus an Tálaidh, 160, 263
lus an torranain, 130, 263
lus an t-saoidh, 139, 263
lus beathaig, 121, 263
lus caolach, 138, 263
lus chasgadh na fala, 186, 263
lus Ghlinne Bhrácadail, 136, 263
lus Máiri, 128, 263
lus míosach, 138, 263
lus na caithimh, 184, 263
lus na fala, 170, 174, 263
lus na Frainge, 177, 263
lus na Spainnte, 161, 263
lus nam bansíth, 142, 263
lus nan cluas, 150, 263
lus nan cnapan, 141, 263
lus nan grán dubh, 119, 263
lus nan laugh, 124, 263
lus nan leac, 138, 263
lus-leíghis, 155, 177, 263
Lycopodium clavatum, 131
Lycopodium selago, 131
Lyme disease, 154
lymph glands, 128

M

Mabon, 29, 263
Mabon vab Modron, 29, 263
MacAlastair, 252
MacCrimmons, 251
MacDonalds, 53, 225
MacDonnells, 52
Macha, 29, 207, 214, 263
Machrie Moor, 58
Mackays, 251
Mackintoshes, 53
MacLachlans, 104
Macleods, 251

MacNeill, 251
MacPherson, 251
madadh-allaidh, 216, 263
Madog, 206, 264
Maes Howe, 7, 58
Maetae, 14, 264
Magic, 7-9, 11-13, 19, 23, 30, 38-41, 43-
   46, 53-58, 60, 63, 67, 81-82, 86-88, 91,
   96, 98, 115, 160, 188, 191, 193, 196,
   198, 206-207, 211, 214, 217, 219-229,
   233, 237, 243, 249, 270
Magic And Luck, 12, 224

Magic Cups, 60
Magic Wand, 67, 88
magical aids, 193
magical helper, 198
magical horse, 29
magical pigs, 209, 215
Magical Practices, 12, 41-42, 219
magical prohibition, 205, 219, 229
Magical Protection, 12, 53, 56, 99-100, 125, 193, 205, 237
magical quests, 209
magical seership, 215
magical staff, 26
Magical woods, 198
magician, 85, 206-207
Magna Mater, 25
magnesium, 146
magpie, 103, 207
Maidenhair Fern, 140
Maiden-Mother-Crone, 23
Maighdeann Uaine, 242, 264
Mairi Nic Iain Fhin, 251
malaria, 124
Male Fern, 140
Maleficium, 220
malevolent Spirit, 64
malt, 25, 74, 101, 147, 157
Malus domestica, 120
Malus sylvestris, 120
Manawyddan Ap Llyr, 29, 264
Mannies an Horses, 73, 270
Maponos, 28-29, 264
Marag Dubh, 68, 264
Marcachd Shith, 248, 264
Marc-raineach, 140, 264
mare, 72-73, 84, 95, 198, 214
Mare's milk, 214
Marigold, 125, 151, 153
Marjoram, 120, 153
Marne river, 29
Marriage, 11, 13, 35, 72, 78, 82, 89-91, 93-95, 99, 107-108, 151, 155, 160, 187, 224, 251
marriage ba, 94
marriage bed, 99, 155, 251
Marriage Divinations, 90
Marrubium vulgare, 149
marry, 39, 50, 73, 86, 90-92, 107, 187, 196, 244

Mars, 24-26, 28, 30, 206, 215-216
Marsh Violet, 124, 180
Martinmas, 67
Mary, 31, 51, 68, 71, 87, 95, 188, 269
Mary, Queen of Scots, 68, 95
Mary's Nut, 51
Marymas, 87
maternity, 26, 29
Matres, 23, 29, 264
Matricaria chamomilla, 144
matron of honor, 94, 97
Matrona, 29
Matunos, 209, 264
Matunus, 29, 264
May Butter, 82
May Day games, 82
May Tree, 145
Maypole, 80
meacan dubh, 132, 264
Meadow Rue, 169
Meadow sorrel, 175
meadow-pipits, 103
Meadowsweet, 166
meant, 40, 75, 86, 95, 153, 179, 236, 264
measles, 128, 162
meat, 16, 65, 78, 86, 102, 209, 215, 233
medicine woman, 232
meilbheag, 164, 264
melancholy, 178, 202, 229
Melancholy thistle, 178
Melissa officinalis, 153, 174, 178
memory aid, 133
Menhir, 58
menopausal hot flashes, 161
menopause, 155
menses, 119, 153, 156
menstrual disorders, 170
menstrual pads, 176
menstrual pain, 141
menstruation, 125, 129, 131, 141, 144-145, 149, 151-152, 154, 162, 164, 170, 174-175, 179, 183, 186
Mentha piperita, 153, 186
Mentha pulegium, 154, 162
Mentha spicata, 153, 156
Mentha spp, 124, 129, 138, 153-154, 166, 202
Menyanthes trifoliata, 124, 153, 166
meóir Mhoire, 181, 264
merchants, 15, 26

Mercurialis perennis, 136
Mercury, 28, 136, 215-216
Merfolk, 243
Mermaid, 241, 243
Mermaids, 241, 243-244
Miach, 27, 29, 264
Miadhach, 206, 264
Miaran na Mna Sithe, 248, 264
Mice, 102, 154, 215, 232
Michael, 6, 29, 66, 85, 88, 196
Michaelmas, 66, 85, 88
Midmar Kirk, 57
Midsummer, 44, 57, 83, 90, 108, 120, 137, 146, 170, 223, 244
Midsummer's Eve, 146, 244
midwife, 46, 75-76, 100, 105-106, 121, 126, 230
Midwinter, 7, 57-58, 70
midwinter Sunset, 58
migraine, 133, 173, 184, 213
Military God, 206
milk, 21, 24-25, 34, 43-44, 50-51, 56, 58-59, 63, 65, 75, 78-79, 81, 85-86, 92, 95, 100, 110, 116, 119, 123, 125-126, 135, 138-139, 143-147, 151, 154, 161, 164, 169, 174, 180-181, 198-199, 202-203, 210-211, 213-214, 220, 222, 225, 236, 240, 242-243, 247-248, 250
milk offerings, 21
milk pail, 51, 125, 145, 151, 198, 236
milkwort, 125, 151
mill, 241, 245
millers, 243
mílsean monaidh, 124, 264
Minerals, 11, 49, 161, 172, 182, 212
Minerva, 24
Mint, 120, 124, 129, 138, 153-154, 166, 202
missionaries, 18, 38, 56
Mistletoe, 27, 39, 69, 104, 154-155, 159, 209, 223, 225
Mither, 29, 31, 78, 87, 264
Mither O' the Sea, 29, 31, 78, 87
Moccus, 209, 264
Modron, 28-29, 263-264
Mogons, 29, 264
molasses, 93, 176, 232
Mole, 215
Molingus Globe, 53
Molluca bean, 99

Molluka Beans, 51
Molluka Nuts, 235
Money, 12, 64, 68, 71, 82, 91, 93, 105-106, 185, 193, 201, 228, 230, 245
Monkshood, 155
Monostroma grevillei, 172
Monsters, 12, 239
Moon, 11-12, 20, 33-36, 39, 49, 51, 55, 57-58, 77-78, 82, 85, 90-92, 100, 110, 115, 125, 180, 184, 195, 220, 223-225, 229-231, 236, 246, 249
Moon Magic, 12, 223
moor of Rannoch, 13
Moray, 31, 73, 112
morning sickness, 167
Morrigan, 264
Mórrígan, 206-207, 211
moth, 103
Móthan, 99, 124-125, 180, 248, 264
Mother Goddess, 24, 29
Mother Goddess of Fertility, 29
Mother Goddesses, 216
Mother Goose, 28, 206
Mother Ocean, 43
Mother of the Gods, 25
Mother of the stars, 35
Mother River Goddess, 43, 86, 211, 223
motherhood, 24, 30, 75, 135, 207
Motherwort, 154-155
mound-dwarf, 242
Mountain Holly, 148
Mountain sorrel, 175
Mountain Speedwell, 143
Mountain Thyme, 179
Mountain Yew, 151
Mouse, 72, 103, 215, 248
mouth, 88, 100, 105, 108, 110, 122-123, 125, 148-150, 153, 162, 167, 174-175, 180-182, 185, 231, 243
mouth inflammations, 122, 182, 185
mouthwash, 122, 167, 179
mucus congestion, 133, 164
mugwort, 82, 107, 156
Mugwort, 82, 107, 156
muir-droighinn, 118, 264
múisean, 133, 264
mullein, 156
mumps, 59
murder, 103, 110

múr-dhroigheann, 118, 264
mur-druidheann, 118, 264
muscle pain, 129
muscle strain, 183
muscles, 128
Mushroom, 146, 165
music, 29-30, 74-75, 88, 91, 93, 105, 107,
245, 247, 249-251
musicians, 20, 88, 91, 251
mussels, 16
Mustard, 156-157
Myrica cerifera, 125
Myrica gale, 125
Myristica fragrans, 178

N

nail, 50, 99, 191, 196, 198, 226
Naming Ceremony, 96, 102
Nantosuelta, 30-31, 207, 264
násad, 85, 264
Nasturtium officinale, 182
natural magic, 220, 223
Nature Spirits, 34, 69, 223
nausea, 119, 142, 154, 162, 179
Need-fire, 45-46, 222
Neimheadh, 21, 264
Neith, 26
Nemain, 207, 264
neóinean, 134, 264
Nepeta glechoma, 144
Neptune, 28
nerve conditions, 158
nerve tonic, 167
nerves, 126, 147, 153, 163, 176, 178-179, 182
nervous afflictions, 170
nervous conditions, 56, 147, 154, 165, 170, 182, 184
nervous irritability, 155
nettle–cloth, 158
Nettles, 6, 86, 134, 156-158, 182, 223
neuralgia, 155, 184
neuritis, 155
new grain, 66, 84-88, 223
New Moon, 20, 34, 49, 77, 90, 223-225
New Year, 37, 71-74, 84, 151
New Years, 39, 70, 222
New Years Eve, 70, 222
newborn, 46, 100-102, 121, 226, 248-249
newlyweds, 59, 208
newt, 232

nicotine, 179
Nighean, 56, 264
night hag, 207
night sweats, 170
night's portion, 225
nightmares, 179
nine mothers meat, 233
Nine Sacred Woods', 45, 81, 118, 121, 184, 191
nion, 120, 264
Njuggle, 243, 264
Nodons, 30, 212, 264
Norse, 6, 13-15, 23, 27-28, 30, 69-70, 79, 91, 111, 197, 242, 245, 253, 255-257, 261-262, 267
Northern Lights, 241
Norway pine, 163
Norway Spruce, 176
nosebleed, 150, 186
nosebleeds, 157
Nuada, 27-28, 220, 264
nuallach, 143, 264
Nuckelavee, 243, 264
Nudd, 28, 264
nursing, 53, 119, 139, 147, 161, 167, 174, 214, 247
nursing mothers, 119, 139, 147, 161, 167, 174, 214
nut milk, 146
nutmeg, 78-79, 81, 178
nuts, 65, 108, 135, 146, 201, 215, 235-236
Nymphaea alba, 152, 183, 189, 272
Nymphaea odorata, 152, 183
nymphs, 26
Nyuggle, 243, 264

O

O'Neills, 17
Oak, 26, 38, 41, 46, 82, 104, 145, 154-
156, 158-159, 191, 207, 209, 225, 229
oak and ash and thorn, 159

Oak galls, 158
Oak King, 82
oatcakes, 65, 86, 95, 106, 202
oaths, 23, 47
Oath Stones, 59
oatmeal, 64-65, 67-68, 70, 81-82, 100-
    101, 135, 157, 159, 192, 202-203, 222,
    232, 267, 272
Oatmeal Bannock, 64, 101, 272
Oats, 15, 65, 85, 133, 159, 170, 202
Ocean Spirits, 239
Ocelus, 30, 265
odhar, 37, 59, 111, 258, 265
Odin, 27, 30, 69, 207, 261, 265, 271
Odínn, 30, 265
Oenach Tailten, 86, 265
Oengus Og, 30, 89, 265
offerings, 21, 38, 40, 42-44, 58-60, 70,
    82-83, 86, 192, 198, 222-223, 242-
    243, 250
Ogham, 16, 30, 236-237, 265
Ogma, 30, 265
Oimelc, 20, 24-25, 39, 42, 63-64, 67, 74-
    77, 90, 135, 151, 195, 216, 221-222, 265
Oisín, 211, 265
Old Growth Forests, 249
Old Hogmanay, 73
Old Samhuinn, 67, 88, 221
old sores, 136, 171

omens, 66, 75, 81, 86, 103
Onion, 67, 142, 159-160
onions, 36, 68, 159-160
Onopordon acanthium, 178
opium poppy, 164
oragan, 153, 265
Orcades, 209
Orchids, 160
Orchis maculata, 160
Origanum vulgare, 153
Orkney, 9, 13-15, 21, 23, 31, 57, 70, 72-73,
    78, 84, 90, 165, 188, 197-198, 206, 209,
    216, 224, 240, 243-244, 246, 268, 270
Orobus tuberosus, 181
orphans, 194
Osmunda regalis, 140
Otherworld, 20, 28-29, 59, 66, 103, 120,
    206, 208-211, 214-215
Otherworldly feasts, 209
Otherworldly islands, 209
Otter, 192, 215
Outer Hebrides, 15
Owein, 207, 265
Owl, 207
Owre-Boggie Wedding, 97
Oxalis acetosella, 185
ox-eye daisy, 134
Oxyma digyna, 175

P

palsy, 133
Palug's Cat, 210
Papaver rhoeas, 164
paper, 40, 78-79, 116, 158, 185, 220
paralysis, 159, 161, 179, 248
parasites, 152, 163, 174, 182
Parsley, 36, 161, 164, 167
parsnip, 202
Passover, 78
P-Celtic, 14
peabar, 162, 265
pearls, 241
pearlwort, 180, 198, 271
pearsal, 161, 265
peat, 15, 26, 36, 44-46, 63, 73, 83-84, 90,
    97, 100, 102, 199, 209-210, 213, 221,
    223, 227, 229, 244-245

Peerie-Folk, 141, 245
peighinn pisich, 34, 265
peighinn ríoghail, 162, 265
Pellitory of Spain, 161
Pen medi bach caseg, 214, 265
Penannular brooches, 16
Pennyroyal, 126, 154, 162
Pepper, 67-68, 127, 146, 162, 177, 232
peppermint, 153-154, 186
Periwinkle, 162
periwinkles, 16
pest control, 36
Petasites albus, 127
Petasites vulgaris, 127
philosophers, 21, 219
phlebitis, 132
Phoenicians, 15

phosphorus, 146, 241
photo-sensitivity, 170, 186
physicians, 20, 213
physicians of Myddfai, 213
Picea excelsa, 176
Pictish, 13-17, 23, 34, 51, 56, 68, 73, 187, 203, 205-206, 209, 211, 215-216, 269
Pictish symbols, 51
Picts, 8, 13-17, 19, 61, 102, 147, 165, 186, 202, 253, 265, 270
Pig, 79, 139, 192-193, 209-210, 212, 215, 221, 232
piles, 15, 126, 130, 141, 158, 162-164, 179-180
Pimpinella anisum, 119, 202
pimples, 118, 171
pin of the plough, 169
pin-chrann, 163, 265
Pine, 35, 42, 46, 69, 111, 163, 232
Pinguicula vulgaris, 99, 124, 151, 188, 271
pink eye, 138
Pinus spp, 163
Pinus sylvestris, 163
Piob Shith, 248, 265
piper, 66, 74, 94, 105, 146, 162, 170, 249, 251
Piper methysticum, 170
Piper nigrum, 146, 162
pipes, 42, 88, 105
placenta, 119, 173
pláigh na carra, 171, 265
Plant, 8, 35-36, 57, 84, 115-117, 119, 121-122, 124, 126, 128-129, 131-132, 134, 136-138, 140-142, 144-145, 147-156, 158, 160-161, 164-175, 177-182, 184-189, 205, 271-272
Plantago major, 163
Plantago spp, 130
Plantain, 90, 130, 163-164
Pleiades, 80
pleurisy, 132, 157
Pliny, 131, 223
Plow, 12, 21, 33, 75, 195-196, 223
plow feast, 223
plowing, 20, 29, 36, 195
Pluto, 28
PMS, 156
pneumonia, 157, 159
pocan cheann, 232, 265
poetic arts, 215
poets, 20, 87, 184, 206, 212, 219, 233, 239, 269
poison, 51, 136, 156, 158, 187, 210

pole Star, 58
Polygala vulgaris, 125, 151
Polygonum amphibium, 122
Polygonum bistorta, 122
Polypodium vulgare, 139
Polypody Fern, 139
pónair chapaill, 124, 265
Pond Lilly, 152
pony, 243
Poppy, 164, 220
Porphyra umbilialis, 172
Poseidon, 28
Pot Marigold, 153
potassium, 146
Potato, 164-165
Potentilla anserina, 174
Potentilla erecta, 180
Potentilla tormentilla, 180, 230
pot-herb, 135
pottery, 16
poultice, 116, 118, 120-122, 124-126, 128-132, 135-136, 141-144, 147-148, 150-153, 156-157, 159-161, 163-166, 169-171, 173, 175, 179, 181-183, 186, 215
praiseach gharbh, 156, 265
prayer, 44, 54, 59, 81, 115, 151, 179, 220-221, 235
Prayers, 12, 42, 44, 52, 54, 66, 69, 219
preas nan airneag, 123, 265
preas súbh chraobh, 166, 265
predictions, 66
Preen-Tail Day, 79
pregnancy, 59, 115, 119, 166, 177, 182
preserve foods, 162
priests, 20
Primrose, 122, 165
Primula officinalis, 122, 133
Primula vera, 133
Primula vulgaris, 165
Procumbent Pearlwort, 180
prolapsus ani, 174
prophecy, 98, 108, 111, 207, 236
prophesy, 206
prophetic powers, 111, 215
prostatitis, 183
protection, 12, 24, 29, 31, 38, 43, 50, 53, 56, 60, 82, 99-100, 104, 106, 125, 151, 168-169, 193, 198, 205, 220, 226-227, 233, 237, 239, 248, 251

protection from drowning, 193
Protective Magic, 12, 223, 225
Protective Stones, 56
protector deities, 24
Protectress of Horses, 27
protein, 146, 178
Prunella vulgaris, 119, 143
Prunus avium, 142
Prunus spinosa, 123

Puffball, 15, 165
puinneag, 175, 265
puinneagan, 175, 265
purgative, 122-123, 136, 140, 145, 150, 177, 181, 232-233
purification, 71, 83, 85-86, 91, 93, 103, 151, 220, 247
pyromancy, 221
Pyrus malus, 120

Q

Q-Celtic, 14
quail, 103
Quarter Days, 12, 57, 221
Quarter Days and Fire Festivals, 12, 221
quartz, 42, 51-52, 164, 203, 227
Quartz stones, 52
queen, 13, 20, 24, 29, 35, 68, 71, 82-83, 85, 95, 112, 166, 206-207, 210, 213, 219, 228, 242, 249-250
Queen Mary, 71
Queen of Elfame, 249
Queen of Summer, 82
Queen of the Fairies, 112, 242
Queen of the Meadow, 166
Quercus alba, 158
quern, 87, 265

R

rabbit, 193, 231
Rabbits, 44, 213
ragweed, 127
Ragwort, 166, 252
raiders, 13, 15, 83
rainbow, 98, 103
raineach ríoghail, 140, 265
raise a storm, 54, 193
Ram, 24, 68, 85, 215-216
Ram horns, 24, 215
ram-headed serpent, 26
ram-headed snakes, 26
ram-horned deity, 26
ram-horned serpent, 216
Ramsons, 142
Ranunculus auricomus, 128
Ranunculus ficaria, 130
Ranunculus flammula, 175
rash, 133, 135, 142, 150, 156, 162
rashes, 141, 167
Raspberry, 124, 153, 162, 166, 178
raspberry leaf, 166, 178
rat, 192-193
Rata, 30, 265
rathadach, 224, 265
Ratis, 30, 265
Rattles, 226

Raven, 25, 30, 103, 191, 206-208
Raven Goddess, 30, 207
reapers, 87, 196
reaping, 36, 198, 245
recumbent stone, 57
red hair, 221, 224
Red Swine of Derbrenn, 209
red thread, 50, 53, 81, 99, 137, 169, 191, 225, 235
red-haired woman, 192
reed, 247
refuge stones, 60
reincarnation, 20
Reindeer, 16
Réitach, 90
Remi, 215, 265
respiratory conditions, 182
Reverend Robert Kirk, 110
revulsion for alcohol, 179
Reyes syndrome, 184
Rheum palmatum, 167
Rheum rhaponticum, 167
rheumatic complaints, 157, 179
rheumatic limbs, 51
rheumatic pains, 147
rheumatic parts, 118, 128, 165
rheumatism, 53, 120, 130, 133, 135, 137,

147-148, 151, 156, 159, 165-166, 169, 171, 179, 183, 187, 215, 229, 232

Rhubarb, 36, 167

Rhus glabra, 156

Ribes grossularia, 144

Ribes nigrum, 164

rice, 94, 157

rickets, 59, 233

rideag, 125, 265

Riding the Marches, 83

Rig Veda, 197, 214, 270

Rigisamus, 30, 265

Ring of Brodgar, 57-58

Ring of Stenness, 57-58

ringworm, 49

ritual, 21, 26, 33, 38-39, 41-42, 44, 46-47, 56-60, 66, 69, 74, 78, 80, 83-85, 87, 91, 94-95, 97, 101-102, 104, 107, 118, 151, 169, 192, 196-197, 210, 212, 215, 222-223

ritual cake, 223

ritual circle, 33, 56, 102

ritual fire, 60, 74, 118, 192, 196, 210, 222-223

ritual hunt, 210

ritual of consecration, 42

Ritual tools, 104

rituals, 12, 20-21, 34, 42, 45, 58, 80, 95, 98, 186, 196, 210, 219, 221

river, 29-31, 41, 43, 56, 77, 85-86, 207, 211, 223, 229, 236, 239-240

River Goddess, 31, 43, 86, 211, 223

river stones, 56, 236

river–hag, 240

rivers, 24, 43, 172, 212

river-sprite, 240

Robert Burns, 73-74, 108, 271

Robert the Bruce, 61

Robin Hood, 37, 69, 82

Robin Hood Games, 82

Rock crystal, 52

Rocking, 59, 89, 98, 102

rocking stone, 59

Ro-ech, 28, 266

Roman, 14-15, 17, 24-25, 27, 30, 94, 159, 206, 213-214, 266

Romano-British, 16

Rooster, 215, 243

ropes, 70, 77, 86, 158, 191, 197

rós, 167, 266

Rosa spp, 167

rosadach, 224, 266

Rose, 31, 51, 94, 116, 167-168

rosemary, 105, 213

roundworm, 129

Rowan, 40-41, 53, 55, 58, 69, 77, 81, 87, 99-100, 111, 116, 120, 137, 151, 168-169, 202, 210, 213, 223, 225, 227, 234, 237, 248

Royal Fern, 140

rú beag, 169, 266

Ruad Rofhéssa, 27, 30, 266

ruamalach, 183, 266

Rubus fructicosus, 126, 151

Rubus idaeus, 166

Rubus spp, 153, 162, 178

Rue, 154, 169

ruis, 137-138, 261, 266

Rumex acetosa, 175

Rumex crispus, 135

Rumex obtusifolius, 135

Rumex spp, 175

Running the Broose, 95

rushes, 75-76

Ruta graveolens, 154

rye, 157, 196

S

Sacred Animals, 12, 209

Sacred Birds, 12, 205

sacred grove, 21

Sacred Spring, 46, 56

sacred three, 45, 75-76

sacred tree, 21, 40-41, 56, 188, 269

sacred warrior, 24, 27, 30

sacred water, 34, 42, 49, 55, 85, 211, 214, 229

sacred wells, 25, 213, 216

sacred woods, 44-45, 81, 118, 121, 184, 191

sacrifices, 19, 80, 86

Sage, 161, 169-170

Sagina procumbens, 180, 198, 271

Saighead Shidh, 248-249

sail chuach, 181, 266

Saille, 183, 266

sailors, 84, 88, 191, 193, 226-227

Saining, 46, 49, 220

Saint Andrew's Day, 68

Saint Brighid, 77

Saint Brigid's Well, 52
Saint John's Eve, 170
Saint John's Wort, 43, 86, 121, 143, 170, 223
Saint Patrick, 59
sáiste, 169, 266
Saitada, 30
salads, 121, 134-135, 142, 152, 175, 178, 182, 185-186
Salix alba, 183-184
Salix spp, 183
Salmon, 16, 146, 201-202, 215-216
Salmon of Linn Feic, 215
Salmon of Wisdom, 146, 215
Salt, 47, 49, 64-65, 67-68, 71, 77-79, 81-82, 91-93, 98, 100, 104, 129, 135, 163, 174, 182, 193, 195, 202, 220, 232, 235, 242
salve, 116-117, 121, 129-130, 132-135, 137, 150, 157, 163-164, 216
salves, 116-119, 128, 130-134, 137, 139-141, 143, 149-150, 161-162, 164-165, 170-171, 179-180, 182, 186
Salvia officinalis, 161, 169
Sambucus nigra, 130, 137, 154, 164, 186
samh, 175, 266
samhan, 151, 266
samhnag, 66, 266
Samhuinn, 20-21, 25, 39, 42, 57, 63-67, 72, 81, 88, 118, 137, 141, 151, 155, 184, 192, 208, 221-224, 250, 266
Samthain, 64, 266
Sanctuary Stones, 60
Sanicula europea, 184
saoghal thall, 103, 266
Sarothamnus scoparius, 127
scabies, 118, 123, 141
Scabiosa pratensis, 171
Scabiosa succisa, 171
Scabious, 171
scabs, 118, 135
Scandinavian Spruce, 176
Scandinavians, 13
scarecrow, 198
Sceólang, 212, 266
Schiehallion, 249
Sciatica, 136, 161, 202, 231
Scone, 23, 61, 220
scones, 70-71, 95, 101, 137, 272
Scota, 61
Scotch pine, 163

Scotch thistle, 178
Scots Dragoon Guards, 61
Scotti, 14, 17, 61, 266
Scottish Oatcakes, 65
Scouring Rush, 149
scrofula, 49, 53, 118, 128, 141, 160, 184, 228, 231
Scrofularia nodosa, 198
scurvy, 134-135, 171, 187
Scurvy-Grass, 171
Scutellaria lateriflora, 154
Sea, 8, 12, 16, 25, 28-29, 31, 33-34, 43, 49, 54, 56, 60, 65, 78, 84, 87-88, 90, 106, 135, 152-153, 163, 172, 182, 187, 191-194, 205-206, 208, 210-211, 214, 222, 227, 229-230, 232, 234-235, 239, 241-244, 246, 248, 270
Sea God, 28, 206, 211, 214, 248
Sea Lettuce, 172
Sea Lovage, 152
sea monster, 239, 243
sea sickness, 153
seagulls, 194
Seal, 43, 59, 91, 117, 193, 201, 215, 227, 244
Seal oil, 215
Seal Women, 244
sealbhad, 175, 266
sealbhag nam fiadh, 175, 266
sealbhag nan con, 175, 266
seals, 241, 244
sealskin, 231
seal-women, 216
seamrag, 185, 266
searraiche, 130, 266
Seasonal Affective Disorder, 170
Sea-Tangle, 173
Sea-Trows, 243-244
seaweed, 106, 172-173, 192-193, 215, 222, 237, 246
Second Sight, 11, 100, 108, 111
sedative, 122, 133, 136, 163, 165, 184
Sedum acre, 177
Sedum album, 167
Sedum telephium, 108
Seed, 12, 15, 63, 78, 94, 119-120, 126, 130, 139, 161, 178, 195-196, 223
Seefer, 244
Seer, 52, 59, 108-109, 111-112, 146, 224
Segais, 146, 266

seilcheag, 266
seilistear, 141, 266
Seine, 30, 212
Selchie, 244
Self Heal, 119
Selkie, 244
Selkies, 84, 216, 244, 266
Selkirk Common Riding, 83
Sempervivum tectorum, 130, 150, 164
Senecio jacobea, 166
Senecio vulgaris, 145, 189, 272
Senna, 154, 173-174
Sennachie, 21, 266
Sequanna, 30
Serpents, 26, 31, 216
Serpent Beads, 51
Serpent Glass, 51
Serpent Stones, 51
Setlocenia, 30, 266
seventh daughter, 231
seventh son, 110, 217, 228, 231
seventh son of a seventh son, 110, 217, 231
Seventh sons, 228
Severed heads, 55
sexual desire, 152, 160
sgeallag, 156, 266
sgiach, 145, 266
sgitheach, 145, 266
Shamrock, 185
shamrocks, 185
Shave Grass, 149
Sheep, 16, 24, 51, 58, 65, 67-69, 80, 89, 91,
    98, 109, 121, 145, 170, 174, 182, 185,
    187, 202, 204, 216, 222, 230, 247, 249
sheiling, 250, 266
shellfish, 201
Shelly-Coat, 244
shepherd, 57, 87, 174
Shepherd's Purse, 174
Shetland, 9, 13, 15, 23, 31, 70, 74, 78, 96, 141,
    188, 197, 199, 224, 231, 243, 268, 270
Shiant Islands, 239
Shiehallion, 13, 266
Shieling Feast, 83
Shielings, 80
shingles, 150, 159, 179
shiubhaile, 103, 266
Shony, 192, 222
shortbread, 71, 96, 105-106, 222

shortness of breath, 149, 155
Shoupiltin, 243
Shriften E'en, 77
shrine, 21, 26, 56, 214
shroud, 104-105, 109
sick children, 44, 146, 184, 233
sickle, 86, 196, 214
Sídh Chailleann, 249, 266
Sifan, 244
Silures, 30, 210, 266
Silvanus, 28, 30-31, 266
Silver, 27, 31, 34, 38, 41, 43, 49, 51-54, 74,
    84, 92, 100, 102, 108, 121, 157, 180, 188,
    193, 207-208, 213, 225-226, 234-236,
    241, 245, 248, 251, 270
Silver bullets, 49
Silver the water, 38, 193, 226
silvered water, 225, 235
Silverweed, 82, 174
sinews, 153
singers, 20
Sisymbrium officinale, 156
siunas, 152
sixth day of the Moon, 223, 225
Skeely Woman, 43, 235
Skekil, 244
skin, 51, 72, 108, 116, 118, 120, 122-123,
    126, 128-131, 133, 135, 137, 141-143,
    148-150, 152, 157, 159, 161-164, 167,
    170-171, 174-175, 177-179, 181, 183,
    185-186, 193, 199, 206, 213, 215-217,
    231, 241, 243-244
skin cancer, 148, 162, 177
skin irritations, 149-150, 152, 157, 162,
    174, 183, 185
skull, 27, 39, 54-55, 70, 229
skullcap, 154
Sky God, 28, 30
Sky World, 34, 38, 44
Skye, 52, 147, 197, 242, 251
slachdan, 67, 75, 88, 266-267
Slachdan Druidheachd, 88, 266
Slachdan Geasachd, 88, 267
Slake, 172
slánlus, 163, 267
slaves, 19
sleep, 92, 120, 131, 133, 137, 146-147, 158,
    164, 201, 224, 243
slippery elm, 116, 129, 132, 140, 152, 183

slócan, 172, 267
Sluagh, 244, 267
Smáladh, 45, 267
small pox, 232
Smertae, 14, 267
smith, 24, 27-28, 50, 75, 97, 110, 196, 198, 203, 228
smith craft, 24, 75, 110
smith-God, 50
Smooring the fire, 45
Smyrnium olusatrum, 119
Snail, 216, 224
Snail-Stones, 51
Snake, 75, 120, 151, 216, 231-232
snake bite, 151, 216, 231-232
Sneezewort, 175
sneud, 93, 267
snuff, 6, 141, 144, 147
sóbhrag, 165, 267
Socrates, 148
soil, 15-16, 36, 63, 172, 195, 229
Solanum tuberosum, 164
Solar Cross, 51, 79, 81, 126, 169, 245
soldiers, 15, 24, 26, 71
Solidago spp, 119, 121, 143, 170
Solidago virgaurea, 143
solstice, 39, 55, 58, 69, 72, 83, 115, 137, 155, 158, 170, 196, 222
Soma, 211
Sonchus oleraceus, 178, 271
Sorbus americana, 168
Sorbus aucuparia, 151, 168
sorcerers, 125, 193, 217
Sorceress, 54, 220
sorcery, 49-51, 53, 55, 81, 84, 137, 145, 150, 168, 180, 191, 236
sore breasts, 131, 182
sore eyes, 49, 51, 119, 128, 144, 159, 232
sore knees, 142
sore lips, 180
sore nipples, 186
sore throat, 125, 138, 145, 152, 158, 163, 170-171, 174, 182-183, 185
sores, 118, 121, 124-125, 128, 132, 136, 141, 144, 149, 153, 163, 167, 171, 174-175, 180
Sorrel, 82, 175, 185
soul, 103, 210
source of a river, 56, 229
sovereignty, 24, 95, 214

sow the seed, 196
Sow thistle, 178, 271
sowans, 69, 222, 267
Sowans Nicht, 69, 222
Spaewife, 108
sparrows, 103
Spear of Lugh, 220
spearmint, 153, 156
spears, 220
Spearwort, 175
Speerin' Bottle, 90
spells, 12, 21, 25, 30, 160, 183, 197, 223, 230, 236, 248
Sphagnum cymbifolium, 176
Sphagnum Moss, 176
Spider, 216, 247
Spinewort, 175
spinners, 242
spinning, 69, 89, 240, 252
spirit animal, 103
Spirit of the Waters, 38
Spirit of Winter, 31
Spirits, 12-13, 20, 34, 37-38, 40, 43-44, 47, 55, 60, 65, 69-70, 74, 78, 81-82, 86, 94-96, 104, 106, 137, 191-192, 194, 203, 220-223, 225-228, 230, 234, 239, 241, 243-244, 250
spit, 43, 192, 227, 232
spleen, 119-120, 141, 186
Spleenwort, 140
Spoonwort, 171
sporran na fala, 174, 267
Sprain, 53, 116, 212, 232-233
sprains, 121, 128, 141, 165, 179, 185, 228
Spring, 27, 31, 33, 41-42, 46, 52, 56, 75, 77-78, 82, 108, 116-117, 122, 124, 127, 130, 134-135, 139, 145, 156-158, 160, 171, 178, 182, 185-186, 195, 197, 222, 233, 235, 244, 248, 250
Spring Equinox, 31, 78, 222
spring tonic, 122, 124, 157, 171
springs, 24, 28, 31, 42, 88, 215-216, 230
Spruce, 176, 232
Spruce Beer, 176, 232
Spurge, 177
St. Michael, 88
Stachys officinalis, 121, 154, 178
staffs, 123, 169
Stag Horn Jelly, 212

Stag Night, 93
stag worshippers, 211
stags, 28, 209, 211-212
stamh, 173, 267
Standing stones, 34, 56, 58, 86
stang, 195, 267
Stars, 20, 35, 55, 80, 92, 125, 180
Stellaria media, 131, 136
sties, 49, 144
stings, 128, 132, 135, 144, 150, 153, 164, 169
Stirlingshire, 110
stitch in the side, 52
stomach, 67-68, 119, 121, 123-124, 128-129, 134-135, 139, 143-144, 149-150, 155, 157, 160, 162, 164, 171, 173, 175, 178, 182-186, 193, 210
stomach cramps, 119, 123, 128, 139
stomach flu, 186
stomach pain, 143, 184-185
stomach ulcers, 124, 135, 149-150, 164
stone, 16, 21, 23, 25-26, 28, 38-40, 42, 51-53, 55-61, 72, 74, 86, 90, 97-98, 102, 106, 111, 115, 131, 159, 169, 193-195, 198, 203, 215-216, 220, 228-231, 235-237, 240-242, 246, 249-250, 271
stone circles, 57-58, 60, 249
Stone Magic, 57
Stone of Destiny, 23, 61, 220, 271
Stone of Fal, 220
Stone of Offering, 59
Stone of Scone, 23, 61, 220
stone seat, 86
Stonecrop, 108, 167, 177
stones, 11, 15-16, 34, 39-42, 44, 49, 51-52, 55-60, 63, 67, 86, 106, 123, 143-144, 148, 175, 184, 203, 205-206, 209, 211, 215-216, 220, 229-231, 236, 240-242, 246, 250, 269
Stones of Power, 11, 55, 58
Stoor Worm, 244
Storm Hag, 240
stormy petrel, 191
story telling, 44, 80
Strath Eireann, 31, 267
straw dog, 84, 197
straw man, 198
Straw Men and Scare Crows, 198
streams, 25, 43, 45, 75, 88, 172, 231, 242-243
strep infection, 126, 148, 167

stress, 126, 153, 160
strewing herb, 125, 177
struan, 66, 267
Styes, 231
styptic, 15, 123, 131, 152, 162-163, 186
Sucellos, 30, 212, 267
súgh dharaich, 154
sumac, 156
summer, 20, 24-25, 29, 31, 33, 39, 41, 55, 63, 65, 72, 75, 78, 80, 82-84, 115, 124, 137, 141, 158, 170, 196, 210, 241-242, 245, 250
Summer Lord, 82
Summer Queen, 82
Summer Solstice, 39, 55, 83, 115, 137, 158, 170, 196
summertime, 227
Sun, 7, 11, 24, 33-35, 40, 42, 46, 49-51, 55, 57, 69, 77, 80, 82-83, 85-87, 91-92, 109-110, 116, 125, 133, 170, 172, 180, 192, 195-196, 208, 213, 220, 222-223, 242, 252
Sun deity, 24
sunais, 152
sunburn, 133, 149-150, 178
Sunhoney Farm, 57
Sunrise, 39, 57-58, 83, 92, 146, 160, 215, 223, 225, 244
Sunset, 39, 54, 58, 80, 82, 244
sunwise, 33, 40, 46, 83, 87, 90, 96, 220, 222
supernatural sight, 216
suppuration, 164
surgery, 20, 174
swallows, 191, 235
Swan, 28, 30, 208
sweat baths, 228
Sweat Houses, 229
Sweet violet, 181-182
Sweet Woodruff, 184
swellings, 118, 129-130, 132, 134, 136, 141, 145, 173, 179, 202, 228
swollen glands, 231
sword, 60, 88, 220
Sword dances, 88
swordsman, 85
sympathetic magic, 58, 82, 98, 191, 193, 196, 220, 222
sympathetic resonance, 220
Symphytum tuberosum, 132
syphilitic sores, 175

T

Taezali, 14, 267
Taghairm, 108, 267
Taibhsear, 108, 267
Taibnsearachd, 109, 267
Tailie Day, 79
Tailtiu, 29, 85-86, 267
Táin Bó Cuálgne, 210, 267
Talismans, 11, 49, 76, 84
Tam Lin, 112
Tanacetum vulgare, 177
Tanarus, 28, 267
Tansy, 177
tape worm, 140
Tara, 61
Taran, 31, 267
Taranis, 28, 31, 206, 267
Taraxacum leontodon, 134
Taraxacum officinale, 127, 178
Taraxacum spp, 125, 151, 198
Tarbfeis, 210, 267
Tarnach, 31, 267
tattoos, 14, 186
taxol, 187
Taxus baccata, 187, 189, 272
Tay, 8, 13, 187
Tea, 118-145, 147-159, 161-171, 174-187, 232
teething, 129, 154, 164
teimheil, 38, 267
Teine, 45, 248, 267
Teine Sith, 248
Tein-eigin, 45, 267
Temple of the Moon, 57
Temple of the Sun, 57
Teran, 29, 31, 78, 87, 267
territorial Goddess, 25
Teutates, 26, 267
Thalictrum alpinus, 169
Thalictrum minus, 169
The Black Faulie, 47
The Blessing of the Circle, 46
The Brahan Seer, 52, 111-112
The Broose, 95
The Cailleach, 23-25, 31, 37, 56, 67, 196, 206, 211, 223, 230, 237, 270
The Cattle Raid of Cooley, 210
the Connra bull, 206
The Coracle of the Fairy Woman, 248

The Daghda, 25, 30, 75, 89, 207, 220
the dead, 16, 20, 29, 36, 43, 50, 58, 65, 67, 103, 106, 111, 122, 169, 187, 208-209, 220, 222, 234-235
The Druid's Chair, 58
The Druid's Herb, 154
The Druids, 11, 14, 19, 26-27, 75, 121, 131, 155, 187, 208, 223
The Fairies, 12, 21, 34, 38, 40, 44, 47, 50-51, 58, 81, 84, 87, 92, 98-99, 101, 110-112, 115, 141-142, 169, 197-198, 201, 203, 221, 224, 226, 228, 230, 241-242, 247-252
The Fairy Hill of Aberfoyle, 249
The Fire Festivals, 11, 23, 33, 42, 45, 63-64, 107, 169, 192, 249
The Fires of Life, 66, 69, 75
the Good People, 110
The Good Striker, 31, 212
The Green Lady, 242
The Green Woman, 27
The Gudeman's Croft, 47, 197
The Hill of Piping, 249, 251
The Horned God, 28
The Horned Goddess, 28
The Knocking Stone, 60
The Lame Goat, 242
The Land of the Ever Young, 248
The Land of the Living, 248
The Land of Youth, 248
The Lore of Boats, 12, 191
The Old Gods, 11, 23, 220
The Plow, the Seed and the Grain, 12, 195
the poor, 40, 66-67, 82, 193, 198
The Red One of great wisdom, 30
The Red Stone of Ardvorlich, 52
The sacred Three, 45, 75-76
The Secret Commonwealth of Elves, Fauns, and Fairies", 110
The Seely Court, 247
The Sight, 109-110, 137, 213, 251
The Straiking, 104
The Thimble of the Fairy Woman, 248
The Triple Mothers, 29
The Unseely Court, 247
The Wake, 105
The Washer at the Ford, 30, 207, 239, 245
The Weeping One, 240

The Year in Scotland, 11, 65
thinning hair, 122
Thistle, 178, 271
Thomas of Ercildoune, 112
Thomas Randolph, the Earl of Moray, 112
Thomas the Rhymer, 112
Thomas the Rhymer and Tam Lin, 112
thorn, 127, 145, 159
Three Worlds, 34, 100, 102, 125, 158, 229, 236
throat inflammations, 123
thrush, 119, 150, 164
thunder, 28, 30-31, 95, 146, 206, 259
thunder deity, 28, 31
Thunder God, 206
Thyme, 179, 202
Thymus serpyllum, 179, 202
thyroid, 161, 173, 179
tí, 178, 267
Tigh na Cailliche, 56, 267
Tillia spp, 154
tinea capititis, 162
Tir nam Béo, 248, 267
tired eyes, 178
Tiree, 242
Tir-Na-N'Og, 248, 267
toad, 232
Tobacco, 124, 156, 179
Tocher, 91, 93
tombaca, 179, 267
tombs, 21, 58, 216, 250
Tom-na-hurich, 111, 249
Tomnaverie, 57
tonsillitis, 163-164, 168, 170-171
tonsils, 184
tools, 16, 39, 47, 75, 94, 104, 141, 168, 229, 250
Tooth Fairy, 215
toothache, 58, 164, 183, 230
torc, 24, 26, 28
Tormentil, 180, 230
torranan, 141, 267
totem plant, 145, 205
trace minerals, 172, 182

Trailing Pearlwort, 180
transformation, 31, 210
Transplant, 36
travel, 14, 29, 37-38, 65, 166, 192, 217, 230, 241, 244, 252-253
travelers, 15, 125
trees, 11, 15, 21, 34, 36, 38, 40, 45, 58, 69, 111, 115-117, 155, 158, 187-188, 220, 225, 229, 271-272
Trefoil, 170
trial marriage, 93
tribal law, 20
tribal protector, 27, 215
Tribal Protector Gods, 215
tríbhileach, 124, 267
Trickster God, 206
Trinouxtion Samonii, 65, 267
Triple deities, 23, 34
triple deity, 29, 31
triple Goddess, 25, 27, 29, 207
troll, 244-245
Trolls, 199, 244, 249
Trout, 41, 88, 201, 216
Trowist, 248
Trows, 70, 99, 141, 230, 244-246
True Thomas, 112
trusgan, 152, 267
tuaithiuil, 33, 56, 66, 90, 92, 192, 213, 268
Tuatha Dé Danann, 27, 169, 248, 250, 268
tuberculosis, 53, 119, 124, 128, 140-141, 149, 153, 157, 160, 175, 184, 228, 231, 233
Tuberous Vetch, 181
tumors, 121, 129, 141, 144, 154, 160, 166, 178-179
Tumuli, 58
Turnera aphrodisiaca, 170
Turnip, 68
Tussilago farfara, 132, 156
Twelve Winds, 37
twine, 69, 158
typhoid, 154
typhus, 185

U

Ubhall, 120, 268
Uí Néill, 17
uil'- íoc, 154, 268
uinnean, 159, 268
Uisge-beatha, 202, 268

ulcerated throats, 180
ulcers, 118, 121, 123-124, 127-128, 130, 132, 135, 141, 144, 149-150, 152, 158, 164, 175, 177-178, 180, 183, 185-186
Ulmus fulva, 132, 140, 183

Ulva lactuca, 172
Undead, 49
Underworld, 34, 38, 220, 245
Up Helly Aa, 268
ura bhallach, 171, 268
úrach bhallach, 160, 268
urinary antiseptic, 151
urinary bleeding, 186
urinary stones, 148

urinary tract infections, 228
urine, 84, 137, 144, 151, 159, 195, 214, 227
Urisk, 239-240, 244-245
Ursa Major, 33
Urtica dioica, 156
Urtica spp, 182
Urtica urens, 157
Uruisg, 245, 268
uterus, 129, 167

V

Vaccinium myrtillus, 123
Vaccinium spp, 202
vaginal discharge, 152
Valentines Day, 78
valerian, 144, 154
Valeriana officinalis, 144, 154
Vampires, 49
varicose veins, 128, 140
Vates, 108, 268
Vedic, 197, 213
Veiled One, 67, 196, 240
venereal diseases, 171
venison, 201-202
Venus, 25, 57
Verbascum thapsus, 156
Verbeia, 31, 211, 268
vermifuge, 177, 185
Veronica chamaedrys, 143
vertigo, 170, 213
vervain, 170

Vetch, 181
Victoria, 25, 83
Victoria Day, 83
Vikings, 8, 15, 171
Vinca minor, 162
vinegar, 118, 120, 129, 135-136, 150, 152, 163, 167-168, 174, 182-183, 202, 212
Vinotonus, 31, 268
Viola canina, 181
Viola odorata, 158, 181-182
violet, 124, 158, 180-182
Violets, 181, 213
Virgin Mary, 71
Viscum album, 154
Vitamin C, 116, 134, 168, 171, 182
Vitris, 31, 268
vomiting, 143, 164, 181, 184
votive, 56, 212, 214
Vulcan, 27

W

Wall Pepper, 177
wand, 59, 67, 88, 169
Waning Moon, 36, 91, 100, 195, 223, 236
War goddesses, 24
war leader, 27
Warrior God, 24, 26, 30, 206
Warrior Goddess, 24
Warrior Gods, 24, 215
Warriors, 19, 25, 28, 30, 60, 74, 83, 102, 106, 143, 202, 205, 207, 209, 211, 215, 225, 242
warts, 54, 128, 135-136, 144, 150, 159, 177, 232
Washer at the Ford, 30, 207, 239, 245

wassail, 71
wasting disease, 230
Water Cow, 245
Water Kelpie, 243
Water Lilly, 183
Water Magic, 11, 38, 82
Water Spirit, 230
Watercress, 134, 182, 202, 231
waterfall, 56, 108, 239, 245
Water-Horse, 240, 246
Waterlilly, 183
watermill, 169
Waters of Life, 202, 222
Waulkin O' the Fauld, 89
waulking song, 251

Waxing Moon, 35-36, 58, 100, 184, 223
weak eyes, 44
weather, 55-57, 67, 69, 72, 75, 80, 85, 87, 191, 237, 252
Weather Magic, 237
weaver, 158
weaving, 6, 16, 72, 197, 240
wedding, 50, 89-97, 107, 207, 251
wedding band, 50
wedding cake, 96, 107
Wedding Feast, 93, 95
wedding ring, 50, 94
wee ane, 247, 268
Wee Mindings, 91
Weed, 36, 117, 230
Weet the Heid O' the Bairn, 101
weight loss, 131
well, 21, 25-26, 33-34, 38-43, 46, 52, 54-56, 58, 64-65, 67, 73, 79, 81-82, 86, 94, 96, 98, 100, 105, 108, 111, 115, 143, 146, 180, 202-203, 206-207, 212-215, 220, 224-225, 227, 229, 236, 241, 243, 245, 247, 253
Well Dressing, 39
Well of Segais, 146
Well of the Head, 54
Well of Youth, 25, 67
Well ritual, 38, 42
Wetting the Baby's Head, 101
Whale, 16, 243-244
whalebone, 15
wheat, 12, 36, 116, 161, 197-198, 208
wheat grass, 161
Whirl of Fairies Wind, 241
whirlpools, 242
whirlwind, 241
whisky, 12, 34, 56, 70-71, 73-75, 83-84, 90, 94-95, 98, 100-101, 105, 117, 123, 130, 157, 177, 192, 195-196, 201-203, 212, 221-222
whistlebinkies, 96
white deer, 211
White heather, 147
White Helleborine, 147
White Horehound, 149
white horse, 66, 89, 213
White Oak, 158
White Pond Lilly, 152
White Stone of the Fairies, 51
White Waterlilly, 183

White Willow, 183-184
Whitethorn, 145
Whitsunday, 80
whooping cough, 124, 126, 144, 162, 164, 179, 214-215, 231
Whuppity Scoorie, 78
Wicked Wichts, 247
widdershins, 33, 42, 90, 213
widows, 194
wife stone, 58
Wild Cherry, 142
Wild geese, 191
Wild Hunt, 69
Wild Mustard, 156
Wild Thyme, 179
William the Lion, 84
Willow, 15, 35, 45, 98, 166, 183-184
Wind, 29, 31, 37-38, 52, 54, 193, 221, 237, 241, 243
winds, 11, 37-38
wine, 56, 100, 102, 120, 127, 131, 133, 135, 137, 146, 164, 167, 171, 178, 221, 243, 247
Winter, 23-25, 31, 33, 36-37, 58, 63, 65, 67, 69, 72, 75, 82, 87-90, 99, 124, 136, 155, 196, 198, 214, 216, 222, 227, 245, 250
Winter Solstice, 58, 69, 72, 155, 222
Winter Sunday, 88
Wise Man, 54
Wise Woman, 54
wish, 39, 50, 52, 55, 57, 73, 194, 201, 222, 224-225
Witch, 51, 137, 179, 199, 213, 236, 246
Witchcraft, 112, 151, 155, 188, 191, 227, 235, 270
Witches, 8, 12, 33, 50, 55, 125, 127, 160, 166, 168-170, 206, 208, 213, 219, 239, 253
Wizard's Tree, 168
Woad, 14, 186, 189, 272
Woden, 57
Wodin, 27
Wolf, 16, 30, 64, 69, 155, 216
Wolf's Bane, 155
wood betony, 154, 178
Wood Sanicle, 184
Wood Sorrel, 82, 185
Wood violet, 181
Woodbine, 151, 184, 229
Woodruff, 184

wood-worm, 103
wool, 53, 84, 86, 105, 141, 184, 186, 232, 241
World Serpent, 244
worming agent, 125, 130
worms, 121, 139-140, 142, 164, 169, 173, 179
Wormwood, 89, 185
wound healing, 124

wound wash, 122, 136, 143-144, 158, 163, 179, 186
wounds, 59, 121, 123, 125, 128-132, 134, 137, 141-142, 144, 149-150, 152, 155, 157-161, 163, 165-167, 170-171, 174-176, 179-184, 186, 202, 209, 211, 232
wrang-gaites, 33
Wren, 208
wrinkles, 133

Y

Yarrow, 144, 154, 175, 186-188
Yew, 8, 41, 46, 56, 59, 111, 151, 187, 249
yonder world, 103
Yule, 27, 69-70, 74-75, 194, 222, 244-245

Yule Eve, 69
Yule Log, 69
Yule's End, 74

Z

Zeus, 26, 31

Zingiber officinale, 173

Available through
www.PendraigPublishing.com
by Peter Paddon

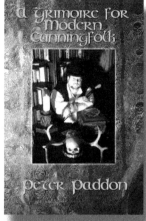

**A Grimoire for Modern Cunningfolk
A Practical Guide to Witchcraft
on the Crooked Path**

The Crooked Path is a way of Crafting based on experiencing the Mysteries of Ancestors and the Sacred Landscape first-hand, and Peter guides the seeker through the basics with competence and humor.

$10.95   **978-0-9843302-1-8**

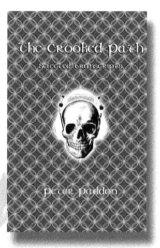

The Crooked Path

Selected transcripts of the Crooked Path Podcast hosted by Peter Paddon.

$10.95   **978-0-9843302-0-1**

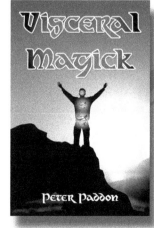

**Visceral Magick
Bridging the Gap
Between Magic and Mundane**

This book explores a set of basic experiences, ideas and techniques that used to be at the heart of every magical Tradition, but which are frequently overlooked or ignored in modern times. But they are the very things that breathe life into magical systems, the secret key that makes the magic actually work.

Coming Soon   978-0-9843302-3-2

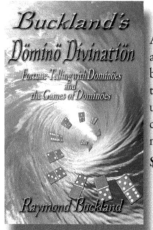
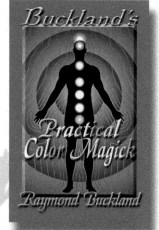
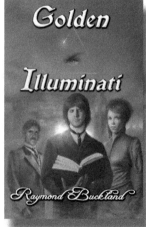